IMMEDIATE EYE CARE

AN ILLUSTRATED MANUAL

Nicola K Ragge
MA, MRCP, FCOphth
Registrar in Ophthalmology,
Bristol Eye Hospital

David L Easty
MD, FRCS, FCOphth
Professor of Ophthalmology,
University of Bristol

with photographic assistance of Mrs Gill Bennerson
and watercolours by Mr Terry Tarrant

Wolfe Publishing Ltd

Copyright © N. K. Ragge and D. L. Easty 1990
Copyright © Line Illustrations. Wolfe Publishing Ltd 1990
Published by Wolfe Publishing Ltd 1990
Printed by BPCC Hazell Books Ltd, Aylesbury, England
ISBN 0 7234 1574 9

A CIP catalogue record for this book is available from the British Library.

For a full list of forthcoming titles and details of our surgical, dental and
veterinary atlases, please write to Wolfe Publishing Ltd, 2–16
Torrington Place, London WC1E 7LT.

Contents

Foreword

It gives me much pleasure to write a Foreword to this book which provides for those whose needs lie somewhere between the medical student's and the fully trained ophthalmologist's. It contains current information expressed in a clear, concise and understandable manner.

The scope is much more comprehensive than the title suggests and a full range of ophthalmic conditions is included, with their recognition and management. There is much recent information which establishes a substantial basis of knowledge for those beginning a study of ophthalmology, but this information is also needed by those whose aim is towards other branches of medicine. It should be used as a manual in clinical situations which present to all doctors involved in acute clinical care. These doctors have considerable responsibility for the recognition and early management of eye conditions, and yet many of them feel that their training is deficient in this field. Their burden will increase with the coming substantial changes in primary health care.

A publication such as this is a ready source of information and easy reference, assisted by its division of contents, the large number of illustrations and a good index. Its division into two distinct sections is useful. The first describes conditions affecting the individual tissues, and the second their wider associations. The high quality illustrations are particularly useful in the recognition of eye signs and help the reader to validate a provisional diagnosis. The adjacent text gives further confirmation and indicates the appropriate investigations and therapy. As far as possible the description, symptoms, signs, differential diagnosis and management of a particular condition are placed on the same page spread as the illustration.

There are numerous ophthalmic conditions which do not require immediate care and those are correctly given limited space. The brief outline description of the later management of these conditions expresses a conservative rather than a radical approach, especially in respect of surgery. Such an attitude is wise for those gaining experience and provides sound guidance which the readers should be cautious to modify.

Nicola Ragge has entered ophthalmology with enthusiasm and early success. She has had a sound basis in her earlier training in medical sciences and pathology, followed by experience in many paediatric subspecialties, intensive therapy and general emergency work. She has gained higher qualifications both in medicine and ophthalmic surgery and has taken up a Fellowship in Paediatric and Neuro-ophthalmology supported with the award of the Keeler scholarship by the College of Ophthalmologists.

David Easty is an authority on many aspects of external eye disease and is highly respected for his many contributions to clinical ophthalmology, both before and after his appointment to the Chair of Ophthalmology in the University of Bristol. He is frequently invited to speak at ophthalmic society meetings and teaching courses. The combination of the talents of these two authors is admirably suited to the preparation of this book and should make it particularly useful to the intended readers. The authors have had the advantage of an abundant source of clinical material and willing co-operation from many colleagues, who have provided illustrations which greatly enhance the usefulness of the book.

The detailed explanatory text goes further than merely assisting in diagnosis, providing a source of reference and guidance. The immediate management is clearly set out and an indication given of which conditions need to be referred, the degree of urgency and to whom the referral should be made. The key coding will be particularly helpful in this respect. Suggestions for further reading are helpful in finding sources of more information. These will be important to those whose interest is stimulated to seek further knowledge in this attractive and increasingly important speciality.

M.J. Roper-Hall
Birmingham

Preface

Doctors often find it difficult to diagnose and manage eye disease. This is unfortunate because the prevalence is high. The fear of blindness, which may be allayed eventually, but only after clinical examination, impels patients to seek an immediate opinion. Some patients will indeed need treatment, others referral to an expert, while many will just require reassurance. It is the responsibility of the general practitioner and casualty officer to make these decisions.

There appear to be a number of reasons why medical graduates worry about their patients with eye disease. Firstly, ophthalmology is not taught effectively because, despite the enthusiasm of university departments, the teaching time allocated to the speciality is regrettably short. The emphasis of the content is rather theoretical and the students have limited time to develop their practical skills.

There are other reasons. The anatomy of the eye and orbit is complex and quickly forgotten. The eye itself is miniature and requires special methods of examination. Many of the diseases are specific to the eye and have their own peculiar nomenclature. Most health centres and casualty departments are not equipped for the care of eye disease and even when the equipment is available, doctors are unfamiliar with its use.

The aim of this book is to provide an illustrated text and atlas for general and family practitioners, hospital casualty officers and emergency physicians, eye hospital casualty departments and ophthalmologists in their initial training. It is a book that medical students will find helpful and interesting in their undergraduate years and in their subsequent careers.

The book sets out to cover all the diseases of the eye which may require an immediate opinion, although experience shows that urgent action is not always necessary. The first half contains a systematic approach to disorders of the eye with each part of the eye described in separate chapters. The second half builds upon this initial section, covering topics of special interest such as tropical eye disease, industrial eye disease, paediatric ophthalmology and drug effects on the eye. Since there is a need for donor corneas for transplantation, a section on eye removal is included.

The book is designed as a manual to be used in the acute clinical situation. Each topic is sub-divided into a short description, symptoms, signs, differential diagnosis and management. The advice on treatment is organised to indicate what degree of therapeutic responsibility can be taken and when referral, urgent or otherwise, must be made. Coded recommendations of levels of care and when to refer are provided to speed and focus the reader on the treatment which they could provide (see Key). Simple therapeutic procedures are shown step-by-step and, where possible, exact dosages of drugs are given. The approach is necessarily didactic, providing a selected method of treatment, although others may be acceptable.

It is hoped that this illustrated guide to immediate eye care will achieve its aims of improving the confidence of medical students and doctors who read it to deal with eye disease, and of heightening their awareness of, and interest in, this vital speciality of medicine.

Key

Ⓟ Family Practitioner and Casualty Officer or Emergency Physician

Ⓡ Eye Casualty Officer or Resident in Ophthalmology

Ⓢ Ophthalmologist or Specialist

Acknowledgements

The authors are grateful to many people for their assistance in preparing this book. In particular we are indebted to Mrs Gill Bennerson for her photographic assistance, Mr Terry Tarrant for his magnificent artwork, Mr Rob Ellis for preparing many of the line diagrams, Mr Patrick Delarue for his photographs of ophthalmic equipment and Dr Juan Salinas for providing the Glossary. We should like to thank the consultants at the Bristol Eye Hospital for allowing us to photograph their cases. Some of the photographs are kind donations from colleagues and we have endeavoured to acknowledge them individually under each photograph. We should like to thank Mr Christopher Dean Hart, as head of the Photographic Department, for allowing us to use some of the photographs from his collection. In addition, we would like to acknowledge with thanks photographs taken of cases at Moorfields Eye Hospital. Our thanks are also due to Sister Jane Fox and the rest of the staff of the Bristol Eye Hospital Casualty department for their cooperation and help with the cases. Many associates have given us assistance in specialist areas including Dr Gavin Goodman, Employment Medical Adviser, Health and Safety Executive (occupational eye disease) and Mr John Sandford-Smith (tropical eye disease). Our thanks are also due to those people who have offered us helpful criticism of the text, in particular Mr Frank Larkin and Dr Mandy Sharpe. Finally, we should like to thank Mr Jonathan Black, the first author's husband, for advice and support throughout the preparation of the book.

Glossary

Abduction – Outward rotation of one eye from the primary position

Aberration – Optical defect in which the rays from a point object do not form a perfect point image after passing through an optical system

AC/A Ratio – Accommodative convergence to accommodation ratio is the measure of accommodative convergence in prism dioptres for each dioptre of initiating accommodation

Accommodation – Ability to increase the convexity of the crystalline lens in order to obtain a clear image of a near object

Accommodative spasm – Spasm of the ciliary muscle

Addition, Near – The difference in spherical power between the distance and near corrections. Abbreviated: add

Adduction – Inward rotation of one eye from the primary position

Amaurosis Fugax – Temporary visual loss similar to a descending curtain; fleeting blindness

Amblyopia – A condition characterised by low visual acuity which is not the result of any clinically demonstrable anomaly of the visual pathway, without any apparent lesion of the eye and which is not correctable by optical means

Ametropia – The ametropic eye has an abnormal type of refraction so that parallel rays of light entering the eye do not come to focus on the retina

Angiography, Fluorescein – A technique used for the examination of the retinal and choroidal circulation, facilitated by the intravenous injection of a fluorescent dye

Angle Kappa – Angle between the optical and the visual axis

Anisocoria – Pupils are of different size

Anisometropia – The refraction of the two eyes is different

Anterior Chamber – Space within the eye, bounded anteriorly by the cornea and posteriorly by the iris and lens

Aphakia – Absence of the crystalline lens. It may be congenital, but usually it is due to surgical removal of a cataract

Aqueous Flare – Scattering of light seen when a beam of light is directed into the anterior chamber, occurring as a result of increased protein content in aqueous humour

Aqueous Humour – Clear fluid formed within the processes of the ciliary body by filtration

Astigmatism – Refractive condition of the eye in which the refracting power is not uniform in all meridians

Asthenopia – Eyestrain, symptoms associated with the use of the eyes

B.d. – Twice a day

Binocular Vision – The ability to use both eyes simultaneously

Binocular Single Vision – The ability to use both eyes simultaneously so that each eye contributes to a common single perception

Biomicroscope – An instrument designed for detailed examination of the eye. Contains a magnifying system and a slit lamp

Break-up Time Test – Test for assessing the precorneal tear film stability

Canal, Schlemm's – Circular venous sinus located in the corneo-scleral junction

Canaliculi – Part of the lacrimal drainage system. Short vertical segments that begin at the puncta, turn through a right angle to form horizontal segments that fuse, and empty into the lacrimal sac

Canthus – Angle formed by the upper and lower eyelids at the nasal or temporal end

Cataract – Opacities in the crystalline lens that disturb vision

Central Fixation – The reception of the image of the fixation object by the fovea

Chalazion – Localised swelling of the lid due to blockage of the duct of a Meibomian gland

Chemosis – Severe oedema of the conjunctiva

Chromatopsia – Condition in which the objects appear falsely coloured

Coloboma – A portion of the structure of the eye is lacking, typically affecting the iris, choroid and retina or eyelid

Concomitance – The two eyes move as a unit, maintaining a constant angle between them for all directions of gaze

Concomitant Strabismus – The angle of deviation remains the same in all directions of gaze, whichever eye is fixing

Confusion – The simultaneous appreciation of two superimposed images owing to the stimulation of corresponding retinal points by two different images

Convergence – Movement of the eyes toward each other or inward

Cover Test — Test for determining the type of strabismus

Crossed Fixation — Either eye is used to fixate in the contralateral field

Crowding Phenomenon — Difficulty in discriminating small visual acuity tests when they are presented next to each other in a row, typically seen in amblyopia

Cycloplegia — Paralysis of the ciliary muscle resulting in a loss of accommodation, usually accompanied by dilatation of the pupil, due to the effect of a cycloplegic drug

Cycloplegic Occlusion — The embarrassment of vision by using a cycloplegic drug (as might be used in the treatment of childhood amblyopia)

Cup/Disc Ratio — The ratio of the vertical diameter of the physiological cup to the vertical diameter of the optic disc

Cyclitis — Inflammation of the ciliary body

Dacryoadenitis — Inflammation of the lacrimal gland

Dacryocystitis — Inflammation of the lacrimal sac

Dioptre — Unit of lens power. It is the reciprocal of the focal length of the lens in metres

Dioptre, Prism — A unit specifying the amount of deviation by an ophthalmic prism. A prism of one prism dioptre power produces a 1 cm linear apparent displacement of an object situated at 1 m

Diplopia — Double vision

Distichiasis — Double row of eyelashes in the lid margin, one row being normal and the other turning inward toward the eye

Divergence — Movement of the eyes outward

Drüsen — Colloid bodies, small, discrete, yellow-white, slightly elevated spots on the retina

Ductions — Rotary movements of one eye from the primary position

Ectasia, Corneal — A forward bulging of the cornea as in keratoconus

Ectopia Lentis — Dislocation of the lens relative to the pupil

Ectropion — Outward turning of the eyelid

Electro-oculography — Measures the standard action potential which exists between the cornea (positive) and the back of the eye electrically (negative)

Electroretinography — Record of an action potential produced by the retina when it is stimulated by light of adequate intensity

Emmetropia — Ideal refractive state of the eye, in which with accommodation relaxed, an object at infinity is focused on the retina (the conjugate focus of the retina is at infinity)

Entropion — Inversion of the eyelid

Enucleation — Removal of the eye from its socket

Epicanthus — A fold of skin partially covering the inner canthus

Esophoria — Inward turning of the eye from the active position when fusion is suspended

Esotropia — One or the other eye deviates nasally

Evisceration — Removal of contents of the eye as in endstage endophthalmitis

Exenteration — Removal of the eye and orbital clearance as seen in malignant conditions

Exophoria — Outward turning of the eye from the active position when fusion is suspended

Exophthalmos — Abnormal protrusion of the eyeball

Exotropia — One or the other eye deviates temporally

Focimeter — Lensometer. Optical instrument for determining the vertex power, axis direction and optical centre of an ophthalmic lens

Fusion — Sensory. Ability to perceive two similar images, one formed on each retina, and interpret them as one

Gaze Palsy — Loss of conjugate gaze which may affect horizontal or vertical versions

Glaucoma — Rise in the intraocular pressure that is associated with damage to the optic nerve head and visual field loss

Gonioscope — Instrument used to observe the angle of the anterior chamber

Guttata, Cornea — Dystrophy of the endothelial cells of the cornea

Heterochromia — Difference in colour of the two irises or of different parts of the same iris

Heterophoria — Both visual axes are directed toward the fixation point but deviate on dissociation

Heterotropia — One or other visual axis is not directed toward the fixation point

Hippus — Small rhythmic variations in the size of the pupils

Hypermetropia (Far Sight) — Refractive condition of the eye in which distant objects are focused behind the retina when the accommodation is relaxed

Hyperphoria (Hypophoria) — A vertical deviation occurring on dissociation in which one eye rotates upward and the other downward depending upon the fixation

Hyphaema — Haemorrhage into the anterior chamber

Hypopyon — Pus in the anterior chamber

Incomitant Strabismus — The angle of deviation differs depending upon the direction of gaze or according to which eye is fixing

Intraocular Lens Implant (IOL) — A lens inserted in the eye to replace the crystalline lens after cataract extraction

Intraocular Pressure — The pressure within the eyeball

Iridectomy – Surgical removal of part of the iris

Iridodonesis – Tremulous movements of the iris as seen in aphakia

Iris Bombé – Forward bulging of the iris due to an increase of aqueous humour in the posterior chamber

Keratic Precipitates – Cellular deposits on the corneal endothelium

Keratoconus – Thinning disorder of the central and paracentral cornea of unknown aetiology. The cornea bulges forward in a cone shaped fashion

Keratoglobus – Rare bilateral enlargement of the cornea in which it assumes a globular shape

Keratomalacia – Pathological changes in the cornea due to Vitamin A deficiency

Keratoplasty – Excision of corneal tissue and its replacement by a cornea from a human donor

Leukoma – Dense, white corneal opacity caused by scar tissue

Myopia (Near Sight) – Refractive error of the eye in which distant objects are focused in front of the retina when the accommodation is relaxed

Nystagmus – Repetitive oscillatory movement of one or both eyes

O.d. – Once a day

Ophthalmoplegia – Paralysis of the ocular muscles

Ophthalmitis, Sympathetic – Bilateral inflammation of the uveal tract which usually follows perforation of one eye

Orthophoria – Both visual axes are directed toward the fixation point and do not deviate on dissociation

Orthoptics – Study, diagnosis and non-operative treatment of anomalies of binocular vision, strabismus and monocular functional amblyopia

Pachometer – A device used to measure the corneal thickness

Papillitis – Inflammation of the optic nerve head

Papilloedema – Bilateral optic disc swelling, secondary to raised intracranial pressure

Penalisation – Treatment of amblyopia or eccentric fixation by optical reduction of form vision of the non-amblyopic eye at one or all distances of fixation

Perimetry – Determination of the visual field

Phacoemulsification – Removal of the lens by emulsifying and aspirating the contents of the lens with the use of a low frequency ultrasonic needle

Polycoria – Two or more pupils in one iris

Posterior Chamber – Space in the eye filled with aqueous humour and bounded by the posterior surface of the iris, the ciliary processes, the zonule and the anterior surface of the lens

Presbyopia – Refractive condition in which the accommodative ability of the eye becomes insufficient for satisfactory near vision

Proptosis – Exophthalmos

Ptosis – Drooping of the upper eyelid

Q.d.s. or **q.i.d.** – Four times a day

Retinal Detachment – Separation of the neuroretina from the retinal pigment epithelium by an accumulation of subretinal fluid

Retinoscopy – Determination of the refractive state of the eye by means of a retinoscope

Rubeosis Iridis – Neovascularisation of the iris

Saccade – Involuntary fast movement of the eyes usually to take up fixation or in response to command

Scotoma – Area of partial or complete blindness surrounded by normal visual field

Seclusio Pupillae – Adhesion of the entire pupillary margin of the iris to the capsule of the lens

Snellen Chart – Situated 6 m from the patient, it is made up of letters of graduated sizes with the distance at which each size subtends an angle of 5′ (minutes) indicated along the side of the chart

Symblepharon – Adhesion between the palpebral and bulbar conjunctiva

Synechia, Anterior – Adhesion of the iris to the cornea

Synechia, Posterior – Adhesion of the iris to the capsule of the lens

T.d.s. – Three times a day

Trabecular Meshwork – Connective tissue located at the angle of the anterior chamber in a meshwork pattern

Trichiasis – Inward misdirection of the lashes

Vergence – Movement of both eyes in opposite directions

Version – Rotary movements of both eyes from the primary position in the same direction

Vestibular Nystagmus – Resulting from stimulation of the labyrinth

Visual Acuity – Test of macular function determined with different charts. Capacity for seeing the details of an object distinctly

Vitreous Detachment – Posterior vitreous separation from the retina

Xerophthalmia – Extreme dryness of the conjunctiva and cornea due to failure of the secretory activity of the mucin-secreting goblet cells of the conjunctiva due to trauma, exposure or Vitamin A deficiency

Dedication

To Jonathan and Božana – our respective partners

1 Methodology

Basic optics of the eye

In order to understand the basic principles of optics, it is helpful to define a few terms.

Refraction of light is the change in direction of a ray of light when it passes from one medium to another of a different density. Snell's law relates the change in angle of incidence to the angle of refraction at the boundary of the two media to their refractive indices by the equation: $n_1/n_2 = \sin i/\sin r$, where n_1 is the refractive index of the first medium, n_2 is the refractive index of the second medium, i is the angle of incidence and r is the angle of refraction. Thus rays of light passing from a less dense medium, for example air, to a more dense medium, for example cornea, will be deviated towards the normal. The effect of multiple rays of light being refracted in the eye is to focus the light on the retina.

Reflection of light occurs when light waves strike a smooth surface and bounce off rather than pass through. Some reflection occurs at the corneal surface as seen when a pen-torch is shone towards the eye.

Rays of light from an object of interest are refracted firstly by the cornea and then by the lens to become focused on the retina. The aqueous and vitreous humour provide clear optical media, but do not themselves contribute to the focusing power. The cornea provides two-thirds of the refracting power of the eye owing to the large difference in index of refraction between air (1.0) and cornea (1.376). The power of refraction is measured in dioptres (D) and the cornea contributes 43D to the refracting power of the eye. The lens provides the remaining power of refraction. It is a more powerful refracting surface in air, but is surrounded by aqueous which reduces its refracting power in the eye to 20D. During accommodation, contraction of the ciliary muscle relaxes the zonule fibres surrounding the lens thus allowing the lens to adopt a more spherical shape, increasing its refracting power for close objects. The combined refracting power of the eye is 58.6D (not a simple sum of the 2 refracting surfaces because they are separated in the eye).

The pupil is an important component of the optical system, acting as an aperture. When the pupil is small, chromatic and spherical aberration are reduced by allowing only paraxial rays through. In addition, the depth of focus is increased. In conditions of dim illumination the pupil enlarges allowing more light into the optical system.

Refractive errors and their correction

Refractive errors are the most common cause of loss of visual acuity. A pin-hole acuity helps to eliminate much of the loss due to refractive error (see p. 14).

Emmetropia is the ideal refractive state of the eye, in which, with accommodation relaxed, parallel rays of light, from an object at least 6m away, are focused at the plane of the retina.

Ametropia is any refractive state of the eye that is not emmetropia. It may occur because the optical elements of the eye are weaker or stronger than normal (refractive ametropia) or because the eyeball is larger or smaller than normal (axial ametropia).

Hypermetropia (far-sightedness) is the condition whereby the focused image is formed in a plane behind the retina; i.e. the eyeball is too small or the optical elements too weak. In mild cases, this may be corrected by accommodation before the onset of presbyopia, when this ability is reduced. Constant accommodation to correct for hypermetropia may cause symptoms of tiredness and headache. In children, similar accommodation may be one of the causes of convergent strabismus due to the close relationship between accommodation and convergence. Hypermetropia is corrected with a convex (plus) lens in the spectacles. The correction required is stated in dioptres, for example Right Eye +3.00DS, where D refers to dioptres and S refers to spherical (that is non-astigmatic) correction.

Myopia (near-sightedness) is the condition whereby the focused image is formed in a plane in front of the retina; i.e. the eyeball is too large or the optical elements are too strong. High myopia is associated with a greater incidence of retinal detachment and also chorioretinal degeneration which may involve the macula.

Myopia is corrected with a concave (minus) lens. Thus a typical correction in a low myope might be: R. eye −2.50DS, L. eye −3.00DS.

Astigmatism is the condition in which the refracting power is not uniform in all meridians. Minor astigmatism is extremely common in the general population and if necessary is corrected with spectacles or contact lenses. Greater degrees of astigmatism may be associated with corneal irregularity as seen, for example, in keratoconus (see p. 102). Treatment with a hard contact lens is often of benefit here.

Astigmatism is corrected with a cylindrical (toric) lens that has no power in one meridian and maximum power in the meridian usually at 90° to this. It is often necessary to combine spherical and cylindrical lenses for optical correction when a prescription might read: R. eye +3.50DS/−1.00DC × 175°, where the spherical correction is +3.50D and the cylindrical correction is −1.00D axis (of no power) 175°.

Aphakia is absence of the crystalline lens, usually as a result of surgical removal of a cataract. Here the refracting power of the eye is greatly reduced leading to refractive hypermetropia. Occasionally in high myopes, removal of the lens may bring the subject close to emmetropia. Correction of aphakia with spectacles produces a magnified image that may be difficult to fuse with that coming from the other (phakic) eye. In addition, since high-powered lenses are often needed to correct the vision in aphakia, distortion of images may occur, leading to considerable difficulty in adapting to the spectacles. For these reasons, a contact lens is often preferable.

Presbyopia is the refractive condition in which the accommodative ability of the eye becomes insufficient for satisfactory near vision. It often starts around the fifth decade in emmetropes, but tends to occur earlier in hypermetropes who require more accommodation, and later in myopes who require little or no accommodation. It is corrected either by using two pairs of spectacles, one for distance and one for reading vision, or by using bifocal spectacles. In bifocals, a lens usually +2.50–3.00D, over and above the standard spectacle correction is incorporated in a lower or reading segment. Alternatively, trifocals or a graduated lens may be used to avoid the sudden division between near and distance vision.

Refraction is the name used to describe various testing methods to measure refractive errors of the eye. These methods include:

- retinoscopy, where a light reflected from the patient's retina is viewed as an illumination at the pupil and movement of this light is neutralised by concave or convex lenses placed in front of the eye as appropriate

- subjective refraction when lenses are placed systematically before the eyes until the best corrected visual acuity is reached

- automated refraction, which is a fast, sophisticated, if expensive approach.

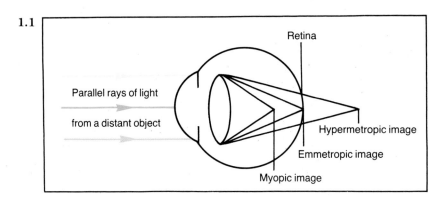

1.1

Fig. 1.1 Refraction of the eye in hypermetropia, emmetropia and myopia

History

(P) An ophthalmic history includes details of the presenting complaint, past ocular history, family history of ocular disease including glaucoma, cataract, macular disease and inherited disorders, general health and past medical history, especially diabetes, hypertension and cardiovascular disease, medications, allergies, smoking and alcohol intake, and social circumstances, including occupation.

Examination

Visual acuity

Visual acuity records the minimum angle subtended at the eye required to resolve two images. It is a test of the visual system from cornea to cortex. It requires patient cooperation and comprehension, clear ocular media, correct focusing, convergence, good retinal function, intact visual pathways and occipital cortex, and the ability to recognise the forms displayed. When all of these functions are intact it is a good test of macular function. Distance vision tests require no accommodation, thus presbyopia does not diminish distance acuity.

The Snellen chart (*Fig. 1.2(a)*) is most commonly used. Each letter height subtends 5′ (1′ is equal to ⅟₆₀°) of arc at a given distance from the eye and each part of the letter, e.g. the arm on an "E", subtends 1′ (*Fig. 1.2(b)*). The distance at which a person with normal vision is able to stand away from the chart to see a particular letter is recorded under each line. The test is carried out at 6m or, if the space is not available, by using a special chart for 3m or a reversible 6m chart situated behind the patient's head with a mirror placed at 3m. The patient covers one eye at a time and his acuity is tested first without, then with spectacles and then looking through a pinhole if necessary.

Recording visual acuity: A person with normal visual acuity will be able to read the 6m line at 6m. This is recorded as 6/6 vision (or 20/20 vision in imperial units). Thus, the numerator is the distance of the patient from the chart and the denominator is the lowest line read. If only the top letter is seen, which can be read normally at 60m, the visual acuity is recorded as 6/60 (20/200) and so on. If the top letter cannot be seen at 6m the patient is brought closer to the chart until it can be identified. The distance of the patient from the chart, e.g. 3m becomes the numerator and the visual acuity is therefore 3/60.

1.2(a)

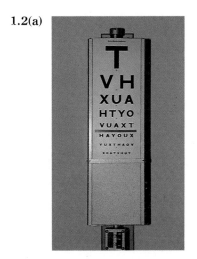

Fig. 1.2(a) Snellen chart

1.2(b)

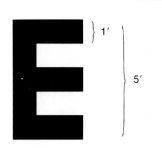

Fig. 1.2(b) Diagram of an 'E' demonstrating that each arm subtends 1′ and the whole 'E' subtends 5′ at the retina

Use of pinhole: If the monocular visual acuity is worse than 6/12 a pinhole is used (*Figs. 1.3 & 1.4*). This corrects any refractive error. If, however, there is a very large refractive error, for instance in aphakia, it will only be partially corrected. It is especially useful if the patient has never had a refraction test or has left his spectacles at home. The new visual acuity is recorded as, e.g. 6/18 U/A (unaided), 6/9 with pinhole. If the pinhole does not improve vision, this is recorded as PHNH (pinhole no help).

Vision less than 1/60: If the top letter cannot be seen at 1 m, the vision is tested for the ability to **count fingers (CF)** (usually at 1 m), to see hand movements or to perceive light. If there is **perception of light (PL) only**, it is useful to record if there is **projection**, that is, if the patient can determine which quadrant the light is coming from. This is recorded as '+' if present, in each of the four quadrants, and is an indication of retinal function in the presence of dense, medial opacity preventing light reaching the retina. If there is **no perception of light** this is recorded as **NPL**.

Other tests of acuity include the **Landholt broken ring test**, where the position of the gap is identified, and the **Illiterate E test** (*Fig. 1.5*), where a cut-out letter E is orientated by the patient in the direction of the E indicated on the chart by the examiner. These tests are useful in patients who are unable to read and can be used in children after the age of 3 years.

Tests used in children: The **Catford Drum** (*Figs. 1.6(a) & (b)*) consists of a drum with a range of different sized dots on it that is rotated in front of the infant. If the infant can see the particular dot size, his or her eyes will be seen to follow the target. The visual acuity scores obtained by this method are a rough guide only. A more accurate test of visual acuity is **preferential looking** (*Fig. 1.7*), where the infant or young child is presented with a series of gratings adjacent to similar sized, plain patches (controls) and the eyes are seen to move towards the patterned side. Thus, the visual acuity is measured by the finest grating size that is reliably discerned. This method of testing appears to be more accurate, but is not yet widely available. Stycar rolling balls are also used in basic assessment of visual acuity, e.g. by health visitors. **Kay picture tests** are used in the 18 month to 3 year age-group and are based on ability to identify pictures. **Sheridan-Gardiner cards** (*Figs. 1.8(a) & (b)*) may be used in the 3–5 year age-group. Here the examiner stands at 6 m and holds up different sized letters in turn. The child is asked to select that letter from a number of letters on the card he is holding. The visual acuity is recorded as for the Snellen chart.

Tests of near vision: Books are available with print of different sizes to test reading ability. This is usually recorded as N or J numbers. In the population aged over 45 years it is important to consider presbyopia as a cause for decreased near visual acuity especially if the distance visual acuity is normal.

1.3

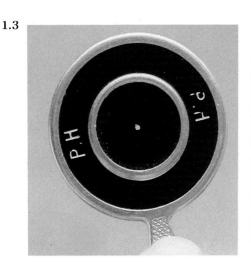

Fig. 1.3 Pinhole

1.4

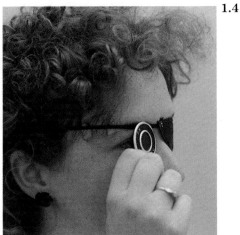

Fig. 1.4 Pinhole in use

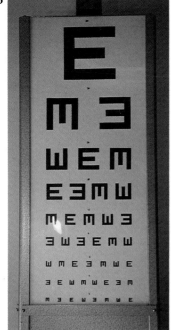

1.5

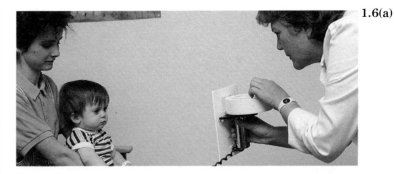

1.6(a)

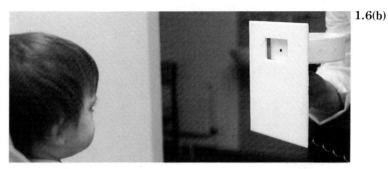

1.6(b)

Fig. 1.5 Illiterate E test   **Figs. 1.6(a) & (b)** Catford Drum

1.7

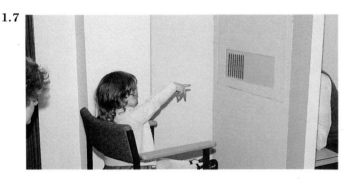

Fig. 1.7 Preferential looking – the infant selects the patterned side (Courtesy of Mr. A. Chandna)

1.8(a)

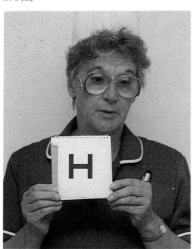

Fig. 1.8(a) Sheridan-Gardiner: the nurse is holding up a large letter 'H' three metres away from the child . . .
Fig. 1.8(b) The child then selects the letter he sees

1.8(b)

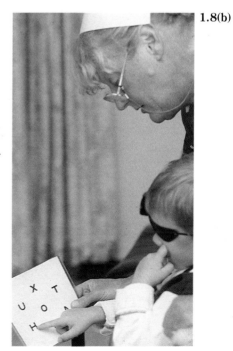

Basic examination of the eye

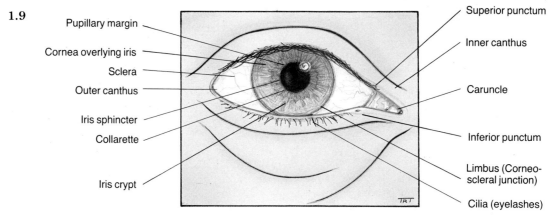

1.9

Pupillary margin
Cornea overlying iris
Sclera
Outer canthus
Iris sphincter
Collarette
Iris crypt

Superior punctum
Inner canthus
Caruncle
Inferior punctum
Limbus (Corneo-scleral junction)
Cilia (eyelashes)

Fig. 1.9 External appearance of the eye

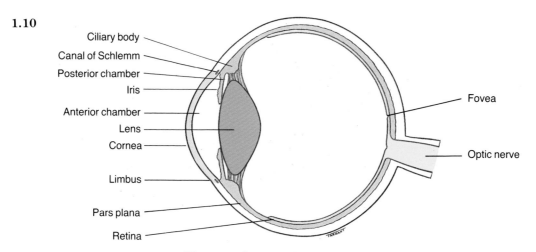

1.10

Ciliary body
Canal of Schlemm
Posterior chamber
Iris
Anterior chamber
Lens
Cornea
Limbus
Pars plana
Retina

Fovea
Optic nerve

Fig. 1.10 Cross-section of the eye

Ⓟ *Figs. 1.9 & 1.10* give guidelines for the non-ophthalmic specialist. The external eye examination should be performed with the aid of a good pen-torch and magnifying loupe (*Fig. 1.11*). The order of examination is lids and lashes, conjunctiva (pattern of inflammation and discharge), cornea (a bright corneal reflex is seen normally), pupil size and regularity, reactions and fundoscopy, preferably after dilation if indicated.

Instillation of drops or ointment (*Figs. 1.12(a) & (b)*) is most easily achieved by asking the patient to look up whilst gently pulling the lower lid down and instilling a drop, or a 1cm length of ointment, in the lower fornix.

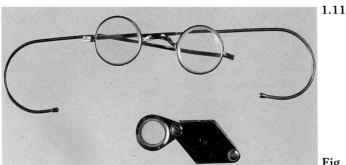

1.11

Fig. 1.11 Magnifying loupe and spectacles

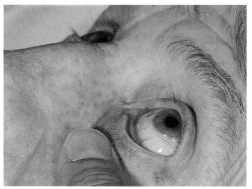

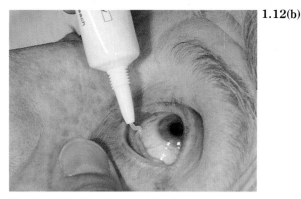

Fig. 1.12(a) Instillation of ointment – the patient is asked to look up

Fig. 1.12(b) The ointment is instilled in the lower fornix

Eyelids

These are examined for malposition – entropion or ectropion, ptosis or lid retraction, misdirected lashes (trichiasis), (*see Fig. 2.25*), scales at the bases of the lashes (blepharitis), eczema and lumps.

Eversion of the upper lid is necessary to look for follicles in viral conjunctivitis or subtarsal, foreign bodies.

● The patient is asked to look down and the upper lid margin and lashes are held between the finger and thumb of the left hand and pulled downwards away from the globe.

● The end of a glass rod or cotton tip, held in the right hand, is placed on the crease of the upper lid (*Fig. 1.13(a)*) at the top edge of the tarsal plate and pushed downwards whilst the edge of the lid is flicked upwards to evert the lid (*Fig. 1.13(b)*).

● The edge of the everted lid is supported with the end of the glass rod until the examination is complete. A subtarsal foreign body is most easily removed with a cotton tip.

● Double eversion is necessary to look for foreign matter in the upper fornix. For this, single eversion is performed, the everted lid supported and the process repeated.

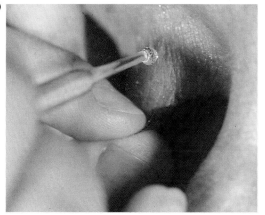

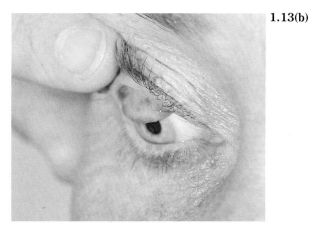

Fig. 1.13(a) Eversion of the upper lid – the rod is placed in the upper lid crease

Fig. 1.13(b) The lid is everted

Conjunctiva

The conjunctiva is a transparent membrane overlying the sclera (bulbar conjunctiva) and the inner surface of eyelids (palpebral conjunctiva). It is examined for injection due to dilatation of the superficial blood vessels either in a ciliary (perilimbal) or conjunctival distribution. The episclera is a deeper layer which may become inflamed and show a deeper dilatation of blood vessels in a radial pattern often as an isolated patch (see p. 76). Conjunctival abrasions can be seen with fluorescein staining.

Cornea

The cornea usually has a bright corneal light reflex (*Fig. 1.14*). If diseased, or in the presence of acutely raised intraocular pressure, it will appear dull and more opaque (*Fig. 1.15*). Corneal sensation (mediated via the fifth nerve) is tested by drawing out a wisp of cotton wool, asking the patient to look up and touching the fine end of the cotton wool on the cornea. A blink reflex (motor via the seventh nerve) is usually observed. Clearly this test is invalid if local anaesthetic drops have been given or if the patient is unable to blink normally.

Absence of corneal reflex is a sensitive and early indicator of pathology involving the fifth cranial nerve. The cornea may be stained by using fluorescein drops or a fluorescein paper strip. This causes yellow staining of any ulcer or abrasion, which is even more obvious under a blue filter when it appears as a brilliant green.

1.14

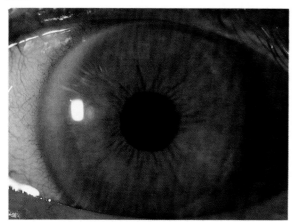

Fig. 1.14 Bright corneal light reflex

1.15

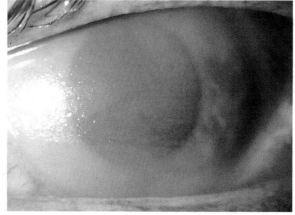

Fig. 1.15 Dull and opaque corneal light reflex

Anterior chamber

A hypopyon (pus in the anterior chamber) (*Fig. 1.16*) or hyphaema (blood in the anterior chamber) (*see Fig. 12.3*) may be seen on inspection with a pen-torch, but for more detailed examination a slit lamp is required. The level of hyphaema is graded according to how much of the anterior chamber is filled, e.g. 1/3 hyphaema signifies blood in the inferior third.

1.16

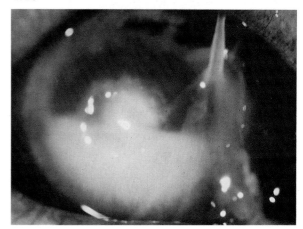

Fig. 1.16 Hypopyon ulcer

Intraocular pressure

A rough estimate of intraocular pressure may be obtained by gently palpating the eyeball through the closed lids using the two index fingers. This method is not very reliable in inexperienced hands and is best reserved for use in suspected acute glaucoma. It is never used after ocular trauma with a suspected ruptured globe.

The Schiotz tonometer is sometimes used for intraocular pressure measurement. It consists of a plate which rests on the anaesthetised cornea and various weights are applied which indent the cornea. A pointer indicates the resistance encountered. There is a calibration scale for each set of weights and a graph for conversion of the reading to mm mercury (mm Hg). Optometrists tend to use a non-contact, air-puff tonometer. The Goldmann and Perkins hand-held tonometers are discussed later (see p. 26).

Lens

Lens opacities are best seen on basic examination using an ophthalmoscope. The dial is set to +10 which allows the ophthalmoscope to be focused on the lens. The lens opacities are seen silhouetted against the red reflex. This is useful even for early lens opacities (*Fig. 1.17*).

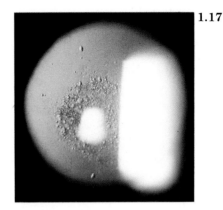

1.17

Fig. 1.17 Early lens opacities against a red reflex

Pupils

The pupils are observed for size, comparing left and right, regularity, reaction to light and accommodation. Normal pupil size is 3–7mm diameter, with less than 0.5mm difference between the two eyes. A pupil diameter of less than 3mm indicates miosis, most commonly due to pilocarpine therapy for glaucoma or senile miosis, but also seen in Horner's syndrome and heroin addiction. A pupil diameter greater than 7mm indicates mydriasis, most commonly due to dilating drops, an Adie pupil, trauma or third nerve palsy. The reaction to light is tested by shining a pen-torch in from the side. There is a direct (same eye) and consensual response (opposite eye), which produce pupils of identical size. The reaction to accommodation is tested by asking the patient to view a distant target and then to focus on a target, for example a finger, placed a few centimetres in front of their nose.

Swinging Torchlight Test: This test looks for a **relative afferent pupillary defect**, which means a difference of afferent input from each eye in testing pupil responses. It is a test of optic nerve function and is very sensitive. In any case of visual loss a relative afferent pupillary defect (also called a Marcus-Gunn pupil) should be tested for before instilling dilating drops to view the fundus.

In a total optic nerve defect there will be no pupil reaction, either direct or consensual, when the torch is shone at the affected eye. This is an **afferent pupil defect** (*Figs. 1.18(a) & (b)*). In a partial optic nerve defect there is a diminished pupil light reaction which is only detectable when compared with the other normal side. The **swinging torchlight test** sets out to detect this and is performed as follows:

• The room should be dimly illuminated.

• A bright light, e.g. from a pen-torch, is shone from below up at the normal eye (in this case the left eye). A brisk direct response is seen in that eye and an identical, consensual response in the right eye (*Fig. 1.18(a)*).

• The torch is quickly swung over to shine similarly into the right (affected) eye. The direct response in the abnormal eye is weaker than the consensual response in the same eye, therefore the pupil on the right will be seen to dilate (*Fig. 1.18(b)*). (Clearly the left pupil will dilate as well, but is not illuminated).

• The torch is swung back to the left (normal) side when the left pupil will be seen to constrict.

• In an afferent lesion, even a total afferent defect, the pupils will be equal in size in normal lighting conditions since the pupil size is determined by the combined afferent input from the two eyes.

• In an efferent defect, e.g. third nerve lesion or iris pathology, the pupils will be of unequal size.

• If there is a normal response to accommodation, but none to light, an Argyll-Robertson pupil (tertiary syphilis) is suggested, especially if the pupils are small and irregular. Diabetes and dorsal mid-brain lesions cause similar, dissociated reflexes. Adie pupils often have no light response and delayed accommodation (*see Figs. 11.2(a) & (b)*).

1.18(a)

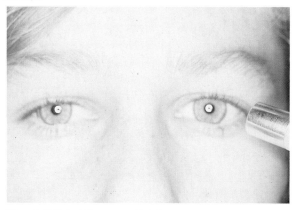

Fig. 1.18(a) Afferent pupil defect – light shone at normal (left) eye. Both pupils constrict

1.18(b)

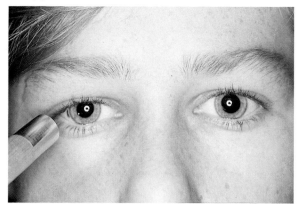

Fig. 1.18(b) Light shone at abnormal (right) eye. Both pupils dilate, but the eye that is being illuminated at the time – here to the right – is observed to dilate

Fundoscopy

The pupils need to be dilated for adequate fundoscopy. For first dilation in adults or children the best dilating drop to use is tropicamide 1%, since it is relatively short acting (about 6 hours) and unlikely to provoke attacks of angle-closure glaucoma in the absence of a suggestive history. There is often a needless reticence to dilate by non-ophthalmologists, but in practice the benefits of dilating far outweigh any risks. When good peripheral examination is required a combination of tropicamide 1% (or cyclopentolate 1%) and phenyl-ephrine 10% drops will usually be effective. Diabetic pupils are often slower to dilate and accordingly a combination of mydriatics, including phenylephrine 10%, is used. It is not recommended to reverse dilating drops with pilocarpine as this **may** provoke angle-closure glaucoma in susceptible individuals and may also cause a headache.

For best results the direct ophthalmoscope (*Fig. 1.19*) should be used in a dimly-lit room with the pupil fully dilated. The ophthalmoscope is held close to the examiner's eye and initially about 15 cm away from the patient to gain a red reflex. The examiner then closes in as near as possible to the patient's eye without touching. The right eye of the examiner is used to view the right eye of the patient with the ophthalmoscope held in the examiner's right hand and *vice versa*. By asking the patient to look at a distant target straight ahead, accommodation will be relaxed and a direct view of the optic disc will be obtained. The view is focused by using a ring of various lenses from −10D to +10D to correct for refractive errors of the patient or examiner. The head of the examiner must not obscure the view of the other eye or the eyes will tend to move. The magnification obtained is about ×15. If there is not a clear view of the fundus, a lens or media opacity is implied.

The disc is examined for size and morphology, swelling of the disc margins, pallor, size of the central cup, character of the blood vessels and so on. The macula is situated two optic disc diameters temporal to the optic disc and slightly below it. It is a deeper red colour and in young individuals has a bright foveal light reflex. It is examined for loss of this reflex, pigment stippling, haemorrhage and exudate. The periphery is examined for haemorrhages, exudates, pigmentation, calibre of blood vessels, A–V nipping, new vessels and so on. Any lesion, e.g. choroidal naevus, is described in terms of optic disc diameters for size and position relative to the optic disc. Red-free light (green) may be used to view blood vessels and the nerve fibre layer more clearly. A small beam of light is useful for small pupils.

1.19

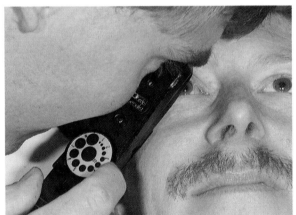

Fig. 1.19 Use of the direct ophthalmoscope

Type of ophthalmoscope

Fundoscopy is one of the hardest areas for the general practitioner or hospital casualty officer to master. Much of this is due to not dilating the pupil or using inadequate equipment. Recent improvements in leading makes of ophthalmoscopes have made them easier to use with improved optics, increased brightness using halogen bulbs, cobalt blue filters incorporated to show up fluorescein staining and a small pinpoint beam included, which is useful for viewing the optic disc. Three manufacturers are highly recommended: Keeler Ltd. (*Fig. 1.20(a) & (b)*), Welch Allyn (marketed via Seward Medical) (*Fig. 1.21*) and Heine (marketed via Albert Waeschle) (*Fig. 1.22*). They all offer a range of ophthalmoscopes from the small, portable type to the sophisticated, specialist instrument. Diagnostic kits are available which combine an ophthalmoscope with an otoscope for a general practitioner or a retinoscope for an ophthalmologist. Welch Allyn offer an especially good, portable ophthalmoscope. The Keeler series and especially The Specialist are well liked by ophthalmologists.

1.20(a)   **1.20(b)**   **1.21**   **1.22**

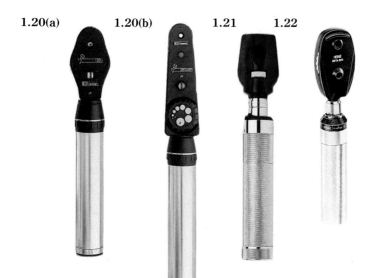

Fig. 1.20(a) Keeler Vista ophthalmoscope (Courtesy of Keeler Instruments, Clewer Hill Road, Windsor, Buckinghamshire, England)

Fig. 1.20(b) Keeler Specialist ophthalmoscope (Courtesy of Keeler Instruments)

Fig. 1.21 Welch Allyn direct ophthalmoscope (Courtesy of Welch Allyn UK Limited, Aston Abbotts, Buckinghamshire, England)

Fig. 1.22 Heine direct ophthalmoscope (Courtesy of Heine – Heine products are marketed through Albert Waeschle, P.O. Box 19, 123–25 Old Christchurch Road, Bournemouth, England)

Other tests of visual function

Field testing

Confrontation field testing (*Fig. 1.23*) will detect large visual field defects, including bitemporal hemianopia, homonymous defects, scotomata and enlarged blind spot. Accurate charting with perimetry is only required to detect more subtle alterations in field, e.g. in glaucoma or small scotomata. A red target is the most sensitive test in suspected optic nerve disease, but if there is decreased visual acuity then a moving finger or, even more crudely, hand movements may be used. One test compares the patient's and examiner's field of view. The examiner sits facing the patient about 1 m away. The patient covers his left eye whilst the examiner covers his right eye. The patient fixates the examiner's nose with the right eye, whilst the examiner fixates the patient's nose. With the left hand the target is slowly brought in from the periphery from eight directions, holding it midway between patient and examiner. The patient indicates when the target is first seen and if it disappears. The blind spot should be mapped. Alternatively, the target may be brought in about 0.33 m from the patient's eye in an arc, when an accurate idea of the visual field may be obtained without comparison of the examiner's field.

Field testing in children is best achieved keeping both eyes open and asking the child to fixate on the examiner's nose. If single eyes are tested the child will inevitably look straight at the target. The examiner holds both arms either side of the child, so that the fingers can just be seen peripherally. The peripheral fields are then tested by asking the child to state on which side the finger is wiggling in several diametrically opposed positions of the arms. Both fingers wiggling simultaneously will test for suppression of one side as in parietal lobe lesions.

(R) **Central field testing** to pick up small scotomas may be accurately performed by the non-ophthalmologist using an Amsler Grid. This consists of a square 10 cm × 10 cm marked off in 0.5 cm small squares with a central spot. The patient fixates on the central spot and can accurately chart any scotomas, distortion etc. in the central 10° of field. It is a very sensitive test of **macula** disease.

(P) **Colour desaturation** is an important sign in optic nerve disease. Use of a red-topped bottle will show up a colour change from bright red to dull red as it passes through an affected part of the vision. There is also a subjective difference in the colour red between the two eyes, the affected one appearing a darker, duller red.

Formal colour testing (*Fig. 1.24*) may be carried (R) out using Ishihara polychromatic plates. These have a series of coloured spots of uniform intensity that form numbers if normal colour vision is present. They are designed to pick up red-green colour defects as seen in optic nerve dysfunction or congenital colour blindness. Ophthalmologists use a more detailed colour test called the Farnsworth-Munsell '100-hue' test in which the patients have to arrange buttons painted with closely graded colours in correct, chromatic order. The results are scored on a chart and a profile is drawn, demonstrating the specific colour defect. This will also pick up macula defects which are typically blue–yellow.

1.23

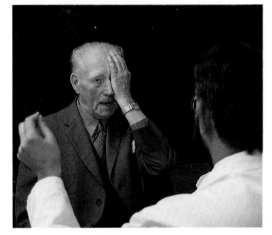

Fig. 1.23 Confrontation field testing

1.24

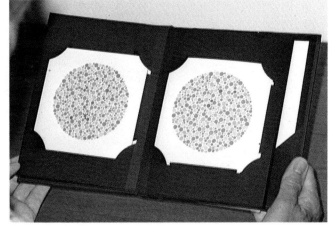

Fig. 1.24 Ishihara colour plates

(P) *Assessment of exophthalmos*

This is best assessed from above and a comparison is made between the two sides. Formal measurement is carried out using an exophthalmometer (see pp. 28–29).

Assessment of extraocular movements

An understanding of the simple anatomy of the extra-ocular muscles is necessary (*see Fig. 13.20*).

The position of the eyes in primary gaze (i.e. straight ahead) together with any asymmetry of corneal light reflexes is noted as a pen-torch is shone at the eyes. If the light reflex is on the nasal side of the cornea, this suggests a divergent or exo- deviation. A cover test (*Fig. 1.25*) is performed to detect a manifest squint. A card is used to cover the straight eye whilst observing the other eye to see if it moves to take up fixation. A movement inwards implies a divergent squint, a movement outwards, a convergent squint (*Fig. 1.26*). This is repeated for the other eye. The test is then repeated on both eyes, but instead of observing the uncovered eye whilst the other is being covered, the covered eye is observed to see what happens when it is uncovered. If a latent squint is present, the eye will tend to drift as it is covered and return to normal as it is uncovered. Again, a compensatory movement inwards suggests a latent, divergent squint and a movement outwards, a latent, convergent squint. Further dissociation of the two eyes can be induced by alternately covering the two eyes in quick succession, which will demonstrate most latent squints (the alternate cover test). The extraocular movements are tested in an 'H' pattern (see p. 190), which tests the individual muscles.

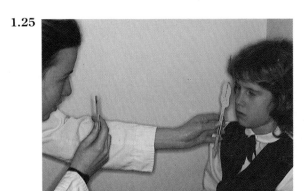

Fig. 1.25 Cover test

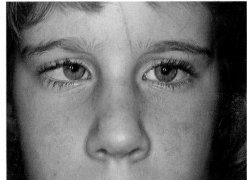

Fig. 1.26 Right convergent squint

Schirmer's test

A quantitative measurement of tear production is obtained by this method, outlined in Chapter 5.

® Further assessment of the eye as in an eye casualty department

Slit lamp examination

The slit lamp biomicroscope allows fuller assessment of the anterior segment, vitreous and fundus of the eye (*Fig. 1.27*). The patient rests his chin on a support, with his forehead against a band. He looks straight ahead as the observer views through the eyepieces. The microscope is positioned by moving a joystick backwards and forwards and from side to side. The eye is usually assessed from the lids progressively inwards. The beam width is adjustable. A wide beam is used to view the surface of the cornea, whereas a narrow, slit beam is used for a cross-section view through the eye, enabling the layers of the cornea and lens to be seen.

1.27

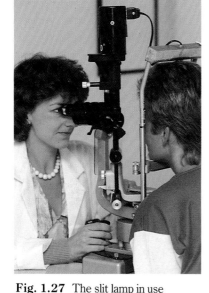

Fig. 1.27 The slit lamp in use

1.28

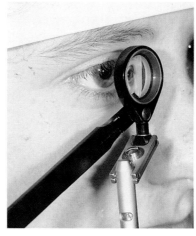

Fig. 1.28 Hruby lens in use

1.29

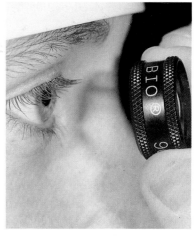

Fig. 1.29 90 D lens in use

Depths of foreign bodies may be accurately assessed, and their removal facilitated using a slit lamp. A pinpoint beam is used to assess flare and cells in the anterior chamber in anterior uveitis. Retroillumination is achieved by using a slit beam directed straight at the eye at 90°, which will demonstrate lens opacities or iris atrophy against the red reflex. After fluorescein stain has been applied, a cobalt-blue filter is used to view the eye for corneal staining, e.g. in abrasions or ulcers. Detailed examination of the disc and macula is carried out using a Hruby lens ($-58.6D$) (*Fig. 1.28*), placed in front of the narrow, slit beam. This produces an upright image. Alternatively, a fundus contact lens is applied giving a similar view. A wider view of the fundus is obtained on the slit lamp using a 90D lens (*Fig. 1.29*), giving an inverted image.

The following three techniques need careful instruction before starting:

Applanation tonometry

This is an accurate and widely used system for measuring intraocular pressure, but it takes practice (*Figs. 1.30(a) & (b)*). Some patients have a tendency to squeeze their eyelids closed. A single drop of a mixture of lignocaine and fluorescein preparation (or benoxinate and fluorescein) is placed in each eye. About 1 minute is needed for the anaesthetic to take effect. A cobalt-blue filter with the brightest, widest beam is used. An applanation tonometer head is then applied to the centre of the cornea such that two, semicircular, yellow lines are seen as demonstrated. The dial is adjusted whilst the tonometer head is in contact with the eye so that these semicircles just interlock as shown (*Fig. 1.31*). The tonometer head is removed from the eye and the pressure is read off directly from the dial.

1.30(a)   **1.30(b)**   **1.31**

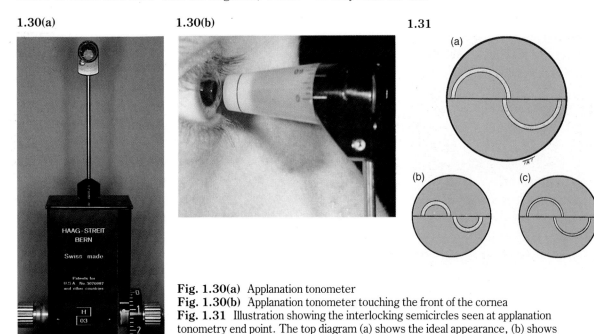

Fig. 1.30(a) Applanation tonometer
Fig. 1.30(b) Applanation tonometer touching the front of the cornea
Fig. 1.31 Illustration showing the interlocking semicircles seen at applanation tonometry end point. The top diagram (a) shows the ideal appearance, (b) shows under applanation or too much fluorescein, (c) shows over applanation or too little fluorescein

Use of Goldmann contact lenses

There are three different types of contact lenses commonly used (*Fig. 1.32*). Again, the application of these lenses is not always easy, depending on the anatomy of the patient and their anxiety, which can lead to uncontrollable blinking.

Each type is applied after first anaesthetising the cornea with 1% benoxinate. The slit lamp is set up to use a narrow slit at 90° to the cornea. The patient is asked to look down (*Fig. 1.33(a)*) and to keep the head forward against the headband. The contact lens cup is filled with about 6 drops of hypromellose or sterile saline. The lower lid is pulled down away from the eye whilst the lower edge of the lens is placed in contact with the lower edge of the cornea using the other hand (*Fig. 1.33(b)*). The lens is tilted to make contact with the rest of the cornea whilst the upper lid is held away. Finally, the patient is asked to look straight ahead and any drops rolling down the cheek are wiped away. The slit lamp is then focused to view the area of interest.

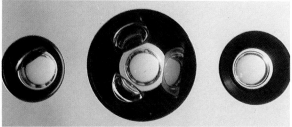

Fig. 1.32 3 fundal contact lenses: left – gonioscopy lens, centre – 3-mirror contact lens, right – plain fundal contact lens

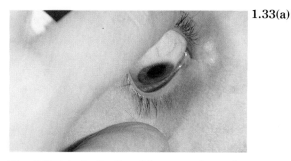

Fig. 1.33(a) Application of the contact lens – the patient is asked to look down

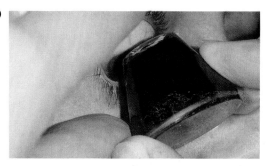

Fig. 1.33(b) The lower edge of the lens is placed on the lower limbus

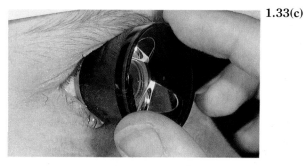

Fig. 1.33(c) The lens in place

The **three-mirror contact lens** (*Fig. 1.33(c)*) is used to view the centre of the fundus through the central lens, and the periphery through three mirrors, each angled to view various zones including the mid-periphery, equatorial and ora serrata/angle. The lens is slowly rotated, whilst the slit lamp is adjusted, to follow a particular mirror until 360° has been completed. Then the next mirror is used and so on. This contact lens is especially useful for viewing retinal detachments and peripheral holes or tears.

The **fundus contact lens** contains an identical lens to the central part of the three-mirror lens. It is easier to use, being less bulky and with better suction to the cornea. It is used for viewing the macula and optic disc in more detail when peripheral views are not required.

The **gonioscopy lens** (*Fig. 1.34*) contains a central viewing lens for the disc and a mirror for viewing the structures of the angle. It is used in glaucoma. Again, the contact lens is rotated through 360° to view the entire angle.

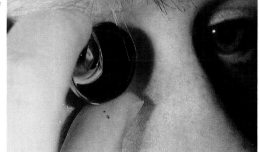

Fig. 1.34 Gonioscopy lens

Indirect ophthalmoscopy

This is a skillful method of viewing the retina which provides a wide field of view and can be used with moderate media opacities (*Fig. 1.35*). It also allows a stereoscopic view, of most value when a three-dimensional impression of an elevated lesion is necessary. It is extremely useful for viewing retinal detachments. The disadvantages are that the image is inverted and back-to-front and that practice is necessary to master the technique.

The examiner wears a headset that contains a light source which should be adjusted so that it is aimed at his thumbnail, held out in front of him. The pupil must be fully dilated. The patient may either be viewed sitting up or lying down. The examiner gently holds the eyelids apart with one hand whilst holding a 20D or 30D lens 5–10 cm in front of the eye until an image is obtained. With the patient sitting, a view of the posterior pole is obtained by asking the patient to look at the opposite ear of the examiner to the eye being viewed. The patient is then asked to look down, down and to the left, across to the left and so on until the entire fundus has been viewed. The direction in which the patient looks throws the equivalent area of fundus into view. For example, looking down and to the left with the left eye demonstrates the inferior temporal fundus (inverted and back-to-front). If the patient is viewed lying down on a couch, with the examiner standing at the top of the head, the image obtained is upright and more easily drawn. For very peripheral lesions, the sclera can be indented using an indentor (*Fig. 1.36*).

1.35 1.36

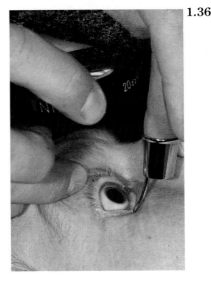

Fig. 1.35 Indirect ophthalmoscopy **Fig. 1.36** Indentation

Measurement of exophthalmos

Viewing the eyes from above is a good way of demonstrating exophthalmos. It may be quantified by using a Keeler exophthalmometer (*Fig. 1.37*). The exophthalmometer is adjusted so that the two curved pieces at the back fit on the lateral orbital rims. The patient fixates first with his right eye on the examiner's left eye. The examiner closes his right eye and lines his left eye up so that the blue marker is directly in front of the mark for 15 mm in the mirror. Then the position of the reflection of the cornea is read off the same scale in millimetres. This is repeated for the other eye. A reading greater than 20 mm, or a disparity of greater than 2 mm between the two eyes, implies a need for further investigation. The distance between the two orbital rims is read off the scale on the bar and recorded for future comparisons.

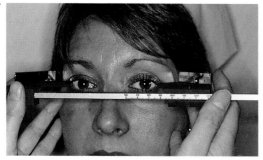

Fig. 1.37 Measurement of exophthalmos

Perimetry – Goldmann and Friedmann Fields

There are two ways of testing visual fields: static and kinetic field tests. The Goldmann perimeter (*Fig. 1.38*), a kinetic test, accurately charts central and peripheral field. The patient rests his chin on a support so that the head is inside a hemisphere with the eye 33 cm from all positions of the target. One eye is covered and the patient asked to fixate on the central target. Small light targets are brought in slowly along meridians and the patient indicates when they are first seen. The position is marked on a chart. The blind spot may be charted, as well as any scotomas. Targets of different sizes and intensities may be used.

Bjerrum fields are another form of kinetic test using a white target on a stick against a flat, black background.

Friedmann analysers (*Fig. 1.39*) are static tests and measure central vision. The patient fixates on a central spot and the visual threshold is obtained. Several light spots are then shone at various positions in the field and the patient recalls those he has seen. Gradually an entire picture of the visual field is built up. A computerised modification of the Friedmann analyser, called the Henson Analyser (*Fig. 1.40*), has now come into use.

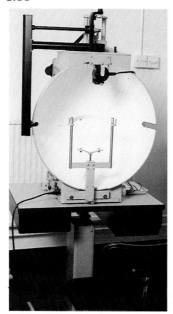

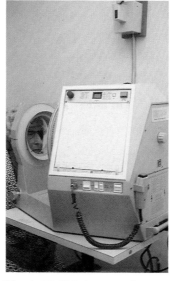

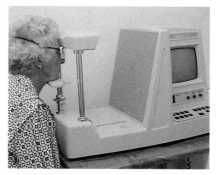

Fig. 1.40 Henson analyser

Fig. 1.39 Friedmann analyser

Fig. 1.38 Goldmann perimeter

Keratometry

The corneal curvatures are measured by keratometry in any contact lens work or prior to insertion of an intraocular lens to calculate the strength required.

Irregularities in the corneal surface, e.g. in keratoconus, may be gauged in the clinic using a Placido's disc (*Fig. 1.41*). Here the examiner views, through a central viewing hole, the corneal reflection of concentric circles produced by the disc. The circles will be more crowded at steeper corneal curvatures. A more accurate picture is obtained using a photokeratoscope.

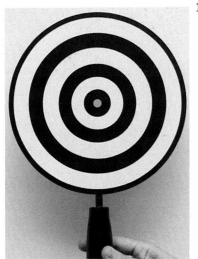

Fig. 1.41 Placido's disc

(S) *Electrodiagnostic tests*

Several different types of electrodiagnostic tests, including electroretinography (*Fig. 1.42*), electrooculography and visual evoked response (potential), are used in ophthalmology, mainly in the diagnosis of inherited retinal diseases, e.g. retinitis pigmentosa. The visual evoked response (VER), however, may also be useful in the acute situation, especially in the diagnosis of retrobulbar neuritis. The VER is the electrical response to the stimulus of a bright flash of light or a checkerboard pattern as measured by occipital electrodes. The wave-form has a characteristic amplitude and latency. Typically, in retrobulbar neuritis, there is a diminished amplitude and increased latency of the first deflection.

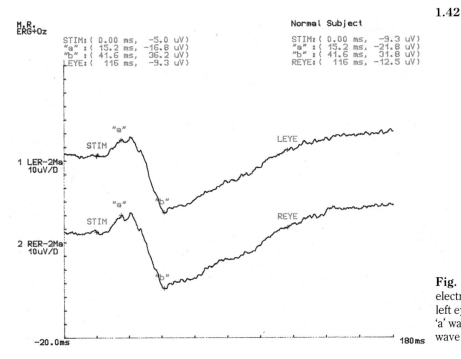

Fig. 1.42 Normal electroretinogram of right and left eye showing typical positive 'a' wave followed by a negative 'b' wave

ⓢ Ultrasound

A sound beam reflected off the various ocular structures can build up a two-dimensional picture of the globe (*Fig. 1.43(a) & (b)*). This is sometimes helpful in the acute situation. For example, in a patient with a vitreous haemorrhage, when there is a poor fundal view, a scan may reveal the presence of a retinal detachment.

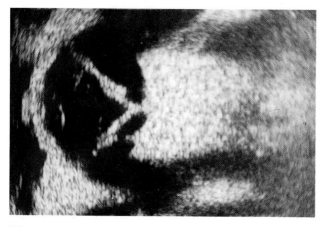

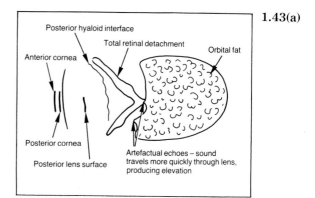

1.43(a)

Fig. 1.43(a) Retinal detachment

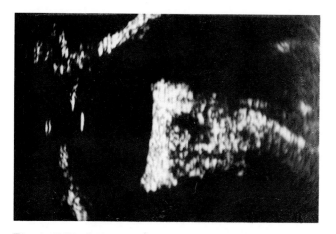

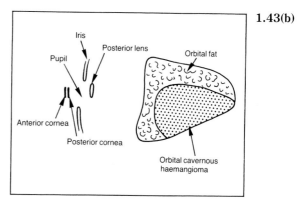

1.43(b)

Fig. 1.43(b) Orbital cavernous haemangioma

ⓢ Fluorescein angiography

This test is useful for further diagnosis of maculopathy, retinal vascular disorders, choroidal tumours and so on. In the context of immediate eye care, the main indication is in acute macular disciform degeneration to determine if the lesion is treatable (see p. 140).

PART I

A SYSTEMATIC APPROACH TO DISEASES OF THE EYE

Key

Ⓟ Family Practitioner and Casualty Officer or Emergency Physician

Ⓡ Eye Casualty Officer or Resident in Ophthalmology

Ⓢ Ophthalmologist or Specialist

2 Eyelid

Normal anatomy of the eyelids and normal appearances

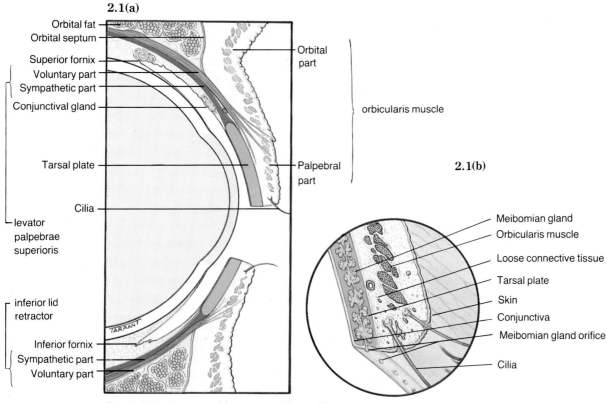

2.1(a)

Orbital fat
Orbital septum
Superior fornix
Voluntary part
Sympathetic part
Conjunctival gland
Tarsal plate
Cilia
levator palpebrae superioris
inferior lid retractor
Inferior fornix
Sympathetic part
Voluntary part

Orbital part
orbicularis muscle
Palpebral part

2.1(b)

Meibomian gland
Orbicularis muscle
Loose connective tissue
Tarsal plate
Skin
Conjunctiva
Meibomian gland orifice
Cilia

Fig. 2.1(a) Anatomy of the upper and lower lid
Fig. 2.1(b) Detail of upper lid

The eyelids (*Fig. 2.1(a) & (b)*) act as protectors of the globe by maintaining a continuously wet surface on the cornea, through blinking and contributing essential elements of the tear film from the glands in the eyelid margin. They open sufficiently to allow light in through the pupil and protect the cornea from foreign matter by maintaining a narrow and variable palpebral fissure and using the eyelashes.

Both eyelids have a similar, layered structure. The most superficial structures are skin, and orbicularis muscle, which can be divided into three sections: pretarsal (lid), preseptal (in front of the orbital septum) and orbital (outermost part). The orbicularis muscle (supplied by the seventh cranial [facial] nerve) is responsible for **closing** the eyelids – the pretarsal part for light blinking and the outer parts for tight closure. During light blinking the tear film is washed over the corneal surface and during tight closure further tears are produced from the lacrimal gland.

Situated deep to orbicularis is the orbital septum, a fibrous supporting structure that lies between the orbital rim and inserts into the levator aponeurosis at the top of the eyelid and the tarsal plate inferiorly. The orbital fat lies behind this structure which also anatomically demarcates a preseptal cellulitis from the more dangerous orbital cellulitis (see p. 170). The stability of the eyelids is maintained by the medial and lateral canthal tendons which are attached to the periosteum.

Superiorly behind the pretarsal orbicularis muscle lie the two parts of the levator palpebrae superioris muscle – the aponeurosis anteriorly, which inserts by finger-like projections into the anterior part of the eyelid, and Muller's muscle, which inserts into the tarsal plate. The levator muscle is mainly supplied by the third cranial nerve, but also by the sympathetic nerves (Muller's muscle). Its main action is to open the eyelids. Damage to either part results in ptosis (see pp. 40–42). In the lower lid there are inferior retractors responsible for depressing the lid on downgaze.

The tarsal plates are fibrous condensations which maintain the form of the eyelids and are situated in the deeper half of the eyelids. They contain about 30 Meibomian glands which open by separate orifices onto the lid margin. The grey line is a visible sign on the lid margin, corresponding to the division between anterior and posterior parts of the eyelid. It is useful for exact alignment of lid structures in lid repair. The eyelashes (cilia) lie anterior to this, together with modified sebaceous glands of Moll and Zeis at their base, and the Meibomian ducts lie posterior to the grey line at the mucocutaneous junction.

Finally, the eyelids are lined with conjunctiva which also contains lymphoid tissue which can enlarge to form follicles.

Specific conditions

Chalazion

A chalazion (*Fig. 2.2*) is a lump in the eyelid that forms owing to inflammation of a Meibomian gland. In the acute stage there is localised hyperaemia, pain and swelling of lid due to acute infection. In the chronic stage Meibomian gland secretions become retained due to blockage of the duct, giving a localised swelling of the lid.

2.2

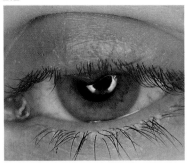

Fig. 2.2 Chalazion

2.3(a)

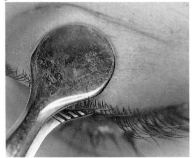

Fig. 2.3(a) Incision and curettage of chalazion – application of eyelid clamp

2.3(b)

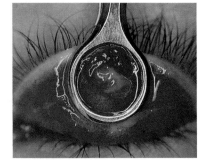

Fig. 2.3(b) Chalazion centred within clamp

2.3(c)

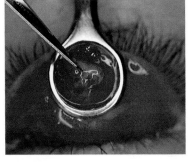

Fig. 2.3(c) Incision of chalazion with scalpel blade

2.3(d)

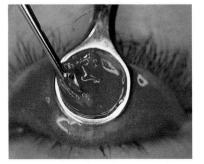

Fig. 2.3(d) Curettage

2.3(e)

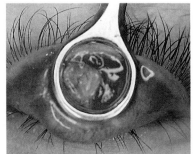

Fig. 2.3(e) Endstage, when all contents have been removed

Symptoms: Range from mild foreign body sensation to pain, together with distorted vision due to pressure on the cornea.

Signs: Swelling of the lid arising from behind the lid margin which may form a granuloma.

(P) *Management:* Early stages: Topical antibiotic ointment four times daily; warm bathing to soften the waxy plug of secretions that is blocking the duct may be helpful. Later stages: incision and curettage is necessary as outlined below (*Figs. 2.3(a)–(e)*). General practitioners can do this after a period of training in an Eye Casualty Department:

- Clean the skin of the eyelid.

(R) • Inject 1–2ml 1% lignocaine and adrenaline subcutaneously around the chalazion.

- Apply eyelid clamp (*Fig. 2.3(a)*) as shown and tighten the screw.

- Evert the lid – the chalazion should be centred within the clamp (*Fig. 2.3(b)*); if not, reposition the clamp.

- Incise the chalazion vertically using a no. 11 scalpel blade (*Fig. 2.3(c)*).

- Curette the contents (*Fig. 2.3(d)*).

- Release the clamp and gently press on the eye for a few minutes to stop any bleeding.

- Use single application of antibiotic ointment and pad the eye for a few hours, as outlined below (*Figs. 2.3(f)–(i)*).

- Continue antibiotic ointment four times daily for one week.

2.3(f)

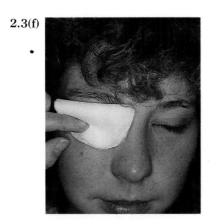

Fig. 2.3(f) A folded pad is placed over the closed eye

2.3(g)

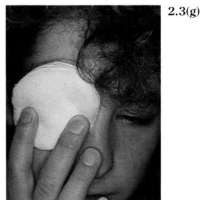

Fig. 2.3(g) A second unfolded pad is placed over the top

2.3(h)

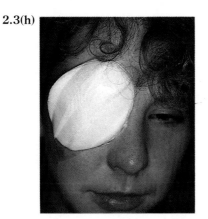

Fig. 2.3(h) Sticky tape is applied along the length of the pad

2.3(i)

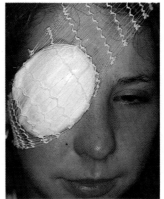

Fig. 2.3(i) An open-weave bandage is fitted to hold the padding firmly in place

Stye (external hordoleum)

This is an acute staphylococcal abscess in the modified sebaceous glands (of Moll and of Zeis) at the base of the eyelashes, or in the follicle itself (*Fig. 2.4*).

Symptoms: A sore, swollen lid for a few days.

Signs: An acute, tender, inflamed swelling in the lid margin, often pointing round a lash follicle. Occasionally multiple swellings may be present.

Ⓟ *Management:* Treatment with 'hot spoon bathing' consists of dipping a wooden cooking spoon wrapped with muslin into boiling water and holding the steaming spoon a few centimetres from the eye (not touching) until the steaming ceases, and repeating the process several times. If necessary, the eyelash associated with the infected follicle may be removed to encourage

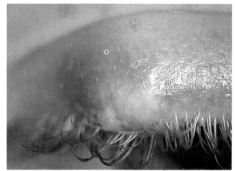

Fig. 2.4 Stye

the stye to discharge. Only occasionally is incision required. Antibiotic ointment q.d.s. to the lid margins is used to prevent spread of infection to other lash follicles.

Primary Herpes simplex virus infection

This may cause a vesicular eruption on the eyelids (*Fig. 2.5*) (see pp. 63, 81).

Ⓟ *Management:* Acyclovir ointment 5% five times daily to the lesions for seven days.

Cyst of Moll

This is a cyst arising from retained watery secretions of an eyelid sweat gland (*Fig. 2.6*).

Symptoms: Slowly enlarging, asymptomatic cyst on the lid margins, usually present for a number of years. Removal is often requested for cosmetic reasons.

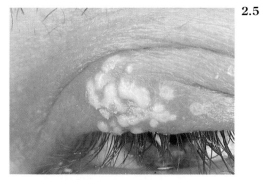

Fig. 2.5 Primary *Herpes simplex* virus infection of the lid

Signs: Translucent cyst on the lid margin.

Ⓟ Ⓡ *Management:* Simple excision or marsupialisation of the cyst under local anaesthetic.

Cyst of Zeis

This is a cyst arising from retained oily secretions of the glands at the base of the eyelashes.

Symptoms: Small, painless lump at lid margin.

Signs: Small, white cyst at lid margin, associated with the base of an eyelash.

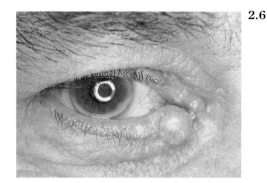

Fig. 2.6 Cyst of Moll

Ⓟ Ⓡ *Management:* Spontaneous resolution is usual over a period of months. Warm bathing may help to loosen the plug of oily secretions. If necessary, it may be excised or marsupialised under local anaesthetic.

Sebaceous Cyst

These cysts, which occur around the eye as elsewhere in the body, are caused by retained secretions from ordinary skin sweat glands (*Fig. 2.7*).

Symptoms: This usually appears as an asymptomatic lump in the skin, but can sometimes become infected.

Signs: Yellow–white lumps in the skin with a central punctum, occasionally inflamed and tender when infected.

(S) *Management:* Simple excision under local anaesthetic. When infected, they should be treated with a course of flucloxacillin prior to complete excision. They should not be incised.

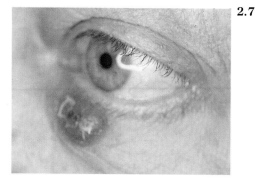

Fig. 2.7 Infected sebaceous cyst

Entropion and Ectropion

Entropion is a congenital or acquired inversion of the eyelid. Ectropion is a congenital or acquired eversion of the eyelid. The main problems encountered are severe discomfort, lacrimation, corneal exposure or erosion, infection, epiphora, and cosmetic. They are often more difficult to treat than is realised.

Entropion

Symptoms: May be asymptomatic. Discomfort due to the rubbing of the eyelashes on the cornea, which may be extreme if a corneal ulcer is present.

Signs: In-rolling of the lid margin and associated punctate, epithelial erosions on the cornea where the lashes are rubbing (*Fig. 2.8*). Occasionally the cornea epithelium is deeply eroded to form an ulcer. This is more likely to occur in an acquired form.

Management:

● **Congenital entropion**

This type of entropion is rare and only involves the lower lid, usually bilaterally. It is caused by hypertrophy of the skin and underlying orbicularis muscle fibres. It is usually mild and self-limiting. If persistent and (S) symptomatic, corrective surgery is aimed at excising the hypertrophic skin and orbicularis and suturing the skin edges to the inferior tarsal border.

Epiblepharon (*Fig. 2.9*) is a different condition in which there is an extra fold of skin in the lower lid margin, but no associated hypertrophy of the orbicularis muscle. It usually resolves spontaneously within 1–2 years. The excess fold of skin may be excised if the lashes are abrading the cornea.

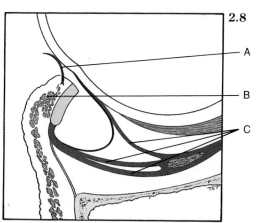

Fig. 2.8 Mechanism of entropion. A – Lash abrading inferior fornix, B – Overriding of orbital part of orbicularis over palpebral part of orbicularis, C – Inferior lid retractors

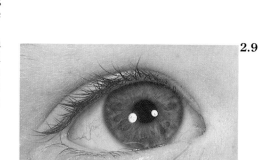

Fig. 2.9 Epiblepharon (Courtesy of Mr. R. Humphry)

• Acquired entropion

The causes are involutional (senile), cicatricial or acute spastic.

(a) Involutional or senile entropion

This is the most common type of entropion and only affects the lower lid (*Fig. 2.10*). It is caused by laxity of the skin and subcutaneous tissues such that they become less adherent to the underlying orbicularis muscle. During lid closure the preseptal (outer) portion of the orbicularis muscle overrides the pretarsal (inner) portion, causing the lower lid to roll inwards.

(P)(R) Treatment of a corneal erosion involves giving a single dose of antibiotic ointment, instilling a drop of homatropine 2%, taping the lower lid onto the skin of the cheek so that the lashes are not touching the cornea and padding the eye firmly overnight.

Daily review with repeated antibiotics and padding is continued until the erosion is healed. Thereafter, until definitive lid surgery can be carried out, the lower lid should be kept taped outwards (*Fig. 2.11*) and lubricating ointment applied to the eye two or three times daily.

Surgery aims to correct the laxity by lid horizontal (S) shortening procedures and prevent overriding of orbicularis muscles by anchoring sutures.

2.10

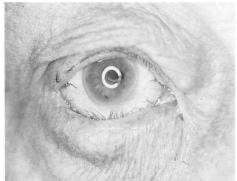

Fig. 2.10 Involutional entropion

2.11

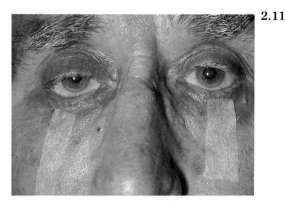

Fig. 2.11 Strapping the lower lid to prevent lashes rubbing in involutional entropion

(b) Cicatricial entropion

In this type of entropion, the palpebral conjunctiva becomes scarred through disease and as the scar tissue contracts, the lid margin is pulled in towards the globe. Both upper and lower lids are involved. It is caused by trachoma, chemical burns (especially alkali), ocular cicatricial pemphigoid and Stevens-Johnson (S) syndrome. The cornea is protected from the ingrowing lashes by regular epilation and surgical lid eversion procedures. Corneal ulceration is managed as in involutional entropion (v.s.).

(c) Acute spastic entropion

Acute spastic entropion occurs when there is increased tonus of orbicularis muscle, as seen in essential blepharospasm or chronic corneal irritation, e.g. by ingrowing eyelashes. Thus an involutional entropion could be exacerbated by a spastic element. Resolution usually follows removal of the source of irritation (e.g. (R)(epilation of ingrowing eyelashes, treatment of corneal ulceration), and eversion of the lower lid by taping it to the skin of the upper cheek until the source of the irritation is removed. Essential blepharospasm is now managed successfully with local injections of botulinum (S) toxin into the skin and subcutaneous muscle in the affected areas. This is carried out as a day-case procedure and needs to be repeated at 3–6 monthly intervals.

Ectropion

Symptoms: Often asymptomatic. Occasionally there is watering of the eye (epiphora) and soreness of the everted lid.

Signs: Lid eversion with resultant displacement of the punctum away from the lacus lacrimalis (*Fig. 2.12*). The exposed conjunctiva becomes hypertrophied and keratinised. The exposed cornea may show signs of drying (e.g. punctate erosions well stained by Rose Bengal) or occasionally scarring in severe cases.

Management:

● **Congenital ectropion**

This is a rare form of ectropion and may affect upper and/or lower lids. It is associated with blepharophimosis. In neonates especially, it may be associated with spasm of the orbicularis induced by crying. If there is (S) a deficiency of skin, a full-thickness graft may be necessary to correct the defect.

● **Acquired ectropion**

The acquired types are involutional (senile), mechanical, cicatricial, or paralytic.

(a) Involutional (senile) ectropion (*Figs. 2.13, 2.14*)
There is general laxity of the lower lid structures including the medial and lateral canthal tendons. Gravity aggravates this, leading to horizontal lid stretching and sagging. Exposure keratitis and corneal drying may (P) result. Temporary measures include frequent instillation of artificial tears (up to every 15 or 30 minutes if necessary), using lubricating ointment at night and taping the eye closed if required. Definitive lid surgery (S) involves lower lid horizontal shortening procedures and tightening the canthal tendons.

(b) Mechanical ectropion
Any form of lid swelling, e.g. a chalazion or a tumour, (R) may produce an ectropion and treatment involves local removal of the lump.

(c) Cicatricial ectropion
This type of ectropion is caused by a deficiency of lid tissues through loss, e.g. trauma or tumour resection, and/or contracture formation, e.g. following burns. (S) Lid surgery aims to resect the scar tissue and extend the skin by Z-plasty or skin graft.

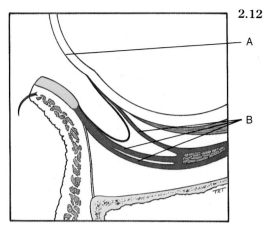

Fig. 2.12 Mechanism of entropion.
A – Exposure of inferior part of cornea,
B – Laxity of inferior lid retractors

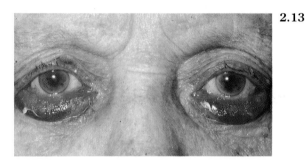

Fig. 2.13 Bilateral ectropion (Courtesy of Mr. S. Cook)

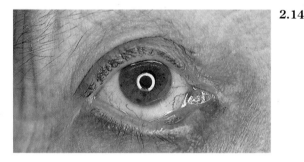

Fig. 2.14 Right medial ectropion

(d) Paralytic ectropion (*Figs. 2.15, 2.16*)

This is caused by facial nerve palsy and consequent weakness of orbicularis muscle with lower lid laxity, incomplete blinking and inability to close the lids (lagophthalmos). The most common complications are corneal drying due to the lack of tear-film maintenance and corneal exposure, especially at night when the eyelids often remain open. Bell's phenomenon, whereby the front of the eye rolls upwards under the upper lid during blinking and lid closure at night, protects the cornea. If the seventh nerve paresis is incomplete and likely to be temporary, e.g. Bell's

palsy, the management consists of frequent instillation (P) (even up to every 15 to 30 minutes initially), of artificial tear drops, use of lubricating ointment and taping the eyelids closed at night. In severe and permanent cases lateral canthoplasty may be used to (S) reduce the palpebral aperture and maintain the tear film. Tarsorrhaphy, where the eyelids are sutured together, usually laterally, is much less acceptable cosmetically, but may be the only way to prevent exposure keratitis.

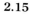

2.15 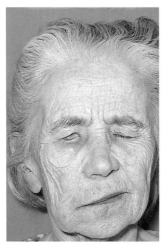   **2.16**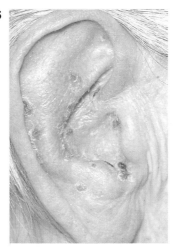

Fig. 2.15 Right facial nerve palsy due to Ramsay-Hunt syndrome, leading to paralytic ectropion (Courtesy of Mr. R. Humphry)

Fig. 2.16 Vesicular eruption in the ear of the same patient in **Fig. 2.15** (Courtesy of Mr. R. Humphry)

Ptosis

This is a congenital or acquired inability to elevate the upper eyelid (*Fig. 2.17*). The eyelid position is determined by upper lid retraction, in turn controlled by levator palpebrae superioris (supplied by the third nerve) and Muller's muscle (which is innervated by the sympathetics). The normal position of the eyelid is 2mm below the upper limbus (see diagram) and the corneal diameter is about 11mm diameter; therefore the position of the eyelid can be determined by

measuring from the lower limbus. The causes may be broadly divided into:

- Neurogenic
- Myogenic
- Aponeurotic
- Mechanical

However, more than one of these factors can play a part in any given condition.

2.17

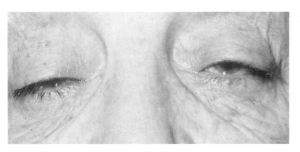

Fig. 2.17 Bilateral ptosis (Courtesy of Mr. S. Cook)

Neurogenic ptosis

This is due to deficient innervation of the levator muscle by the third nerve leading to a complete, or almost complete, ptosis (see pp. 192–93) or by deficient sympathetic innervation, as in a Horner's syndrome, leading to a partial ptosis (see pp. 186–87). There can also be aberrant innervation by the third nerve after trauma where unusual eyelid movements accompany extra-ocular movements. The Marcus-Gunn jaw-winking syndrome is a congenital abnormality, probably originating from the brainstem, which causes an elevation of the ptotic lid during jaw movements – a synkinesis (*Fig. 2.18(a) & (b)*).

2.18(a) 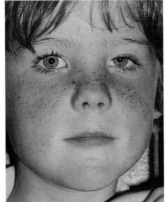 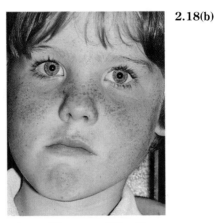 2.18(b)

Fig. 2.18(a) & (b) Marcus-Gunn syndrome (Courtesy of Miss H. Frank)

Myogenic ptosis

Levator dysfunction is associated with a number of muscular disorders including myasthenia gravis (one of the most important conditions to exclude in ptosis), oculopharyngeal muscular dystrophy, progressive external ophthalmoplegia and myotonic dystrophy.

Congenital ptosis

This is caused by a dystrophic levator muscle and is usually unilateral. There is often poor contraction and also defective relaxation of the levator muscle. If the visual axis is obstructed, there is a danger of amblyopia developing and ptosis surgery is indicated without delay. Otherwise, it is wise to defer this until the eye can be more accurately assessed from orthoptic and refraction standpoints and a more definitive approach adopted (usually around four years). Congenital ptosis can also be associated with the autosomally inherited condition, blepharophimosis (*Fig. 2.19*), where there is hypertelorism, epicanthus inversus and ectropion.

2.19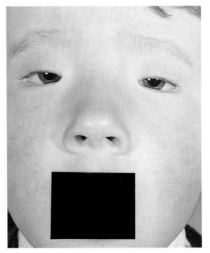

Fig. 2.19 Blepharophimosis (Courtesy of Mr. C. Dean Hart)

Aponeurotic ptosis

Senile ptosis is caused by involutional changes in the levator aponeurosis in older patients. Levator function is preserved. An aponeurotic ptosis may also occur postoperatively, e.g. after cataract surgery, when the aponeurosis may have been stretched, or following occlusion (patching) during the treatment of amblyopia. Trauma to either the levator muscle or aponeurosis results in ptosis, e.g. following laceration.

Mechanical ptosis

Excessive weight on the upper eyelid, such as with an eyelid tumour like a neurofibroma, may lead to a mechanical ptosis (*Fig. 2.20*). Conjunctival scarring, as in benign ocular pemphigoid or Stevens–Johnson syndrome, may lead to a restriction of eyelid movement.

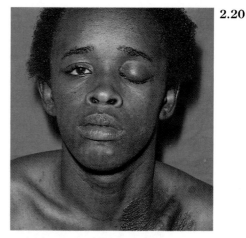

2.20

Fig. 2.20 Mechanical ptosis due to plexiform neurofibroma (left side) (Courtesy of Mr. R. Humphry)

Ⓢ *Management of senile ptosis:* The treatment of this type of ptosis only will be discussed.

Assessment:
• The degree of ptosis is ascertained by comparing the difference between the actual position of the upper lid and the ideal position. This gives a measure of the amount of ptosis surgery required.

• Levator function is assessed by eliminating frontalis action (the thumb is placed firmly on the skin on the eyebrow) whilst asking the patient to look up. The excursion of the upper lid is measured. The following grading is used:

Normal – 15 mm
Good   – 8 mm+
Fair   – 5–7 mm
Poor   – 4 mm or less

If levator function is good, the levator muscle is resected. If it is poor, suspension from the frontalis muscle is carried out.

• Assessment of Bell's phenomenon is performed by asking the patient to keep his eyes closed whilst the examiner tries to prise the lids open. The eye will be seen to roll upwards if there is a good Bell's phenomenon, and the cornea will be better protected following ptosis surgery.

• Dry eyes are tested for using a Schirmer's test. Ptosis surgery should not be performed if there is serious lack of tear secretion.

• Myasthenia gravis should be excluded (see p. 196).

• Corneal sensation is assessed (see p. 18).

• Extraocular movements and pupil size are tested to exclude a third nerve palsy or coincident superior rectus weakness.

• In young patients, test for jaw-winking phenomenon by asking the child to chew and move the chin from side to side.

Treatment, as mentioned, is by levator resection if there is good levator function.

Blepharitis

2.21(a)

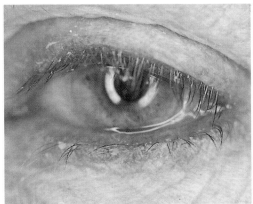

2.21(b)

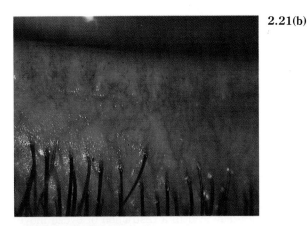

2.22

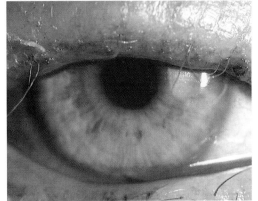

Fig. 2.21(a) Blepharitis – left eye showing erythema of the lid margins and crusting
Fig. 2.21(b) Blepharitis – showing meibomitis
Fig. 2.22 Blepharitis – showing loss of lashes

Blepharitis is a common, usually bilateral, chronic inflammatory disorder of the eyelid margins (*Fig. 2.21(a) & (b)*). It is associated with an increased incidence of dry eyes, marginal ulcers, styes and chalazia. Two main aetiological factors are:

• **chronic infection** of the base of the eyelashes with *Staphylococcus aureus*, or occasionally *Staphylococcus epidermidis*

• **excessive secretion of lipid** by the Meibomian glands. There is often excessive sebaceous gland secretion elsewhere as seen in rhinophyma and acne rosacea.

Symptoms: Chronic irritation of the eyes: burning, stinging and itching most commonly.

Signs: Erythema of the lid margins, crusting at the base of the lashes, trichiasis (malaligned and inverted eyelashes), blanching and sparsity of the lashes (*Fig. 2.22*), papillary conjunctivitis, associated disorders, e.g. stye, chalazion, marginal corneal ulcers and punctate epithelial erosions of dry eyes.

Management:

Ⓟ • **Lid hygiene** twice daily. This consists of cleaning the base of the lashes thoroughly to remove all the crusts with a cotton-tip bud dipped in a weak, soapy solution of sterile water (boiled) with 2–3 drops of Johnson's baby shampoo added.

• **Topical antibiotic/steroid ointment** e.g. oc chloramphenicol H.C.A. applied to eyelids twice daily after lid hygiene until the condition is improved (usually a 2–4 week course). Plain antibiotic ointment should be used in mild cases or if there is any contra-indication to steroid treatment, e.g. past history of herpes simplex eye disease.

• **Systemic antibiotic**, such as tetracycline 250 mg b.d. for 6 weeks decreased to 250 mg daily for maintenance in more deep-seated infections.

• **Mechanical expression** of the Meibomian glands with warm compresses in those with excessive lipid secretion and blocked ducts.

• **Artificial tears** in those with symptoms of burning or signs of the superficial punctate keratitis associated with dry eyes.

Lice infestation

A further cause of chronic blepharitis is infestation of the eyelashes with lice (*Fig. 2.23*), commonly the pubic variety. The individual nits (empty egg cases) and actual lice may be seen on close inspection.

(R) *Management:* The nits and any live lice should be individually picked off with forceps and the eyelashes shampooed with carbaryl 0.5% once daily. Alternatively, physostigmine 0.5% solution on a cotton tip can be used to cause the nits to drop off. Additional treatment is required for clearing the pubic or head area.

2.23
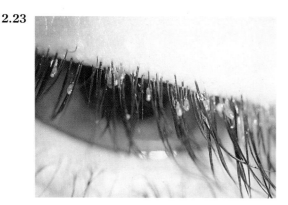
Fig. 2.23 Lice infestation (Courtesy of Sister J. Fox)

Tick

Ticks, commonly picked up from sandy areas, may become buried in the eyelid (*Fig. 2.24*).

Management: Application of Vaseline over the tick (P) deprives it of air and it will spontaneously drop off without leaving its mouthparts behind in the eyelid.

2.24
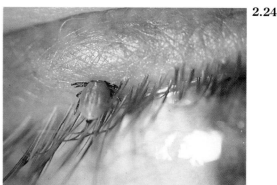
Fig. 2.24 Tick burying in upper lid

Trichiasis

In this condition the eyelashes become disorganised and point in all directions, including inwardly against the cornea (*Fig. 2.25*). It is often associated with chronic blepharitis.

Symptoms: Irritation and lacrimation caused by the lashes rubbing the cornea.

Signs: Punctate epithelial erosions, even confluent erosions on the cornea in the areas abraded by the lashes. In chronic cases, scarring and vascularisation of the cornea may develop.

(R) *Management:* Corneal erosions are healed by application of antibiotic ointment and a firm pad for 24–48 hours. Inwardly pointing lashes are epilated with forceps. This is repeated as the lashes regrow until a more definitive procedure is performed. The permanent treatment consists of either electrolysis of individual hair follicles or cryotherapy of wider areas of the lid

2.25
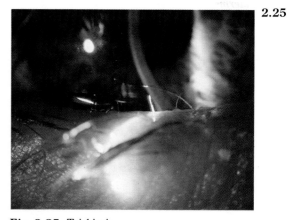
Fig. 2.25 Trichiasis

margin. This latter technique is more effective for extensive trichiasis, but may lead to scarring and depigmentation, especially in darker skinned individuals.

Periorbital and eyelid dermatitis

The skin around the eyes is very susceptible to atopic and contact dermatitis. Being thinner and more distensible than elsewhere, it reacts in a florid fashion. It is also involved in drug hypersensitivity to eye drops.

Atopic dermatitis

This arises as an acute type I hypersensitivity response to an allergen, e.g. pollen, cat or dog fur, horses, drugs, or food in a sensitised individual (*Fig. 2.26*). There is usually a history of atopy (eczema, asthma or hay fever) in the individual and/or the family.

Symptoms: Intense itching of the eyes and surrounding areas with swelling of the lid shortly after exposure to the allergen.

Signs: Periorbital and lid oedema, usually bilateral unless the allergen has been locally introduced into the eye. There is often associated conjunctival chemosis (jelly-like swelling of the conjunctiva) (*Fig. 2.27*) and urticarial reactions elsewhere in the body, especially antecubital and popliteal fossae and lateral neck folds.

(P) *Management:* Symptomatic relief may be obtained with cool compresses and antihistamine eye drops. The patient should be strongly reassured that this alarming reaction will settle. Avoidance of the presumed allergen in future.

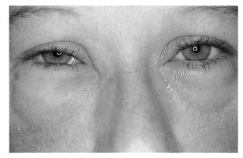

2.26

Fig. 2.26 Acute allergic response – showing periorbital oedema

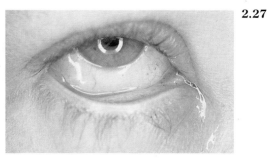

2.27

Fig. 2.27 Acute allergic response in same patient as in **Fig. 2.26** – showing conjunctival chemosis

Contact dermatitis

The skin of the eyelids is often involved in contact sensitivity. Frequently, the allergen concerned is transferred to the area by the fingers, e.g. when irritative washing substances are not properly rinsed off, or eye cosmetics themselves are directly sensitising (*Fig. 2.28*). Sometimes the allergen is well away from the eyes, e.g. the well-documented allergic response to nail lacquer, but the eyelids are more reactive zones.

Symptoms: Irritation of the eyelid and periorbital skin.

Signs: Skin thickening, slight erythema and flaking of the areas involved.

Management: In the short term, that is weeks to a few (S)(P) months, topical hydrocortisone ointment 1% b.d., applied to the skin areas involved, may be used, but not over a prolonged period of time as it may exacerbate the dermatitis. The main therapy lies in elimination of the allergen which may be identified using patch testing.

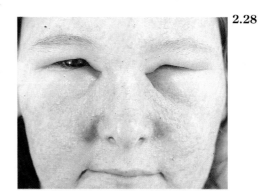

2.28

Fig. 2.28 Contact dermatitis (Courtesy of Dr. G. Burton)

Drug reactions

This is an extremely common problem, ranging from mild ocular irritation following instillation of the drops to severe suppurative reaction if use of the drops continues. There is a high prevalence of hypersensitivity and toxic reactions to commonly used drops, e.g. chloramphenicol, even in those individuals who have never knowingly been exposed to them. This must be borne in mind when there is a temptation to prescribe such drops in conditions such as viral conjunctivitis where their value is doubtful. Records of drug hypersensitivity should be clearly displayed in the patient's notes.

(a) Drug hypersensitivity (see Chapter 16)

This type of reaction arises following initial exposure to the drug, allowing sensitisation, and then either continued exposure or re-exposure at a later date, giving rise to a follicular conjunctivitis and a contact dermatitis. It is also seen in reactions to contact lens solutions and cosmetics.

Symptoms: Itching, burning and sometimes discharge.

Signs: Follicular reaction of the lower palpebral conjunctiva together with swelling and erythema of the lids and periorbital skin, which is worse around the lower lid. Sometimes the upper lid and limbal conjunctiva develop follicles. Occasionally, the dermatitis may become so severe as to mimic erysipelas with severe swelling, redness and weeping of the skin surface.

Management: The most likely source of hypersensitivity (R) is identified and another drug prescribed if treatment is still necessary. If multiple allergies to different drops, e.g. all antibiotic drops, are present, then the likely allergen is the preservative, usually thiomersal or benzalkonium chloride. If treatment is still essential try using ointment or preservative-free drops if available. Many of the 'Minim' drops (sterile single-dose applications) are preservative-free, providing useful sources of dilating drops. Common offenders are neomycin-containing drops, e.g. Betnesol-N and Predsol-N. In general these are best avoided since they contain fairly low levels of antibiotic and commonly lead to allergy. It is better, albeit less convenient, to use separate steroid and antibiotic preparations.

(b) Toxic reactions to drugs

This is a direct, non-immunological response to the drug itself or to the preservative, which is reversible once it is recognised and the stimulus removed. It is often seen as a response to constituents of contact lens solutions, e.g. thiomersal.

Symptoms: Irritation and soreness of the eyes. Sometimes toxic reactions to antiviral agents lead to delayed healing of the cornea in dendritic ulcers.

Signs: Papillary conjunctivitis and superficial punctate keratitis in an inferior distribution. Persistent herpetic ulcers in the presence of antiviral therapy. Longstanding cases of toxic drug reactions can lead to dyskeratotic changes in the conjunctiva.

Management: Removal of the drug or preservative (S)(F) that has lead to the reaction. Use of preservative-free drops and contact lens solutions.

Molluscum Contagiosum

This is a viral infection of the skin, commonly affecting children, which may occur on the face or eyelids (*Fig. 2.29*). It manifests as a raised, shiny, umbilicated skin nodule which may periodically shed viral particles. If the lesion occurs on the eyelid, it gives rise to a follicular conjunctivitis and occasionally a superficial punctate keratitis. It usually resolves spontaneously within 6–9 months.

Management: The skin lesion can be curetted easily under local anaesthetic, but care must be taken not to spread viral particles along the eyelid margin. Following this the nodule should disappear and the follicular conjunctivitis resolve. Alternative procedures are to cauterise the lesion or to excise it.

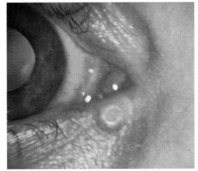

Fig. 2.29 Molluscum contagiosum (Courtesy of Miss H. Frank)

Benign lid tumours

Viral warts (verruca vulgaris)

These are sometimes multiple, filiform warts that occur on the eyelid (*Fig. 2.30*). They are more common in children when they are usually secondary to warts on the fingers. In extreme cases of papillomatosis the lesions need to be excised and the base cauterised.

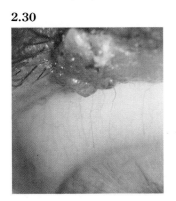

Fig. 2.30 Papilloma

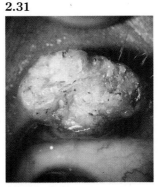

Fig. 2.31 Keratocanthoma (Courtesy of Miss H. Frank)

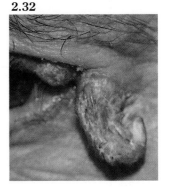

Fig. 2.32 Squamous papilloma with horn (Courtesy of Mr. R. Humphry)

Keratoacanthoma

This rapidly growing tumour starts as a reddish papule and within a couple of months has reached its maximum size. It has a characteristic appearance of a raised, pink nodule with a crater filled with a keratin plug (*Fig. 2.31*). It usually involutes spontaneously, but may leave an untidy, indented scar. For this reason, and its similarity in appearance to a squamous cell carcinoma, it is often best removed.
Differential diagnosis: Squamous cell carcinoma

Squamous papilloma

This is a benign tumour of squamous epithelium (*Fig. 2.32*). It occurs singly as either a sessile or a pedunculated lesion on the eyelid margin. There is often an associated keratinous horn. Treatment is by simple, local excision as a day-case procedure.
Differential diagnosis: Seborrhoeic keratosis, solar keratosis, viral warts.

Seborrhoeic keratosis (basal cell papilloma)

This is an overgrowth of basal epithelium (*Fig. 2.33*). The lesions may be single or multiple and are very common in the elderly. They appear as raised, soft, greasy lesions which are often a grey–brown colour. (S) Treatment consists of excision by shaving off the hyperkeratotic areas, and checking the scrapings histologically.

Solar keratosis (senile or actinic keratosis)

This is a dyskeratotic lesion occurring mainly in the elderly, especially those with fair skins who have received excessive sun exposure. It appears as a dry, scaly, plaque-like area with keratin excess on the surface, sometimes in the form of a horn. It sometimes progresses to Bowen's disease and in 25% of cases to (S) squamous cell carcinoma. Treatment consists of complete excision. Cryotherapy has been successfully used to keep lesions around the eye under control.

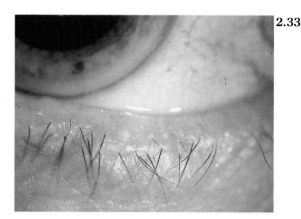

Fig. 2.33 Basal cell papilloma

Naevi

Naevi are birthmarks, but the term is usually reserved for congenital melanocytic lesions that acquire their pigmented appearance around puberty. Those on the eyelids are usually raised and do not undergo malignant (S) transformation. Excision is required for cosmetic reasons or if they cannot be distinguished from more malignant varieties, e.g. lentigo maligna in the elderly.

Xanthelasma

These are subcutaneous fatty deposits around the eye (*Figs. 2.34, 2.35*). They can be associated with hyperlipidaemia.

Bowen's disease (intraepithelial carcinoma)

This is a premalignant stage of squamous cell carcinoma. It appears as a well demarcated, dull red patch on the skin with overlying keratin crusting. It requires complete excision as it is likely to progress to the (S) more malignant form.

Management: They may be excised surgically to (S) improve cosmetic appearances or overlying skin touched with application of trichloracetic acid. They tend to recur.

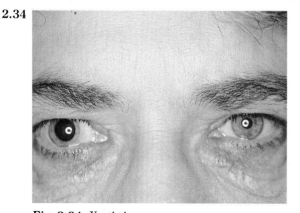

Fig. 2.34 Xanthelasma

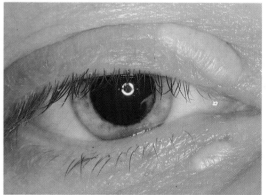

Fig. 2.35 Xanthelasma – advanced

Haemangiomas

'Strawberry naevus'

This presents in the first few weeks of life as a slowly enlarging, plump, red lesion with a pitted surface resembling a strawberry (*Fig. 2.36(a) & (b)*). Sometimes it retains normal skin appearance, but shows a few dilated blood vessels on the surface of the tumour. It continues to enlarge for many months, but usually resolves completely without cosmetic defect by 5–10 years. Elsewhere in the body it is best left alone, but if it occurs on the eyelid and interferes with vision there is a danger of amblyopia developing. If amblyopia is present, prompt correction of refractive errors and occlusion of the other eye is necessary, together with treatment of the lesion. Some instances may be associated with intraorbital extension as in the case pictured here. To date, the most successful mode of treatment is intralesional injection of triamcinolone by a plastic surgeon. If the lesion is inaccessible, systemic steroids can be fairly successful, although the use of steroids in children is not generally encouraged. Radiotherapy, injection of sclerosants and lasers are less effective.

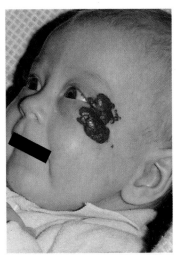

2.36(a)

Fig. 2.36(a) Strawberry naevus (Courtesy of Mr. N. Dallas)

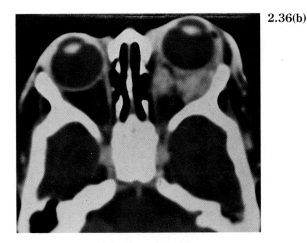

2.36(b)

Fig. 2.36(b) Head CAT scan of same child in **Fig. 2.36(a)** showing orbital encroachment by haemangioma (Courtesy of Mr. N. Dallas)

Naevus flammeus

This causes a red discolouration of the skin, often referred to as a 'port-wine stain' or a naevus flammeus, which is present at birth and permanent (*Fig. 2.37*). If it occurs on the face in the distribution of one of the branches of the trigeminal nerve it may be associated with hemihypertrophy of the involved area. It may also be associated with an intracranial haemangioma, which calcifies and gives rise to the 'tram-track' lines of curvilinear calcification on the lateral skull radiograph and may be associated with seizures and contralateral hemiplegia. This is the Sturge-Weber syndrome. Glaucoma occurs in about 50% of patients with haemangiomas of the upper eyelid, manifesting in childhood (occasionally in infancy), almost invariably on the side(s) of the lesion. Other ocular manifestations include conjunctival and choroidal vascular lesions and heterochromia iridis. Laser treatment is being used to reduce the severity of the skin lesion, but there is no curative treatment. Skin tone cosmetics may be useful.

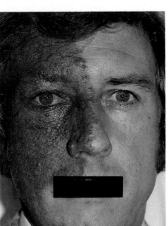

2.37

Fig. 2.37 Naevus flammeus (Courtesy of Miss H. Frank)

Malignant lid tumours

Basal cell carcinoma

This is the most common malignant tumour of the skin surrounding the eye (*Figs. 2.37, 2.38*). It tends to be locally invasive, but does not metastasise. It occurs in two forms:

• **Nodular-ulcerative** type. This is the classical rodent ulcer with a pearly, rolled margin and a shallow, ulcerated, often crusted centre. It is locally destructive, but less likely to recur after treatment.

• **Morphoeic** or **sclerosing** type. This tumour also has a central crusting area, but is flatter, less well-defined and more prone to recurrence.

Management: Local excision for nodular type with a (S) 3mm margin of clearance. In elderly or debilitated patients, or if local excision would lead to excessive loss of tissue, cryotherapy or radiotherapy is used. With medial canthal tumours that can spread deep into the orbital fascial planes, local excision is preferable because the irradiation may be too superficial. Morphoeic type requires more extensive clearance, often with plastic surgical techniques. Both types require histological confirmation of complete removal.

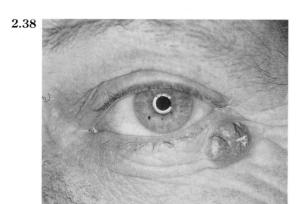

Fig. 2.38 Basal cell carcinoma

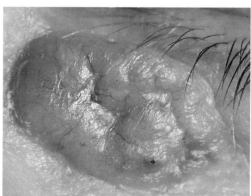

Fig. 2.39 Basal cell carcinoma – detail

Squamous cell carcinoma

This rare tumour (40 times less common than basal cell carcinoma) may arise from an existing area of solar keratosis or *de novo* (*Figs. 2.40, 2.41*). Its appearance may be nodular or ulcerative. Alternatively, it may resemble a papilloma or a keratoacanthoma. It is locally invasive and may also metastasise to the preauricular or cervical lymph nodes.

(S) *Management:* Wide local excision or sometimes radiotherapy.

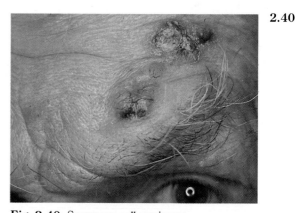

Fig. 2.40 Squamous cell carcinoma

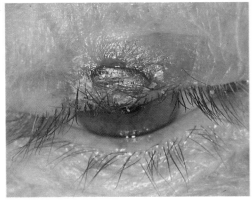

2.41

Fig. 2.41 Intraepithelial carcinoma

Malignant Melanoma

This is a very rare eyelid tumour (*Fig. 2.42*). It arises from a pre-existing naevus, from lentigo maligna (a pre-malignant condition in the elderly) or *de novo*. Any development of ulceration, bleeding, increasing size or pigmentation in a naevus should arouse suspicion.

(S) *Management:* Complete excision. Some lesions may be radiosensitive.

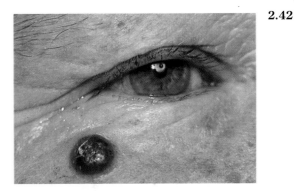

2.42

Fig. 2.42 Malignant melanoma (Courtesy of Miss H. Frank)

Sebaceous gland carcinoma (Meibomian gland carcinoma)

This may arise from either the Meibomian glands or the glands of Zeis. It presents most commonly as a recurrent chalazion, but may also resemble chronic blepharitis if it is of the diffuse, infiltrating type.

Management: Local excision or radiotherapy if the (S) tumour involves a large proportion of the eyelid. Mortality is 15% due to delay in recognition.
N.B. Histology should be requested on recurrent, atypical chalazia.

3 Conjunctiva

Normal anatomy

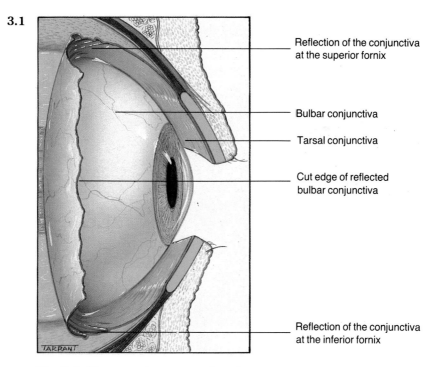

3.1

Reflection of the conjunctiva at the superior fornix

Bulbar conjunctiva

Tarsal conjunctiva

Cut edge of reflected bulbar conjunctiva

Reflection of the conjunctiva at the inferior fornix

Fig. 3.1 Diagrammatic representation of the relationships of the bulbar and tarsal conjunctiva

The conjunctiva forms a continuous layer of mucous membrane starting at the grey line of the lid margin, the mucocutaneous junction, lining the inner aspects of the tarsal plates, and then extending upwards or downwards to form cul de sacs (the fornices), and finally being reflected onto the sclera and Tenon's capsule, to form the bulbar conjunctiva (*Fig. 3.1*). The layer terminates at the limbus, the meeting of the conjunctiva with the corneal epithelium. The fornices are extensive, the upper extending backwards as far as the equator of the globe. Therefore foreign bodies can be trapped in this region and escape detection.

The conjunctiva is composed of columnar epithelium and goblet cells overlying a substantia propria which merges into a layer known as Tenon's capsule. In the normal state it is barely visible because it is a thin transparent membrane overlying the white avascular sclera and the highly vascular tarsal plates.

The conjunctiva is important in the protection of the eye against foreign materials and micro-organisms. Where chronic conjunctival disease exists, the epithelial barrier of the cornea is often compromised by micro-erosions, increasing the risk of infection by invasive organisms.

Conjunctival response to disease

The following responses occur:

- **Hyperaemia** – most prominent at the fornices, tending to fade away at the limbus. In ciliary injection, associated with intraocular inflammation such as uveitis, the pericorneal and episcleral vessels are involved at limbus (*Fig. 3.2*).

- **Subconjunctival haemorrhage** – due to injury, acute inflammation, vascular congestion of the head, local manifestation of systemic disease such as hypertension, and haemorrhagic blood dyscrasias (*Fig. 3.3*).

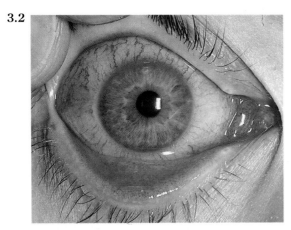

Fig. 3.2 Typical hyperaemia occurring in conjunctivitis (Courtesy of Institute of Ophthalmology)

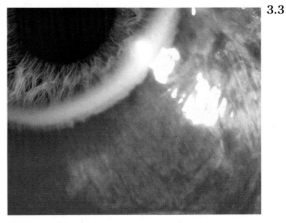

Fig. 3.3 Spontaneous subconjunctival haemorrhage

- **Chemosis or oedema of the conjunctiva.** This is common and characterised by translucent swelling of the membrane (*Fig. 3.4*). It results from increased capillary permeability during inflammation, venous congestion, reduced plasma protein as in the nephrotic syndrome, and in orbital disease.

- **Follicles** are dome-shaped elevations containing collections of lymphocytes. The blood vessels lie on their surface (*Fig. 3.5*).

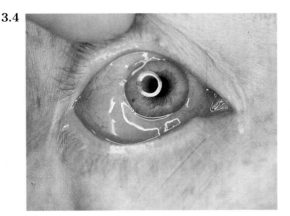

Fig. 3.4 A conjunctival chemotic reaction

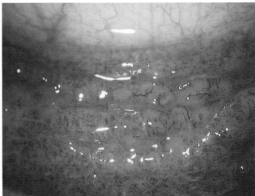

Fig. 3.5 A follicular response in the lower fornix

• **Papillae** are a common response to inflammation and consist of tiny elevations that are tightly packed together, with vascular cores (*Fig. 3.6(a)*). Sometimes they become aggregated to form large papillae, as in vernal catarrh and giant papillary conjunctivitis (*Fig. 3.6(b)–(d)*).

• **Discharge** is one of the main features of conjunctivitis, and is relevant to the history and clinical examination. It is described as purulent (*Fig. 3.7(a)*), mucopurulent (*Fig. 3.7(b)*), serous and watery.

3.6(a)

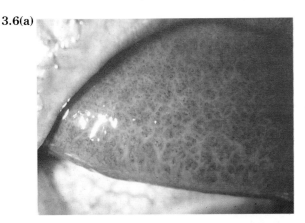

3.6(b)

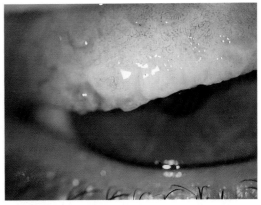

Fig. 3.6(a) A papillary response in the upper tarsal plate

Fig. 3.6(b) Cobblestone papillae in vernal catarrh

3.6(c)

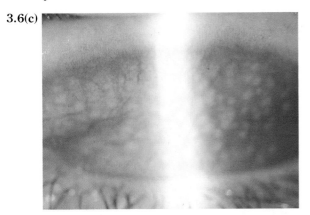

3.6(d)

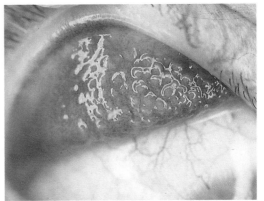

Fig. 3.6(c) & (d) Giant papillary conjunctivitis (GPC)

3.7(a)

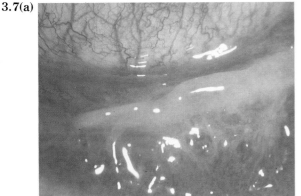

3.7(b)

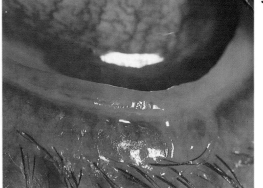

Fig. 3.7(a) Purulent discharge on the lower conjunctival plate (Courtesy of Mr. A. Richards)

Fig. 3.7(b) Mucopurulent discharge in the lower fornix (Courtesy of Mr. A. Richards)

• **Membrane formation** occurs in severe conjunctivitis. It may be adherent to the tarsal plate or non-adherent, in which case it is designated a pseudo-membrane (*Fig. 3.8*).

• **Scarring** of the conjunctiva occurs in certain types of infection or auto-immune disease, inducing in-turning of the tarsal plates or entropion (*Fig. 3.9*).

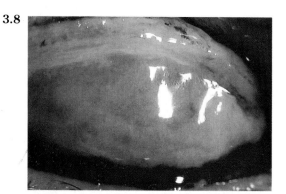

Fig. 3.8 An inflammatory membrane on the upper tarsal plate

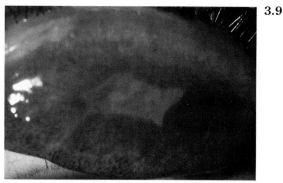

Fig. 3.9 Scarring of the upper tarsal plate following viral conjunctivitis

Conjunctivitis

This must be differentiated from other causes of a red eye, such as anterior uveitis and acute glaucoma (*Table 1*).

Table 1 The red eye

	Conjunctivitis	Anterior uveitis	Acute glaucoma
Symptoms			
Pain	Minor – gritty or foreign body sensation	Present	Severe ocular pain and unilateral, frontal headache
Discharge	Present with stickiness in morning	Absent	Absent
Vision	Unaffected	Blurred	Blurred – rainbow haloes around lights
Signs			
Hyperaemia	Superficial and diffuse – most marked in fornices	Limbal	Diffuse and intense
Discharge	Mucoid, mucopurulent, or watery	Nil	Nil
Pre-auricular lymph node	Palpable	Impalpable	Impalpable
Cornea	Clear	Clear – but KP visible with slit lamp	Oedematous
Intraocular pressure	Normal	Occasionally elevated	High

Symptoms: Discharge, particularly on waking, producing a sticky eye, grittiness, photophobia, or itching. Itching usually means that the patient suffers from some form of allergy.

Signs: Exudate on the lid margins and within the conjunctival sac, hyperaemia of the bulbar and tarsal conjunctiva, which is most intensive towards the fornices, and usually a clear cornea. The pre-auricular lymph node, lying just in front of the tragus, will often be palpable. Routine examination of the external eye includes eversion of the tarsal plates to examine the lining conjunctiva. Since the normal conjunctiva is transparent, the blood vessels within the tarsal plate are visible as vertical arcades, but in inflammatory disease the vessels are often hidden by follicles or papillae.

Conjunctivitis must be considered as a potentially serious condition because of the risk of corneal disease. The causes are bacterial, viral, mycotic, allergic and auto-immune (*Table 2*). Sometimes conjunctivitis can be recurrent or persistent. It is then necessary to exclude chronic infection of the lacrimal sac (dacryocystitis) when there will be a history of watering. Pressure over the lacrimal sac expresses mucopurulent material from the upper and lower canaliculi in chronic disease.

Table 2 Causes of conjunctivitis

	Allergic	**Bacterial**	**Viral**
Symptoms			
Soreness	Present	Present	Present
Photophobia	Present – sometimes severe in morning	Present	Present
Discharge	Watery – mucopurulent in active vernal catarrh	Purulent, mucopurulent, watery	Watery
Morning stickiness	Present	Present	Present
Itching	Present	Absent	Absent
Signs			
Preauricular nodes	Palpable on occasions	Palpable	Palpable
Bulbar conjunctiva	Hyperaemic	Hyperaemic	Hyperaemic. Particularly caruncle in adenoviral infection
Tarsal conjunctiva	Hyperaemic. Papillary reaction	Hyperaemic. Papillary reaction	Hyperaemic. Follicular plus papillary reaction
Cornea	Uninvolved except in vernal catarrh	Punctate epithelial erosions	Punctate epithelial and stromal keratitis in adenoviral infection
Intraocular pressure	Normal	Occasionally elevated	High

Bacterial conjunctivitis

The causes are Gram positive *Staphylococcus aureus*, sometimes mixed with other infectious agents, *Streptococcus pneumoniae*, common in children, Gram negative *Neisseria gonorrhoeae*, and Gram negative Haemophilus species, Proteus species, and *Klebsiella pneumoniae*.

Symptoms: Watering and irritation in one eye, followed shortly in the other.

Signs: Hyperaemia of the tarsal and bulbar conjunctiva, occasionally with petechial haemorrhages. Marginal corneal infiltrates occur in staphylococcal and haemophilus infection. Discharge is scanty and mucopurulent.

Investigation of bacterial conjunctivitis: Laboratory studies must be performed where there is any difficulty in reaching a diagnosis, but are mandatory in neonatal conjunctivitis, hyperacute conjunctivitis, membranous conjunctivitis and in severe and long-standing conjunctivitis.

The following investigations can be made:

(P) • Conjunctival swabs are taken without the use of a local anaesthetic by wiping a sterile, moistened, cotton-tipped applicator along the lower fornix and then plating onto blood or chocolate agar. Where there is evidence of lid margin involvement, cultures must be taken using similar techniques. The swabs must be moistened with sterile saline or culture medium. Both eyes must be cultured, although the infection may apparently be unilateral.

• Scraping of the tarsal plates, following instillation of local anaesthetic, is carried out in order to help determine the diagnosis. Smears are prepared and stained with Giemsa. They are used when information about the type of inflammatory cell, the condition of the epithelium or the presence of inclusions is desired. The inflammatory cell characteristics will allow an early diagnosis of bacterial (predominantly polymorphonuclear), viral (predominantly mononuclear), or allergic conjunctivitis (a few eosinophils).

Management: A broad spectrum antibiotic, e.g. (P) chloramphenicol, is applied as drops four times a day, and as ointment at night. Failure to respond is an indication to discontinue topical treatment and to obtain appropriate laboratory studies.

Acute purulent conjunctivitis

Caused by neisserial infection, most often by *N. gonorrhoeae*, but occasionally by *N. meningitides*. Gonococcal infection is seen mainly in neonates, but occasionally in adolescence and adulthood. The neonatal infection is contracted during passage through the maternal, infected birth canal. Adolescent and adult infection occurs by fomite spread or auto-inoculation from infected genitalia.

Symptoms: Marked swelling of lids, aching pain, excessive discharge and tenderness.

Signs: Lid oedema, marked hyperaemia, chemosis, sometimes an inflammatory membrane, and a tender, pre-auricular lymph node on the affected side. There is a copious, purulent discharge.

Where treatment is not instituted immediately, there is a high risk of corneal ulceration and visual loss since the organism has the capacity to invade the intact corneal epithelium.

Investigations: A conjunctival scraping must be Gram and Giemsa stained. The inflammatory response is polymorphonuclear and, by the third day, Gram negative diplococci are seen within these cells. Chocolate agar is inoculated directly from the eye. The laboratory will distinguish between *N. gonorrhoeae* and *N. meningitides*, as the latter can be systemically spread.

Management:

• Systemic – antibiotics should be used in full doses.

• Topical – Penicillin drops should be instilled every two hours for 48 hours. These organisms will also be sensitive to gentamicin sulphate drops or tetracycline ointment.

Treatment usually results in cessation of the ocular discharge within 24–48 hours. Lid oedema, hyperaemia and chemosis resolve within 7–14 days.

Chronic bacterial conjunctivitis

Chronic bacterial conjunctivitis (CBC) may be caused by the enteric group of bacteria, such as *Proteus mirabilis*, *Klebsiella pneumoniae*, *Serratia marcescens*, and *Escherichia coli*, all of which are Gram negative rods. They may all be isolated from the normal eye in small numbers, but cause symptoms and signs of CBC in large numbers. Gram negative diplococci, such as *Neisseria catarrhalis*, are occasional causes of CBC, as are certain Gram negative diplobacilli, e.g. *Moraxella lacunata*, which can cause blepharoconjunctivitis involving the inner and outer canthal angles. It is essential to exclude chronic infection of the lacrimal sac in chronic conjunctivitis, which may be a cause for extremely persistent conjunctivitis (see p. 175).

Staphylococcus aureus, although a common cause of acute conjunctivitis, is a frequent organism isolated in chronic conjunctivitis. The organisms populate the lid margins and are associated with ocular inflammatory responses caused by a series of exotoxins. They induce:

• chronic blepharitis (*Fig. 3.10*)

• non-specific, conjunctival inflammation and inferior punctate keratitis

• marginal keratitis and phlyctenular keratitis

• recurrent hordolea or styes (infection of the lash follicle) (*Fig. 3.11(a)*)

• chalazia (infection of Meibomian duct) (*Fig. 3.11(b)*) (see pp. 34–35)

3.10

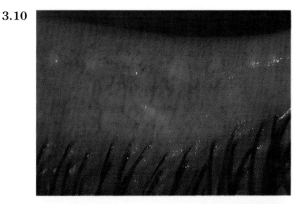

Fig. 3.10 Lid hyperaemia, swelling, and scaling in staphylococcal blepharitis
Fig. 3.11(a) Stye
Fig. 3.11(b) A chalazion affecting the left upper lid

3.11(a)

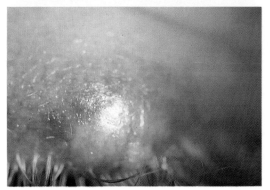

3.11(b)

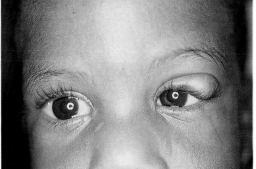

Blepharitis is associated with:

- grittiness on waking
- itching of the lids
- redness of the margins
- crusting of the lid margins and a deposit of froth
- a notched appearance of the lid margins

Where blepharitis is associated with chronic conjunctivitis, there is:

- bulbar and tarsal hyperaemia
- cellular infiltration of the tarsal plates
- inflammation of the Meibomian ducts which are dilated
- inflammation of lash follicles which cause loss or misdirection of the cilia
- occasional eczematous reactions particularly at the outer canthus

Investigations: In chronic blepharoconjunctivitis, laboratory studies yield a heavy growth of *Staph. aureus* or *Staph. epidermidis* from the lid margins and the conjunctival sac.

Management: The management of chronic conjunctivitis is simple and requires a bland, topical antibiotic such as chloramphenicol, framycetin, neomycin, polymyxin B or tobramycin ointment four times daily.

The treatment of chronic blepharoconjunctivitis Ⓟ is more difficult, because it can be refractory and recurrent.

- The lid margins should be cleansed using a moistened, cotton-tipped applicator to remove the scales and exudate.
- A dilute solution of Johnson's baby shampoo for moistening the applicator has proved effective.
- This is followed by an antibiotic ointment to the lid margins twice daily.
- Refractory chronic meibomitis requires expression of the purulent material using a glass rod.
- Low doses of tetracycline are helpful (say 250mg b.d. for six weeks).
- Where marginal ulcer or phlyctenular keratoconjunctivitis occurs, low concentration topical steroid Ⓡ (Prednisolone 0.1% or 0.125%) in combination with a topical antibiotic is effective.

Viral conjunctivitis

The viruses that cause conjunctivitis are adenovirus, *Herpes simplex* virus and *Molluscum contagiosum*. They cause acute follicular conjunctivitis which does not respond to antibiotic treatment (*Table 3*). There is frequently pre-auricular lymphadenopathy.

Table 3 Causes of follicular conjunctivitis

	Discharge	PAG*	Tarsal plates	Cornea
Herpes simplex virus	Purulent	+	Follicles	PEE**, dendrite
Varicella	Purulent	+	Follicles	PEE, disciform
Zoster	Purulent	+	Follicles and haemorrhage	PEE, dendrite, disciform
EBV***	Watery	+	Follicles, haemorrhage, membrane	Disciform
Adenoviruses	Watery	+	Follicles, papillae	Punctate epithelial and stromal keratitis
Molluscum contagiosum	Watery	–	Follicles	PEE, pannus
Coxsackie A	Purulent	+	Membrane	Pannus
Enterovirus 70	Purulent	+	Follicles papillae and haemorrhage	
Chlamydia trachomatis	Watery	+	Follicles papillae	Punctate epithelial keratitis, pannus

*Pre-auricular gland, **Punctate epithelial erosions, ***Epstein-Barr virus

Adenoviral conjunctivitis

There are two syndromes caused by adenoviral infection:

• epidemic keratoconjunctivitis caused most often by adenovirus type 8.

• pharyngoconjunctival fever caused by adenovirus type 3.

Adenoviruses survive for substantial periods on non-living objects and so outbreaks occur by transmission from such objects. One example is the hospital-based outbreak, due to contamination of applanation heads, which must always be sterilised prior to use.

Symptoms: Soreness, watering and a foreign body sensation.

Signs:

• A variable degree of follicular conjunctivitis, particularly involving the lower tarsal plates and fornices (*Fig. 3.12*).

• Often marked papillary response in the upper tarsal plate with follicles at the angle and upper margin.

• Occasionally membranous conjunctivitis occurs.

• The plica and caruncle can often become hyperaemic.

• Petechial haemorrhages can be seen on the everted tarsal plates.

• Keratitis is seen in patients with type 8 infection and has been recorded in other types, e.g. 3, 4 ,5, 7, 9, 11, 21, and 10/19. It begins in the epithelium with punctate lesions which spread to the stroma producing punctate scarring (*Figs. 3.13, 3.14*).

3.12

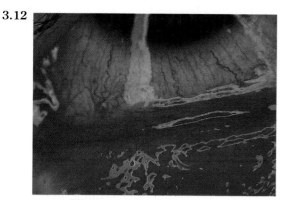

Fig. 3.12 Follicular conjunctivitis in a patient with adenoviral infection involving lower fornix

3.13

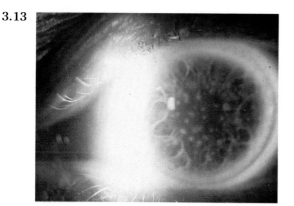

Fig. 3.13 Punctate opacities in the corneal stroma following infection with adenovirus 8

3.14

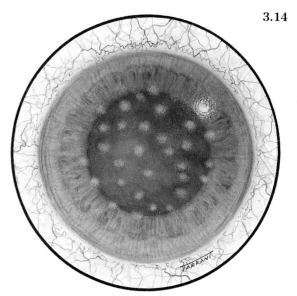

Fig. 3.14 An artist's impression of adenoviral punctate keratitis

Ⓡ *Investigations:*

• Culture on sterile swabs stored in viral transport media.

• Two consecutive specimens of serum to detect a rising antibody titre.

Differential diagnosis: Other causes of punctate keratitis are chlamydial infection, Staphylococcus allergic keratoconjunctivitis and Thygeson's punctate keratitis (*Figs. 3.15, 3.16*).

3.15

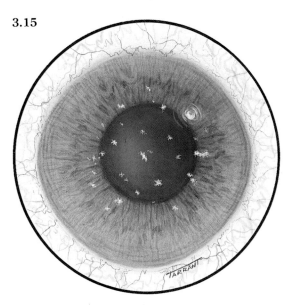

Fig. 3.15 Epithelial punctate keratitis as seen in Thygeson's keratitis

3.16

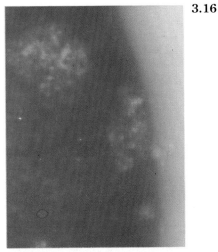

Fig. 3.16 A microphotograph of the epithelial lesions in Thygeson's keratitis (Courtesy of Mr. N. Brown)

Management: There is no recognised treatment of the condition. It is important to identify an outbreak at an early stage so that appropriate isolation measures can be taken to limit the spread:

Ⓡ • Hospital casualties must set up separate clinical areas for the examination of known or suspected cases.

• Separate hand washing and sterilising facilities must be made available.

• Equipment, including slit lamps, must be cleaned following use.

• Intraocular pressure should not be measured on suspect patients unless absolutely necessary.

• Patients should be warned about the highly contagious nature of the virus and advised to take appropriate precautions in their hygiene.

Herpes simplex *virus conjunctivitis*

It is very important to remember that the *Herpes simplex* virus can cause follicular conjunctivitis (*Fig. 3.17*), because incorrect treatment may cause more serious disease. However, correct treatment, if given early, may improve the long-term prognosis. The diagnosis must depend on a high level of suspicion as it is a rare condition. It may be primary or recurrent.

Primary is associated occasionally with a facial eruption (*Fig. 3.18*), but this may be obscure, and the cutaneous lesion can lie hidden amongst the lashes. A primary dendritic ulcer may follow the follicular conjunctivitis.

Recurrent herpes simplex follicular conjunctivitis occurs in the absence of corneal disease.

Investigations: Culture and serial antibody measurement.

Management: Early treatment is ideal and where the ⓟ diagnosis is obvious an antiviral can be given, such as idoxuridine (Kerecid), as ointment or drops, adenine arabinoside ointment (Vira A), or acyclovir ointment (Zovirax). All patients with any kind of ocular herpes simplex infection must be referred to an eye depart- ⓡ ment.

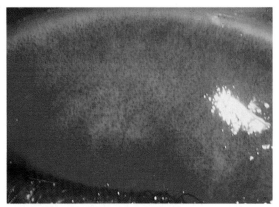

Fig. 3.17 Follicular papillary conjunctivitis due to the *Herpes simplex* virus (Courtesy of Professor S. Darougar)

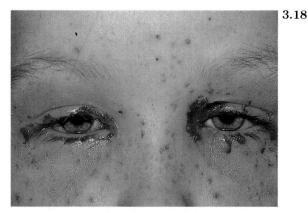

Fig. 3.18 Primary facial herpes (Courtesy of Institute of Ophthalmology)

Enterovirus

Enterovirus 70 causes highly infectious haemorrhagic conjunctivitis (*Fig. 3.19*).

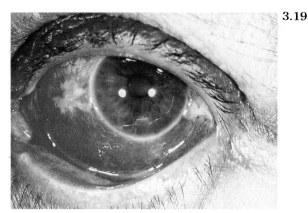

Fig. 3.19 Haemorrhagic conjunctivitis following enterovirus infection (Courtesy of Dr. P. Aspell)

Adult inclusion conjunctivitis

This occurs in young people as a follicular response and is sexually transmitted. The conjunctivitis appears 7–21 days after taking a new partner.

Symptoms:

- Acute or subacute onset of redness

- Mucopurulent discharge

- Photophobia

- Lid droop

Signs:

- Pseudoptosis and lid swelling

- Palpable pre-auricular lymph node

- A follicular response, mostly in the upper and lower fornix, and a papillary conjunctival response in the upper tarsal plate (*Figs. 3.20, 3.21*)

- Superficial punctate keratitis

- Micropannus

A key sign in recognition of inclusion conjunctivitis is the presence of follicles in the upper fornix, examined by using a lid retractor to double evert the upper lid.

Investigations: The diagnosis is made by scraping the ®ᴿ tarsal plates and producing a smear which is then stained with Giemsa to demonstrate the elementary bodies. Organisms can be cultured for isolation using irradiated tissue culture cells (McCoy cells), but this takes some time. A better method employs fluorescent antibody, which is sensitive and quick. The test depends upon the binding of antibody by the cell inclusions that are demonstrable on conjunctival scrapes.

Management: ⓢ

- Systemic treatment is with tetracycline 250 mg t.i.d. for three weeks.

- The sexual consort is treated simultaneously.

- Pregnant women should be treated with erythromycin 500 mg q.d.s. for three weeks.

- Topical treatment is with tetracycline hydrochloride or chlortetracycline ointment q.d.s. for three weeks.

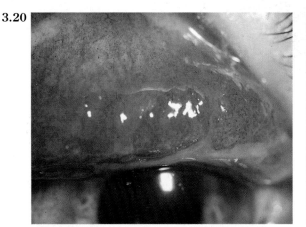

Fig. 3.20 Follicles in the upper fornix due to chlamydial conjunctivitis

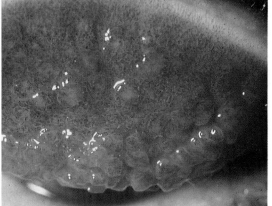

Fig. 3.21 Papillae and follicles in an adult with inclusion conjunctivitis

Allergic Conjunctivitis

Allergic conjunctivitis presents a spectrum of disease ranging from benign hay fever conjunctivitis to the more serious vernal catarrh. Atopic conjunctivitis is seen in atopic, adult patients.

Vernal catarrh

Vernal catarrh is more serious and occurs in children and young teenagers (5–15 years).

Symptoms: Itching, discharge, soreness, and severe photophobia on waking or throughout the day. Young children cannot be examined because of this photophobia, so a general anaesthetic may be required.

Signs:

- discharge within the conjunctival sac (*Fig. 3.22*)

- hyperaemia of the bulbar conjunctiva

- papillae of the tarsal plates, often forming cobblestones (*Fig. 3.23*)

- limbal papillae are sometimes seen (*Fig. 3.24*)

- punctate corneal erosions which signal disease activity due to mediator release from degranulating mast cells, situated in the upper half of the cornea, associated with a superficial vascular ingrowth (pannus)

- severe corneal ulceration (*Fig. 3.25*) can occur due to adherence of sticky mucus to the damaged corneal surface in layers, increasing the severity of the symptoms, and threatening vision

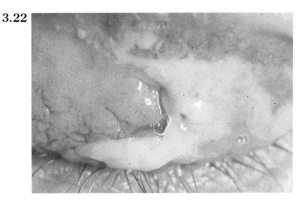

Fig. 3.22 Everted upper tarsal plate demonstrating cobblestone papillae, scarring, and mucus discharge in active vernal catarrh (Courtesy of Institute of Ophthalmology)

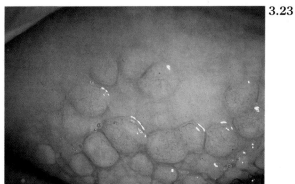

Fig. 3.23 Inactive vernal disease

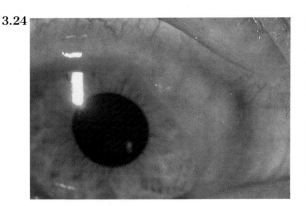

Fig. 3.24 Limbal vernal disease

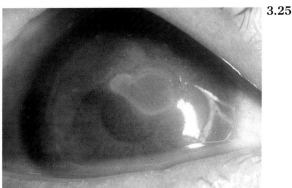

Fig. 3.25 A corneal ulcer in a patient with vernal catarrh

Hay fever conjunctivitis

Hay fever conjunctivitis is minor, but a nuisance and extremely common. Sometimes it is ranked as being more important than the upper respiratory tract symptomatically.

Symptoms: Itching, watering and soreness.

Atopic conjunctivitis

Atopic conjunctivitis occurs in late teenagers and adults, usually with a history of serious atopic disease elsewhere in the form of eczema or asthma.

The conjunctivitis is papillary, usually with the papillae packed together to form a continuous mesh, rather than appearing as cobblestones as in children (*Fig. 3.26*).

It can be associated with other conditions such as persistent blepharitis, ectropion of the lower lids and keratitis, which is sometimes complicated by herpes simplex infection.

Investigations:

• The full history may identify causal allergens. The period when perennial symptoms are maximum will give guidance to the causal allergen.

• Cutaneous prick testing will help in identification of allergens.

• Serum IgE levels are usually raised, together with levels of specific antibody, using the radio-allergosorbent test (RAST).

(P) *Management:*

• The first line treatment must employ mast cell stabilisers, such as Opticrom, or antihistamines, such as Otrivine-Antistin drops. These preparations are effective in low-grade allergic conjunctivitis, such as in hay fever, but will not help in active vernal disease.

(R) • In active vernal disease, topical steroid is suitable for short courses of treatment.

(S) • The serious effects of long-term corticosteroid treatment are seen after prolonged use. The patient therefore requires regular medical supervision to ensure that the intraocular pressure is not elevated, or that an early subcapsular cataract is not forming.

Signs:

• hyperaemia of the bulbar and tarsal conjunctiva

• minimal evidence of follicles or papillae

• chemosis of the bulbar conjunctiva, together with swelling of the lids

3.26

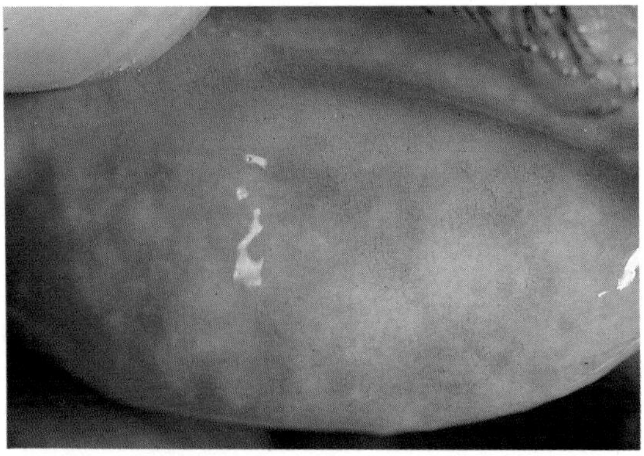

Fig. 3.26 Papillary conjunctivitis in an adult atopic subject with allergic conjunctivitis (Courtesy of Institute of Ophthalmology)

• It is recommended that dilute steroid is used and, if ineffective, the dosage is increased. Initially, prednisolone 0.25% drops may be used. Where control is not obtained within about 24 hours, the concentration can be stepped up to 0.5%, or 1%.

• Sometimes the keratitis is severe enough to warrant admission to hospital. This benefits the patient because medical treatment is fully supervised and the patient is likely to be isolated from causal allergen.

• Where there is a vernal ulcer there is a poor response to corticosteroid treatment. The mucous deposit beneath the ulcer must be removed under general anaesthetic, by careful dissection to minimise damage to basement membrane. Once the mucous plaque has been removed, the corneal epithelium regenerates and the symptoms resolve.

Allergic reactions to eye drops occur (*Fig. 3.27*), when the skin of the eyelid and cheek is involved, with the appearance of contact dermatitis.

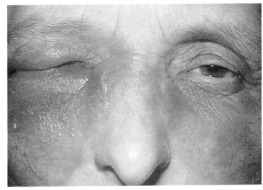

Fig. 3.27 Allergic response to topical ocular therapy

Chlamydial disease

Chlamydiae are intracellular parasites that resemble gram negative bacteria. They are more closely related to bacteria than to viruses because they contain both DNA and RNA. In clinical disease they involve the conjunctival epithelial cell. Elementary bodies, which are intracellular inclusions that stain reddish-blue with Giemsa, are formed. These later develop into initial bodies, which subsequently divide into large numbers within the cell.

The Chlamydiae cause infection of the conjunctiva in three population groups:

• Western, adult communities in which it is known as inclusion conjunctivitis

• Western neonates as a result of infection via the infected, maternal birth canal, when it is one of the causes of ophthalmia neonatorum (see pp. 238–39)

• All age groups in endemic areas within the Third World, where it causes the much more serious condition known as trachoma (see pp. 256–59).

Phlyctenular keratoconjunctivitis

This is common in the developing world and uncommon in Western communities. It is due to hypersensitivity to an antigen, formerly considered to be tuberculous. Where the incidence of tuberculosis is low, phlyctenulosis is uncommon. When it occurs in these circumstances it is often due to staphylococcal hypersensitivity.

Symptoms: Severe pain, photophobia, and watering.

Signs:

• Whitish nodules, which sometimes invade the cornea to form superficial, vascularised, tongue-shaped opacities, form at the limbus (*Fig. 3.28*).

• The lesions sometimes ulcerate.

• There are diffuse, fine, punctate, epithelial erosions.

Diagnosis: Phlyctenulosis must be distinguished from rosacea keratitis, which may, in fact, be similar in aetiology and mechanism. The patient (and his family) must be evaluated for tuberculosis and typical skin lesions must be excluded if rosacea is suspected. It can be distinguished from vernal conjunctivitis by the absence of changes in the tarsal plates in phlyctenulosis. Infective ulcers must also be distinguished, but these are usually more central in distribution.

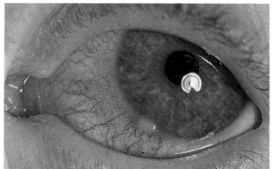

3.28

Fig. 3.28 Phlyctenular keratoconjunctivitis

Management: Topical steroid will generally alleviate ⓢ the condition, but it is important that the patient be regularly examined to ensure that secondary infection does not supervene.

Auto-immune conjunctivitis

Certain disorders of the skin and mucous membranes can involve the eye. They are rare, provide considerable difficulty in management, are liable to secondary infection and may require treatment in emergency departments.

Cicatricial mucous membrane pemphigoid

Pemphigoid is a group of diseases that includes the bullous disorders of the skin and mucous membranes, and features subepidermal bullae rather than the intraepidermal blisters associated with disruption of the intercellular bridges (acantholysis), which are seen in pemphigus.

Symptoms: Cicatricial mucous membrane pemphigoid (CMMP) is a condition that is generally seen in the elderly. Blistering skin involvement is present, but is not a major aspect. It is confined to the extremities or the inguinal areas. Mucous membrane lesions are predominant.

Signs:

• The most frequently involved mucosae are the oral, pharyngeal and conjunctival. Oesophageal and genital mucous membranes are involved less often.

• Blisters appear in the early stages, with long-term clinical disease arising when chronic scarring and shrinkage of the conjunctival sac occurs.

• The caruncle and plica semilunaris are involved in the inflammatory and cicatricial process at an early stage.

- Elevated folds are seen when the lower lid is reflected in routine examination and are a key sign (*Fig. 3.29*).

- There is reduction in the tear secretion, eventually producing total dryness.

- The conjunctival scarring leads to in-turning of the lid margins (entropion), and keratinisation of the inner aspects of the tarsal plates and cornea (*Fig. 3.30*).

- Sometimes the lid margin becomes directly attached to the bulbar conjunctiva, forming a bridge, with maintenance of the fornix beneath it (symblepharon) (*Fig. 3.31*).

- As the condition progresses the cornea becomes subject to multiple epithelial erosions, vascularisation and eventually to scarring.

- There is a risk of corneal bacterial infection.

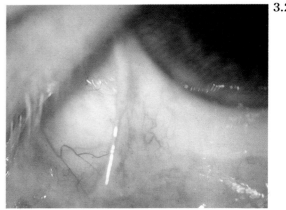

Fig. 3.29 Symblepharon formation in a patient with mucus membrane pemphigoid

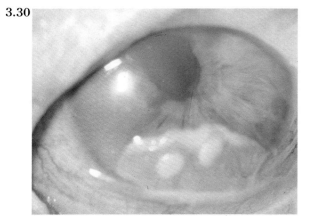

Fig. 3.30 Keratinisation of the lower part of the cornea in a patient with severe cicatricial mucus membrane pemphigoid

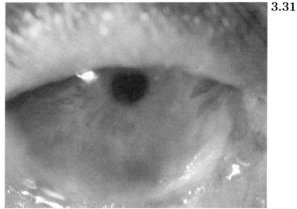

Fig. 3.31 Loss of the lower fornix with symblepharon in a patient with chronic cicatricial mucus membrane pemphigoid

Diagnosis: The diagnosis depends upon the presence of chronic conjunctivitis with ulceration, symblepharon, poor tear secretion and sometimes peripheral corneal infiltrates. The history may indicate involvement of other mucous membranes.

(S) *Management:* The condition varies in its severity, but in general carries a poor prognosis. The principles are:

- Maintenance of the tear film with tear substitutes such as hypromellose or liquifilm drops.

- Avoidance of secondary bacterial infection. Conjunctival and lid margin cultures should be taken regularly, and, where pathogenic organisms are identified, appropriate antibiotics should be chosen.

- When there is active ulcerative disease, topical corticosteroid can be employed carefully, using dilute prednisolone drops (0.1% q.i.d. to begin with) and monitoring the therapeutic effect. Where an improvement occurs, stronger steroid can be used.

- In the early acute phase systemic corticosteroid can be tried. However, it is rare that a significant improvement is obtained and the risk of adverse side effects is increased since many patients are elderly and infirm.

- Where the symblepharon are a serious hazard, attempts at surgical division may be successful for a time. However, the condition inevitably recurs, with eventual loss of the fornices.

- Scleral contact lens shells have been tried and may lead to some amelioration of the condition for finite periods. There is an increased risk of infection when they are used.

- Trichiasis is common, causing damage to the corneal epithelium. Frequent epilation may be necessary, but permanent removal of lashes can be achieved with cryotherapy.

Erythema multiforme

This is an acute bullous disorder involving the skin and mucous membranes. In the major form mucous membranes are involved, while in the minor form there is predominantly involvement of the skin alone. The condition occurs from any time between infancy and 50 years and affects the sexes equally. In children it may be known as Stevens-Johnson syndrome.

It is due to a hypersensitivity to infectious agents such as *Herpes simplex* virus, or Mycoplasma, or to a wide range of therapeutic agents such as the sulphonamide preparations. The immune mechanisms are not understood, but the essential process is a vasculitis. Mucosal blisters form with conjunctival shrinkage, keratinisation and tear deficiency.

Signs:

- Initially there are hyperaemic skin lesions on the extensor surfaces and the distal parts of the limbs. Blistering occurs and is followed by crusting.

- Membranous conjunctivitis occurs.

- Permanent damage to the conjunctiva may later occur including conjunctival shrinkage, keratinisation, tear deficiency, trichiasis and entropion (*Fig. 3.32*).

- Secondary effects on the cornea include vascularisation, epithelial keratitis, stromal opacification and a continuing risk of bacterial infection.

(S) *Management:* This must concentrate on avoidance of secondary bacterial infection and reduction of the inflammatory response in an attempt to prevent the later sequelae of conjunctival scarring and keratinisation.

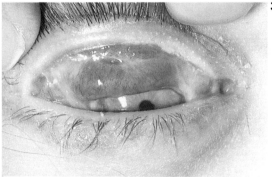

3.32

Fig. 3.32 Everted upper tarsal plate in a child showing severe scarring and keratinisation, following an attack of Stevens–Johnson syndrome

- The patient must be examined twice daily with the slit lamp to ensure that the treatment is not producing further complications during the acute phase. A hand-held slit lamp is extremely useful when the patient is infirm and cannot reach the eye department. A consultant should manage the treatment of the eye disease.

- Regular conjunctival cultures for bacteria must be taken and topical antibiotic given when indicated.

- When the conjunctival sac is sterile, topical steroid can be introduced, using dilute preparations to begin with. This may reduce the risk of permanent effects on the tarsal conjunctiva.

- The long-term sequelae are similar to those occurring in cicatricial mucous membrane pemphigoid. A conservative approach in management is recommended.

Chronic conjunctivitis in sarcoidosis

The most common ocular disease associated with sarcoid is tear deficiency as a result of involvement of the lacrimal gland. In the acute phase of the disease it can be infiltrated and occasionally enlarged. Infiltration with palpable enlargement of the lacrimal gland rarely occurs with salivary gland infiltration or uveoparotid fever. Skin lesions are seen on the lid margins as discrete masses, lupus pernio or millet seed granulomas. Occasionally, conjunctival outgrowths are seen in the lower fornix and biopsy of these can be helpful in diagnosis (*Fig. 3.33*). Other ocular conditions are anterior or posterior uveitis and retinal vasculitis.

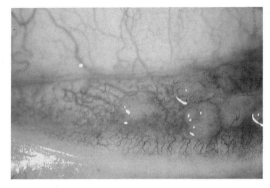

Fig. 3.33 Lower tarsal plate in a patient with sarcoid, demonstrating chronic granulomata

Conjunctival degenerations

Two, common, degenerative conditions of the conjunctiva are pinguecula and pterygium. The former may present to the emergency department because it can become inflamed. The latter is a progressive lesion that encroaches onto the cornea and can affect vision.

Pinguecula is a triangular, fleshy lesion, situated on the bulbar conjunctiva at 3 o'clock or 9 o'clock, the base of which abuts onto the limbus (*Fig. 3.34*). As a rule it remains stationary and is greyish in colour, with occasional yellow spots on the surface. When it is well developed it is conspicuous. It requires no treatment.

Pterygium is a triangular encroachment of conjunctival tissue onto the cornea, usually on the nasal side (*Fig. 3.35*). It is found in hot and sunny regions of the world and is common in out-of-doors workers. It is located within the palpebral fissure and is a fibrovascular connective tissue overgrowth which slowly extends onto the corneal surface.

Management: It can be removed by surgical excision, (S) but many lesions recur. The rate of recurrence can be reduced by postoperative beta-irradiation.

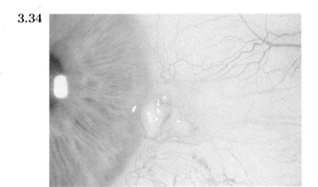

Fig. 3.34 A pingueculum

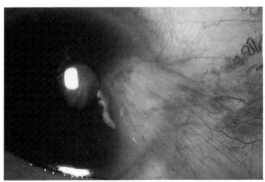

Fig. 3.35 Pterygium

Conjunctival tumours

All the components of the conjunctiva may form tumours. As a rule they are rare and so only the common ones are discussed.

Dermoid choristomas

Dermoid cysts (*see Figs. 13.16 & 13.17*) are usually found in the upper temporal portion of the conjunctival sac, but also occur in the orbit. When situated anteriorly they produce a superficial nodular swelling at the orbital margin. The conjunctival cyst should not be removed if it lies in the upper and outer quadrant, as it is easy to remove the ductules of the lacrimal gland, and cause a permanent dry eye.

    Epibulbar limbal dermoids are most often found at the lower temporal quadrant of the eye and usually overlap the limbus (*Fig. 3.36*). They are sometimes keratinised and contain lash follicles, sebaceous and sweat glands, adipose tissue and cartilage. They are associated with other congenital abnormalities involving branchial arch derivatives such as the oculoauriculo-vertebral dysplasia (Goldenhar's syndrome). They can be easily removed in infancy, but usually a lamellar keratoplasty is required to obtain the best results.

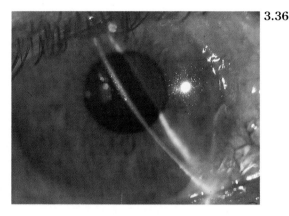

3.36

Fig. 3.36 Conjunctival dysplasia, encroaching onto the surface of the cornea

Epithelial tumours

Papillomas are pedunculated tumours which occur usually at the medial canthus (*Fig. 3.37*). They possess a smooth non-keratinised surface and a vascular core. They can easily be removed, but sometimes may be recurrent.

    Precancerous lesions occur, particularly in association with pingueculae and pterygiums, as abnormal keratinisation (keratosis). Dysplasia, that is, the abnormal maturation of surface epithelium associated with cellular atypia and loss of polarity, may progress to squamous carcinoma.

    ***In situ* squamous cell carcinoma** generally occurs at the limbus as a firm, white plaque with an irregular surface which may be nodular (*Fig. 3.38*). Atypical pleomorphic cells replace the full thickness of the epithelium. Squamous carcinoma may appear papillomatous and tends to spread onto the corneal surface. The neoplasm essentially remains superficial, although malignant cells may occasionally break through the surface. It is rare for lymph node involvement to occur and the prognosis is, on the whole, good.

Management: Recurrence of precancerous and cancerous lesions is always a possibility, and so regular follow-up is necessary.

- Biopsy and microscopic section must be performed.

- Complete excision is necessary.

- Postoperative beta radiotherapy is advantageous.

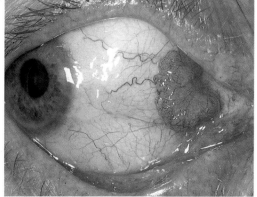

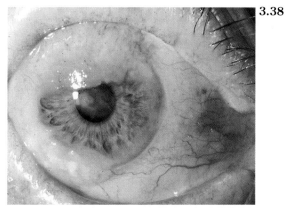

Fig. 3.37 A papilloma on the caruncle

Fig. 3.38 A squamous cell carcinoma of the conjunctiva

Pigmented lesions of the conjunctiva

Conjunctival naevi are common tumours of the conjunctiva (*Fig. 3.39*). The morphology is similar to cutaneous naevi. They are sometimes associated with mucous cysts of the goblet cells, which may enlarge and give the impression of malignant transformation.

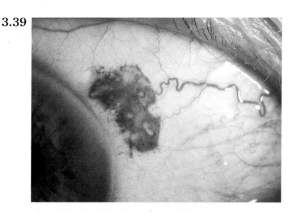

Fig. 3.39 A benign naevus of the conjunctiva

Primary and secondary conjunctival melanosis

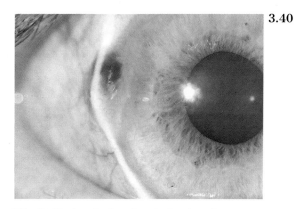

- Endogenous causes include metabolic disease (Addison's), chemical, radiation and chronic disorders such as vernal conjunctivitis and trachoma. Exogenous causes include adrenaline drops, silver, mascara and foreign bodies.

- Primary acquired conjunctival melanosis may be non-progressive but occasionally it is associated with junctional activity (*Fig. 3.40*), leading to superficial and deep invasion. Malignancy rarely occurs. It appears as unilateral, diffuse pigmentation, with a variegated appearance.

Fig. 3.40 Acquired conjunctival melanosis

• Conjunctival, malignant melanoma is a flat, pigmented lesion often seen at the limbus. It may arise from primary, acquired melanosis (*Fig. 3.41*), or from a junctional or compound naevus.

Ⓢ *Management:*

• Biopsy must be performed.

• Local excision can be employed for lesions near the limbus.

• Radical surgery is required for more extensive lesions.

• Lesions arising from acquired melanosis may be sensitive to postoperative radiation treatment, if removal is incomplete.

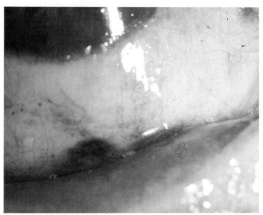

Fig. 3.41 Acquired conjunctival melanosis leading to malignant change

4 Episclera and sclera

Normal anatomy

4.1

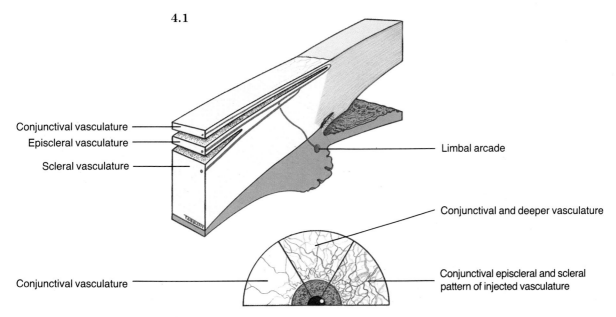

Fig. 4.1 Diagram of the vascular relationships in the conjunctiva, episclera and sclera

The episclera is a layer of loose connective tissue overlying the sclera, and beneath the conjunctiva and the connective tissue sheaths of the extraocular muscles. The sclera is the collagen coat of the eye and is relatively avascular. It is nourished by the vasculature within the episclera and the choroid.

The distribution of the blood vessels in the conjunctiva, episclera and sclera produce different clinical appearances when each layer is involved in inflammatory disease. This helps in diagnosis. Three layers of vessels are detectable on slit lamp examination (*Fig. 4.1*).

● The conjunctival plexus is the most superficial. It is mobile when pressure is applied via the lid margin.

● Beneath the conjunctiva is the superficial and deep episcleral plexus.

a. The superficial layer is radially arranged.
b. The deep layer forms an anastomotic network.

● The third layer is within the sclera, the main vessels emerging near the insertions of the recti.

The conjunctiva and episclera can be blanched with 1/1000 adrenaline.

Episcleritis is an infrequent condition with good prognosis, but scleritis may be much more serious and can carry a poor prognosis. The diagnosis depends upon careful slit-lamp examination to determine the precise layer of vessels that is affected. The red-free filter is useful in accurately determining the layer of vessels involved. Examination of the eye in daylight is useful. A bluish hue to the area of inflammation indicates that the scleral vasculature is involved. In contrast, episcleral hyperaemia has a bright pink colour.

Episcleritis

Episcleritis commonly presents to the general practitioner or casualty as a localised patch of redness overlying the sclera, not associated with systemic disease. It may be simple or nodular.

• In simple episcleritis the congestion is diffuse (*Figs. 4.2 & 4.3*).

• In nodular episcleritis there is localised hyperaemia and swelling which is mobile over the surface of the globe (*Fig. 4.4*).

About 30% of the patients have other systemic conditions such as the collagen disorders, *Herpes zoster*, gout, syphilis, erythema nodosum, Schönlein–Henoch purpura and erythema multiforme.

Management: The response to treatment differs between the simple and nodular types of episcleritis. In both, oxyphenbutazone ointment or prednisolone drops q.i.d. may be used. More potent drops, such as Betamethasone, must be used if the inflammation is not controlled. Resolution of nodular episcleritis is slower than that of the simple form.

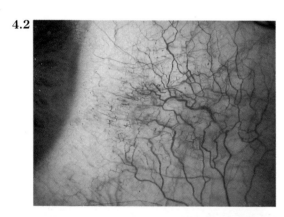

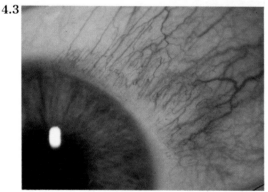

Figs. 4.2 & 4.3 Diffuse episcleritis
Fig. 4.4 Nodular episcleritis

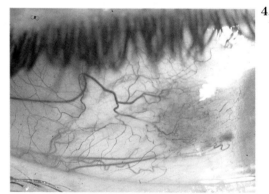

Scleritis

In scleritis the inflammation has a slightly bluish hue compared with episcleritis, indicating that the deeper vessels are involved in the process. The condition is classed as nodular, diffuse or necrotising (where it may occur with or without inflammation). There is a rare form involving the posterior segment. In addition to the lacrimation and photophobia, pain is an important diagnostic feature.

The types of scleritis are distinguished according to their clinical appearance.

• In diffuse scleritis the whole or part of the anterior segment may be involved (*Figs. 4.5 & 4.6*).

• In necrotising scleritis an ischaemic patch is visible. Where there is no clinical evidence of inflammation the condition is known as scleromalacia perforans and the symptoms are less severe than in the other varieties. Yellow infiltrations occur with overt ulceration of the conjunctival surface, eventually sloughing away to expose the ciliary body. Scleromalacia perforans usually occurs in patients with severe rheumatoid arthritis (*Figs. 4.7(a) & (b)*).

With time, increased transparency of the sclera occurs as a result of the inflammation. The uveal pigment becomes apparent as a darkening of the white sclera, generally in patches, on resolution of the

active disease (*Fig. 4.8*).

• Posterior scleritis is uncommon, although it is probably under-diagnosed. It may occur in association with anterior scleritis, or, primarily, as true posterior scleritis without anterior segment signs. Posterior segment signs include:

a. Exudative retinal detachment
b. Cystoid macular oedema
c. Choroidal effusion
d. Swelling of the optic disc
e. Proptosis can occur

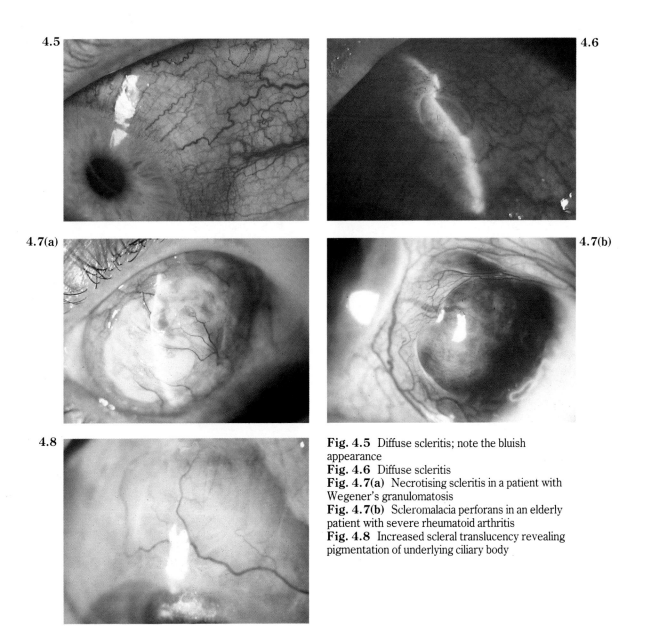

Fig. 4.5 Diffuse scleritis; note the bluish appearance
Fig. 4.6 Diffuse scleritis
Fig. 4.7(a) Necrotising scleritis in a patient with Wegener's granulomatosis
Fig. 4.7(b) Scleromalacia perforans in an elderly patient with severe rheumatoid arthritis
Fig. 4.8 Increased scleral translucency revealing pigmentation of underlying ciliary body

Complications: There are a number of complications that may present as an emergency. These include:

- Scleral thinning (to be distinguished from increased transparency)
- Staphyloma formation
- Uveitis
- Glaucoma
- Cataract
- Retinal detachment

Corneal changes include:

- Acute stromal keratitis
- Sclerosing keratitis
- Limbal guttering

Investigations: Full blood count (FBC), viscosity index, complement levels, rheumatoid factor, immune complexes and auto-immune profile.

(S) *Management:* Since the treatment is sometimes complex the patient with suspected scleritis should attend a consultant-supervised, out-patient clinic. Treatment must depend upon the recognition of disease and accurate documentation of inflammatory activity, so that it can be modified accordingly. Pain is a common symptom which is reduced as treatment takes effect.

- Topical steroid can be tried in the manner of a therapeutic trial, starting with dilute concentrations. The approach must be to taper down therapy gradually as improvement occurs to prevent a rebound of inflammation. On occasions this may lead to a much more severe disease process than was originally witnessed.

- Systemic treatment has a proven effect, but great care is necessary in monitoring the patient for side effects as many are in poor health and do not respond predictably. Where there is bilateral involvement and vision is threatened such treatment can be instituted. Treatment has proved to be beneficial with anti-inflammatory agents such as the prostaglandin antagonist, Indomethacin, which must be prescribed in increasing steps, e.g. 25 mg/day for 2 days, 50 mg/day for 2 days, and 75 mg/day for 2 days. The treatment must be continued until the condition has cleared. Topical steroid is used at the same time.

- Where avascular zones appear, systemic corticosteroid, or immunosuppressive drugs such as Azathioprine, Cyclophosphamide, or Cyclosporin A, can be employed under the guidance of a clinical immunologist, or a physician familiar with the treatment of connective tissue disorders.

5 Cornea

Normal anatomy

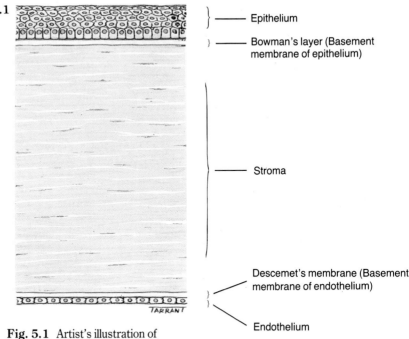

5.1

Epithelium

Bowman's layer (Basement membrane of epithelium)

Stroma

Descemet's membrane (Basement membrane of endothelium)

Endothelium

TARRANT

Fig. 5.1 Artist's illustration of cornea in section, demonstrating epithelium, stroma and endothelium

The cornea is an avascular, transparent membrane that serves as the refracting lens of the eye as well as its protective coat. It is about 11mm in diameter and 0.5mm thick. It is well protected by the conjunctival mucous membrane, the tear film, the lids and the normal immune protection afforded by non-specific and specific immune responses. Loss of the motor nerve supply to the lids, via the facial nerve, can lead to corneal damage due to exposure. Loss of corneal sensation due to damage to the ophthalmic division of the V nerve may also lead to trophic damage to the eye.

The cornea is composed of three layers: the epithelium, stroma and endothelium (*Fig. 5.1*).

The epithelium is about five layers thick and is composed of columnar cells at the base, surmounted by squamous, stratified epithelium superficially. Damage to the surface is quickly replaced by cells sliding into position to cover the deficit.

The epithelium rests on a basement membrane that merges with a thicker layer of collagen material known as Bowman's membrane.

The stroma accounts for about 95% of the corneal thickness. It is composed of a lattice of collagen within a ground substance of proteoglycans. The collagen fibrils are equal in diameter and equidistant from each other. This lattice arrangement accounts for the transparency of the cornea. When the precise arrangement of fibrils is lost the cornea becomes opaque.

The endothelium is a single layer of cells which is important in the maintenance of transparency. A metabolic pump ensures that the corneal stroma does not absorb water. Where the endothelium has lost its function, the cornea swells, becomes opaque and vision is lost. Damage to the endothelium can occur as a result of surgery to the anterior segment of the eye, e.g. during the removal of a cataract, leading to corneal opacification. The endothelium has no capability for cell replication and so this leads to permanent loss of vision.

The endothelium rests on a basement membrane, and a thicker collagen layer called Descemet's membrane.

Corneal response to disease

The cornea responds to insult as follows:

• Corneal oedema due to inflammation or endothelial decompensation (*Fig. 5.2*).

• Vascularisation, either superficial, where the vessels are in continuity with the conjunctival vessels at the limbus, or deep, where they are within the stroma (*Fig. 5.3*).

• Inflammation results in infiltration with polymorphonuclear leukocytes within the stroma (*Fig. 5.4*), which may appear yellowish where there is infection, but otherwise cause a haze which may be difficult to distinguish from oedema. Prolonged inflammation leads to scarring which may be permanent. Punctate sub-epithelial infiltrates may follow punctate epithelial keratitis, and are caused by:

a. Staphylococcal hypersensitivity
b. Adenoviral infection
c. *Herpes simplex* and *Herpes zoster*
d. Chlamydial infection.
e. Onchocerciasis
f. Reiter's syndrome

• Epithelial deficits due to traumatic abrasions, tear film abnormality, or corneal ulcers can be demonstrated with stains such as fluorescein or rose bengal drops. Punctate epithelial erosions are commonly seen (*Fig. 5.5*), and can be of diagnostic significance in the following:

a. Diffuse non-specific punctate erosions occur in early bacterial and viral conjunctivitis.
b. In staphylococcal blepharitis and trichiasis, the lower part of the cornea is involved.
c. In keratoconjunctivitis sicca, ultraviolet light exposure, and inadequate blinking, the punctate lesions occur within the palpebral fissure.
d. In superior limbic keratoconjunctivitis, vernal keratoconjunctivitis and thiomersal toxicity, punctate erosions occur in the upper part.

5.2

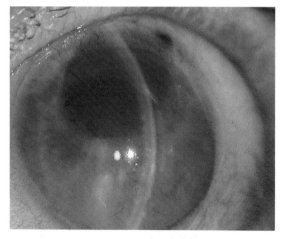

Fig. 5.2 Corneal oedema following the introduction of an intraocular lens implant

5.3

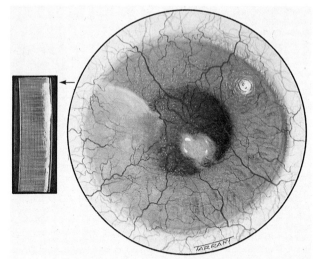

Fig. 5.3 Superficial vascularisation in a patient with a severely keratinised cornea (artist's painting)

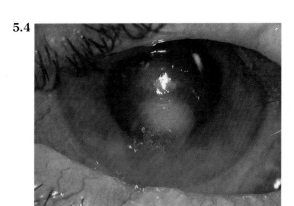

Fig. 5.4 A polymorphonuclear cell infiltration in a peripheral corneal ulcer

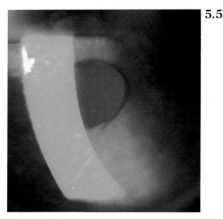

Fig. 5.5 Punctate epithelial staining demonstrated with fluorescein dye in a patient with allergic conjunctivitis (Courtesy of Mr. R. Marsh)

Examination

The cornea in general practice can be examined with indirect illumination using a pen-torch and a ×8 magnifier. Care must be taken to document the clinical signs in as much detail as possible.

The casualty officer must be scrupulous in the documentation of active, corneal, inflammatory disease prior to treatment to determine whether the therapy is effective.

Viral disease

The cornea is affected by *Herpes simplex*, *Herpes zoster* and *Epstein Barr* viruses, together with certain adenoviruses, *Molluscum contagiosum* virus and mumps virus.

Herpes virus infection

Four Herpes viruses produce infection in man: *Herpes simplex*, *Herpes zoster (varicella)*, *Epstein Barr* (EBV) and *Cytomegalovirus* (CMV).

Herpes simplex *keratitis*

The *Herpes simplex* virus (HSV) is a common cause of infectious corneal disease leading to unilateral, and occasionally bilateral, blindness. The condition occurs with greater severity in the immunocompromised, for example organ transplant recipients. It is estimated that there are about 500 patients per million population presenting yearly with dendritic ulcers in Western communities. Below the age of 16 years, infection occurs equally in males and females, while above this age, males are affected more often. The recurrence rate in patients who have experienced a single dendritic ulcer is 40%. Recurrence is usually within six months.

The mouth is the most common site of primary infection with type I HSV. The virus spreads via the sensory nervous system to set up a long-term latent infection in the posterior root ganglion, where it appears to be incorporated into the DNA of the host cell. Recurrence occurs as a result of stimuli such as trauma, exposure to sunlight, emotional stress, upper respiratory tract infection or menstruation.

The eye may be involved in the primary infection (see p. 36, p. 63), or through reactivation and recurrence of the virus within the corneal epithelium to form a dendritic ulcer, or by spread of the virus into the stroma to produce deeply seated disease that leads to loss of vision.

Ulcerative herpes simplex keratitis

The dendritic ulcer is branched and has a zigzag shape, the tips of the side branches being associated with stromal opacity. The ulcer has a vertical edge and stains with fluorescein or rose bengal drops (*Figs. 5.6(a) & (b)*). The infected cells at the edge of the ulcer stain with rose bengal drops.

In patients where corticosteroid has inadvertently been given in treatment, the area of ulceration is much more extensive with the ulcer becoming geographic or amoeboid in appearance (*Fig. 5.7*). The risk of developing stromal disease is increased. Steroid is contra-indicated for treatment of all forms of herpetic keratitis, except in certain patients with stromal inflammation, who are under the supervision of a consultant ophthalmologist.

Ulceration occurs in the form of a trophic ulcer as a result of the anaesthesia induced by *Herpes simplex* virus in the cornea (*Figs. 5.8 & 5.9*). It is often central and extremely persistent. It usually does not bear any resemblance to the dendritic ulcer.

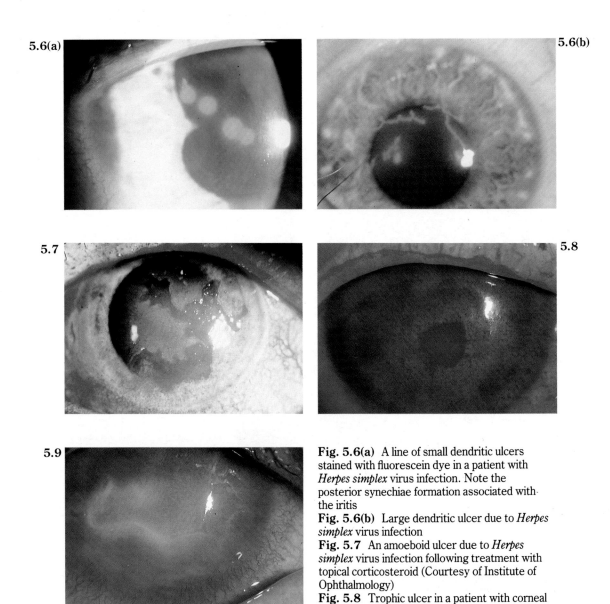

Fig. 5.6(a) A line of small dendritic ulcers stained with fluorescein dye in a patient with *Herpes simplex* virus infection. Note the posterior synechiae formation associated with the iritis

Fig. 5.6(b) Large dendritic ulcer due to *Herpes simplex* virus infection

Fig. 5.7 An amoeboid ulcer due to *Herpes simplex* virus infection following treatment with topical corticosteroid (Courtesy of Institute of Ophthalmology)

Fig. 5.8 Trophic ulcer in a patient with corneal anaesthesia due to *Herpes simplex* virus infection

Fig. 5.9 Trophic herpetic ulcer in a patient with a history of atopic conjunctivitis

5.10

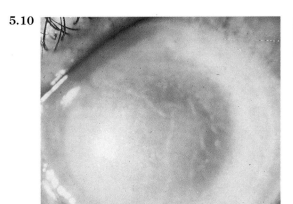

Fig. 5.10 Diffuse herpes simplex stromal keratitis

5.11

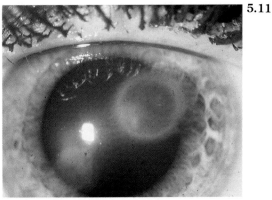

Fig. 5.11 An immune ring occurring in the stroma following ulcerative herpetic keratitis

5.12(a)

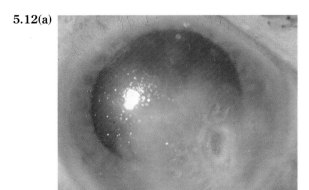

Fig. 5.12(a) Corneal perforation in a patient with a history of herpetic keratitis

5.12(b)

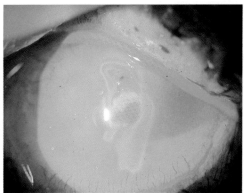

Fig. 5.12(b) Positive Siedel test in the same patient. A rivulet of aqueous humour can be seen emerging at the perforation, clearly visible in the fluorescein- stained tear film

Stromal disease is due to the presence of live virus or viral antigen within the stromal cells, the keratocytes. It is characterised by inflammatory oedema, cellular infiltration and an active process of vascularisation. The inflammation may lead to permanent scarring, sometimes necessitating a corneal graft.

Stromal herpes keratitis presents with a variety of clinical appearances.

● A ghost of a previous dendritic ulcer occurs involving the superficial stroma in a pattern reminiscent of the original ulcer.

● Disciform keratitis involves the central area of the stroma, with oedema, cellular infiltration and sometimes the appearance of folds in Descemet's membrane (*Figs. 5.10, 5.11, 5.12(a) & (b)*).

● Keratouveitis is seen as diffuse corneal oedema and infiltration, with uveitis.

● Limbal keratitis originates in association with a peripheral dendritic ulcer. The keratitis is characteristically persistent. and associated with a persistent epithelial deficit.

• Recurrent anterior uveitis can follow a dendritic ulcer, with large, mutton-fat, keratic precipitates (*Figs. 5.13 & 5.14*).

5.13

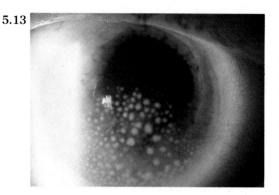

Fig. 5.13 *Herpes simplex* uveitis with large "mutton fat" KP

5.14

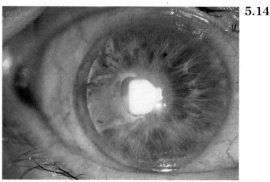

Fig. 5.14 Iris atrophy in a patient with a history of herpes simplex uveitis

Investigations:

• The appearance of a dendritic ulcer is so typical that investigation does not seem appropriate.

• However, it is recommended that the lesion is cultured as other corneal lesions can masquerade as dendritic ulcers.

• Bacterial culture must be carried out because secondary infection is common.

• Rising serum antibody indicates primary infection, but does not change in recurrent disease.

• Where the cause of stromal inflammation is unclear, absence of specific antibody is helpful since it indicates that there can be less danger from the use of topical corticosteroid.

Management of ulcerative disease:

(R) **Dendritic ulcer** – Treatment, which is by debridement and antiviral therapy, must be introduced early to prevent virus spread. Where the trigger for recur-
(P) rence is known, an antiviral must be prescribed for the patient to instil at the earliest opportunity.

Debridement consists of gently removing the virus-infected cell at the edge of the lesion with a cotton wool applicator. A sterile swab can be used and sent for culture for virus, having been placed in a suitable transport medium.

The antivirals available today are acycloguanosine, idoxuridine, adenine arabinoside and trifluorothymidine.

• Acycloguanosine (Acyclovir, Zovirax) is available in ointment form (3%) which has good penetration through the corneal epithelium and low toxicity. Systemic treatment with tablets is also available.

• Idoxuridine (Kerecid) is available as 0.1% drops or 0.5% ointment. The former must be given hourly for 24 hours and then five times a day. The ointment must be given five times daily from the start of treatment. Treatment must be continued until the lesion has healed, usually after 7–10 days. It is toxic to the corneal epithelium and conjunctiva.

• Adenine arabinoside (Vidarabine; Vira-A) is an ointment (3%) that can be instilled five times per day. Toxicity of the corneal epithelium occurs with prolonged use.

• Trifluorothymidine is formulated as 1% drops. It has good penetration through corneal epithelium, but is toxic if used for long periods.

All the antivirals, with the exception of acycloguanosine, can be toxic to the external eye when used for long periods. They induce follicular conjunctivitis, keratinisation of the tarsal conjunctiva, occlusion of the canalicular puncta, tear deficiency, punctate epithelial keratitis and superficial stromal scarring.

The patient must be seen after five days to evaluate the therapeutic effect. When stromal inflammation occurs the patient must be referred to the consultant clinic.

Ⓢ **Management of stromal herpetic keratitis —** Stromal inflammation induced by the *Herpes simplex* virus is treated under the supervision of a consultant.

An antiviral with good penetration is recommended such as acyclovir. The minimal amount of topical corticosteroid, consistent with achieving a therapeutic improvement in the stromal disease, is used. Dilutions of standard corticosteroid preparations may be used, such as prednisolone drops 0.01, 0.1, 0.25 and 0.5%. A therapeutic effect can generally be obtained with prednisolone drops 0.1% four times daily. Where no benefit is obtained a higher concentration is used. Steroid therapy is not used without antiviral cover.

In the case of early primary disease, or where there is severe keratouveitis, or just uveitis alone, systemic treatment with acycloguanosine is indicated.

Topical steroid should never be used for any external eye disease by a general practitioner or an untrained hospital casualty officer.

Varicella zoster

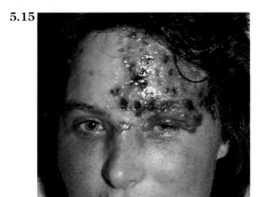

Fig. 5.15 Cutaneous lesions in a patient with *Herpes zoster ophthalmicus*

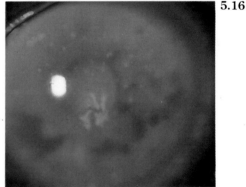

Fig. 5.16 A small dendritic ulcer in a patient with early *Herpes zoster ophthalmicus*

Varicella (chickenpox) has been reported to be associated with disciform keratitis and uveitis.

Herpes zoster ophthalmicus forms a unilateral eruption, confined to the dermatome supplied by the first part of the trigeminal nerve, the ophthalmic division. The lesions within the dermatome may be diffuse or sparse. They extend from the brow into the parietal region, well above the hairline. There are prodromal symptoms of paraesthesia followed by the appearance of a vesicular rash in successive crops. These are followed by the formation of scabs, which can be delayed by the onset of a secondary infection (*Fig. 5.15*). The eruption only rarely extends across the midline, but may occasionally affect more than one dermatome.

Early in the attack the periorbital tissue becomes oedematous on both sides, making ocular examination extremely difficult. A useful sign to determine whether the eye is affected is involvement of the nasociliary nerve, in which the eruption extends onto the side of the nose. Inflammatory disease occurs in the eye during the early stage of active disease, but may persist or recur well after the initial rash has disappeared.

Microdendritic ulcers occur at an early stage of the infection. They are smaller than those seen in herpes simplex keratitis and indicate that there is ocular involvement (*Fig. 5.16*).

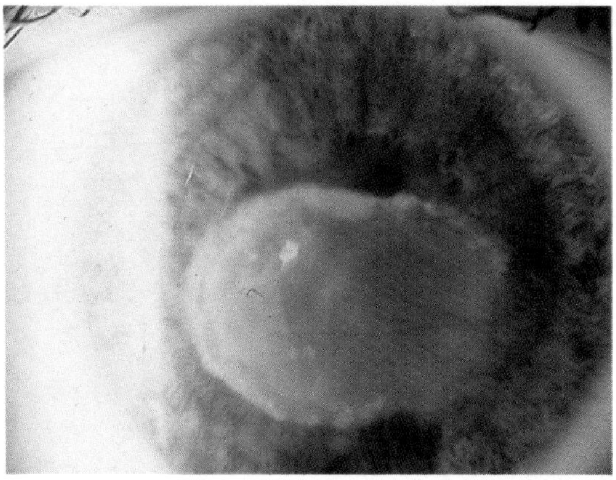

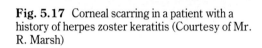

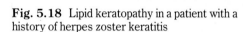

Fig. 5.17 Corneal scarring in a patient with a history of herpes zoster keratitis (Courtesy of Mr. R. Marsh)

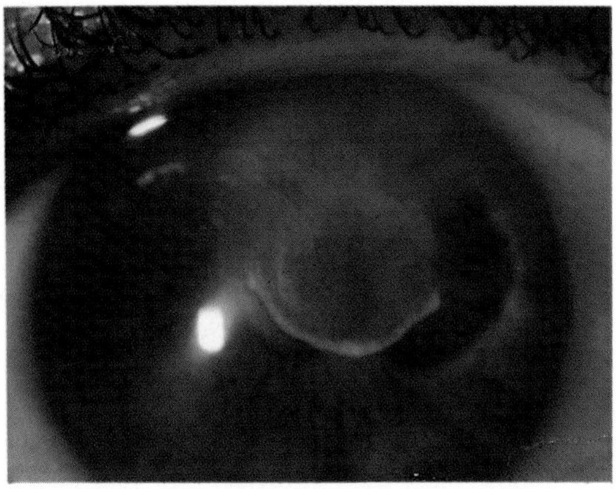

Fig. 5.18 Lipid keratopathy in a patient with a history of herpes zoster keratitis

Mucous plaque keratitis occurs where abnormal epithelial cells cause adherence of mucous. This sometimes forms a dendritic pattern and is raised above the epithelial surface. The whole lesion stains brilliantly with rose bengal and poorly with fluorescein.

Although herpes zoster keratitis is pleomorphic in the same way as herpes simplex keratitis, several forms can be described.

● Punctate stromal keratitis, with the opacities within the superficial layers of the stroma.

● Focal keratitis, with similarities to disciform keratitis in *Herpes simplex*, can affect the central area with oedema and folds in Descemet's membrane (*Figs. 5.17, 5.18, 5.19*).

● Diffuse keratitis, where the complete cornea is oedematous, can occur.

● Punctate keratitis, sometimes with large and persistent corneal erosions when there is corneal anaesthesia.

● Nodular episcleritis or scleritis is common.

● Abnormality of the lid margins resulting from post-zoster scarring.

● Stromal inflammatory responses lead to permanent scarring with vascularisation. On the central edge yellowish and crystalline lipid deposits occur.

● Uveitis occurs, but is not severe. It is associated with sectorial atrophy in the iris due to local vasculitis (*Fig. 5.20*).

Management:

(P) ● Acute rash. Management is aimed at rapid healing of the cutaneous eruption and reduction of secondary bacterial infection. Topical antibiotic–steroid combinations can be used until the crusts have separated. Acyclovir (Zovirax) tablets (800mg five times a day) can be given as they are thought to reduce the severity of the rash and possibly of post-zoster neuralgia if given at the onset of the eruption.

● Anterior segment inflammation can be treated with (S) topical corticosteroid according to the following principles:

a. Steroid should only be used if absolutely necessary.
b. The dilution of prednisolone drops (0.1–0.25 – 0.5–1.0%) which achieves a therapeutic effect is used.

- Ocular muscle palsies, scarring of the skin of the lids, neuroparalytic and neurotrophic keratitis, lid margin deformity and tear-film abnormality are seen. Post-zoster neuralgia is not uncommon.

- Posterior pole manifestations include papillitis, choroiditis and retinal haemorrhage.

- Steroid drops should not be curtailed suddenly because they can excite a rebound of inflammatory disease. They must be reduced over several weeks.

The ocular manifestations of *Herpes zoster* must be managed in a consultant clinic.

5.19

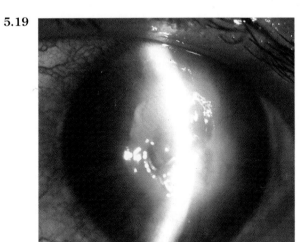

Fig. 5.19 Corneal perforation following herpes zoster keratitis. The cornea was completely anaesthetic (Courtesy of Institute of Ophthalmology)

5.20

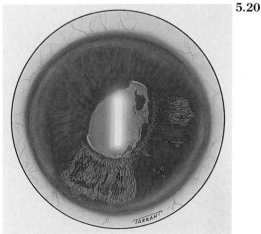

Fig. 5.20 Iris atrophy following *Herpes zoster ophthalmicus*

Bacterial corneal ulcers

Peripheral corneal ulcers

Marginal ulcers occur, associated with chronic infection of the lids and accessory glands by *Staphylococcus aureus*. The ulcers are generally situated at the corneal margin (*Figs. 5.21, 5.22, 5.23*). They are not associated with direct infection of the cornea, but are an immune or toxicity response to antigens produced by organisms residing in the lid margin.

5.21

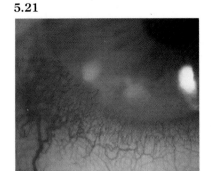

Fig. 5.21 Marginal ulcer in a patient with staphylococcal blepharitis (Courtesy of Institute of Ophthalmology)

5.22

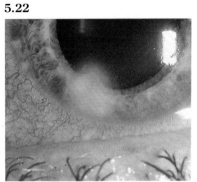

Fig. 5.22 Staphylococcal marginal ulcer

5.23

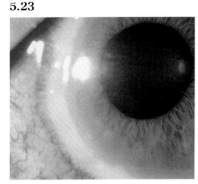

Fig. 5.23 Diffuse marginal infiltration in association with staphylococcal disease of lid margin

Symptoms: Watering, pain and grittiness, photophobia.

Signs: Peripheral, whitish infiltration, which usually stains with fluorescein, and local limbal hyperaemia.

Management: Topical antibiotic for three days, ®︎ followed by a five-day course of topical corticosteroid

Central ulceration of the cornea

Corneal ulceration can be caused by a number of bacteria. This presents a true ocular emergency and requires active steps to limit the spread of ulcers and damage to the eye.

Bacterial ulcers are generally associated with previous external eye disease. They are increasingly seen in contact lens wearers (*Figs. 5.24 & 5.25*).

Corneal ulcers must not be treated until a full laboratory investigation has been made to identify the organism.

Bacterial infection of the cornea may be focal or extend to involve the entire area, leading to permanent scarring and visual disability, or perforation. Management involves identification and elimination of the organism, minimising the destructive effects and promoting epithelial healing.

5.24

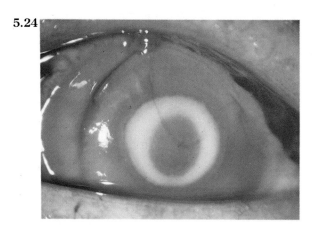

Fig. 5.24 Pseudomonas infection following contact lens wear

5.25

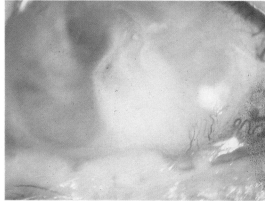

Fig. 5.25 Pneumococcal corneal abscess in a patient with severe rheumatoid arthritis

Pathogens

The main corneal pathogens are the Gram-positive cocci, *Staphylococcus aureus* and *Staphylococcus epidermidis*, *Streptococcus pneumoniae*, *Streptococcus pyogenes*, the Gram-negative diplobacilli, *Moraxella lacunata*, and the Gram-negative rods *Pseudomonas aeruginosa*, *Proteus morganii*, *Klebsiella pneumoniae* and *Escherichia coli*.

Symptoms: Acute photophobia, watering, purulent discharge, pain and visual blurring.

Signs: Conjunctival hyperaemia and lid swelling in severe cases. Clinical manifestations vary according to the infective organism.

● Staphylococcal ulcers occur in compromised corneas following, for example, ulcerative herpetic keratitis or bullous keratopathy.

a. *Staph. aureus* causes a localised infection which remains superficial, with a surrounding area of cellular infiltration. In chronic cases the abscess may become intra-stromal and can be seen with multiple satellite infiltrates.
b. *Staph. epidermidis* produces a chronic, localised infiltration with little inflammatory response within the anterior chamber.

● Pneumococcal ulcers follow injury, with the infiltration starting at a point on the periphery of a corneal abrasion and spreading towards the centre. The inflammatory response in the anterior chamber is marked and a hypopyon usually forms.

● Ulcers caused by beta-haemolytic streptococci are often severe, but are not characterised by typical features, whereas alpha-haemolytic streptococci are chronic and indolent.

● Gram-negative organisms commonly induce rapidly progressing infection and the threat of perforation, sometimes within 24 hours of onset of symptoms.

Severe infection is caused by *Pseudomonas* strains. These organisms are found surviving on fomites, including ophthalmic solutions and ocular cosmetics. The organisms produce proteases and elastases. Infection follows an episode of trauma.

Epithelial and stromal oedema present as a diffuse greyness in the cornea, outside an area of dense cellular infiltration, occasionally in ring form. A greenish-yellow, mucopurulent discharge remains attached to the surface of the lesion prior to treatment.

Gram-negative rods, such as *Proteus, Escherichia coli* and *Klebsiella*, cause indolent ulceration in compromised corneas, with less inflammatory response within the anterior chamber than *Pseudomonas. Moraxella* causes ulcers which are oval, and situated in the lower part of the cornea. They occur in debilitated patients.

● Anaerobes can cause ulceration, usually following soil contamination. *Nocardia* is a Gram-positive organism with branching filaments which may cause indolent ulceration. *M. fortuitum* may also cause slowly progressive ulcers with a cracked windshield appearance to the ulcer base.

5.26(a)–(c)

(a) Local anaesthetic drops   (b) Corneal scrape

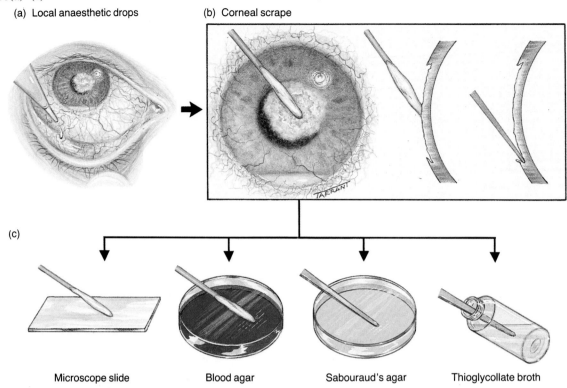

(c)

Microscope slide   Blood agar   Sabouraud's agar   Thioglycollate broth

Fig. 5.26(a)–(c) Diagrammatic presentation of the steps required in taking corneal smear and culture

(R) *Laboratory diagnosis:* The laboratory diagnosis is made by taking cultures from the conjunctival sac and the ulcer itself (*Figs. 5.26(a)–(c), 5.27*). The method is as follows:

- The cornea is anaesthetised with 0.4% benoxinate hydrochloride drops (*Fig. 5.26(a)*).

- A sterile applicator is touched on the central area of the ulcer and streaked onto blood or chocolate agar, and then onto fungal agar (*Fig. 5.26(b) & (c)*).

- The ulcer is then scraped with a sterile spatula and the material is smeared onto a glass slide for microscopic examination using Gram stain (*Fig. 5.26(b) & (c)*).

- Further material for culture should be taken by scraping and inoculated onto solid media.

- In cases where antibiotic therapy has been provided prior to assessment, the organism may have been eliminated from the superficial lesion. However, as it can remain active within the anterior chamber, additional material should be obtained by an anterior chamber tap.

5.27

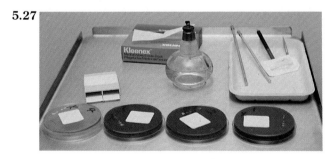

Fig. 5.27 Equipment required for corneal bacterial culture

Management: Antibiotic therapy is guided by laboratory investigation, according to Gram-staining and to culture and sensitivity. Admission to hospital is necessary to investigate the condition. Appropriate therapy should be arranged and its effect monitored.

The fortified antibiotics are more effective than the commercially available ones and must be made up in the hospital pharmacy. Therapy must be given half-hourly to begin with until a therapeutic response is produced. Intensive therapy of this type is more effective than subconjunctival injection.

● Gram-positive organisms should be treated with fortified drops such as cefazolin (50 mg/ml), or vancomycin (50 mg/ml).

● Gram-negative organisms must be treated with gentamicin forte (15 mg/ml).

Gentamicin forte is made up by adding 80 mg (2 ml of intravenous gentamicin) to a 5 ml bottle of commercial genticin drops containing 3 mg/ml. The other antibiotics can be made up to the recommended concentrations in water for injection, normal saline or artificial tears.

● Systemic intravenous or intramuscular antibiotic is rarely necessary unless there is evidence of spread of the organism to produce endophthalmitis. In patients with threatened perforation, subconjunctival injection of antibiotic produces adequate concentrations to prevent intraocular involvement.

Mycotic infection

Fungal keratitis occurs more commonly in subtropical than temperate climates. In subtropical regions up to 20% of corneal ulcers can be due to fungi, the commonest organisms being *Fusarium solani*, *Aspergillus fumigatus* and *Candida albicans*.

Infections occur following minor trauma. Three features should indicate fungal infection (*Figs. 5.28 & 5.29*).

● The stromal infiltrates have feathery edges.

● They tend to be grey and elevated above the corneal surface.

● Satellite lesions occur.

Candida infection can have a collar-stud appearance. Although these characteristics are helpful, it must be remembered that any corneal infiltrate with associated epithelial deficit can have a fungal cause.

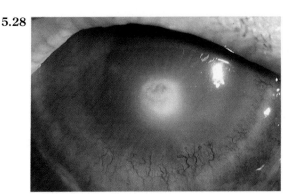

Fig. 5.28 *Candida albicans* corneal ulcer

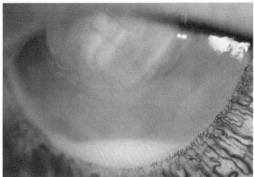

Fig. 5.29 Mycotic infection following trauma due to *Scopulariopsis brevicaulis*

Laboratory investigation: It is routine practice to perform cultures for fungi in the majority of infectious corneal ulcers, usually by taking scrapings from the base of the ulcer in a way already described. The scraped material must be plated onto media that can support the growth of fungi, such as blood agar, maintained at room temperature, and a Sabouraud agar plate, incubated at room temperature. Material is also placed on slides for Gram and Giemsa staining to demonstrate fungal hyphae.

Management: Following the laboratory identification of a fungal aetiology, treatment is initiated with 5% natamycin suspension (50 mg/ml) hourly during the day and two-hourly at night. Where infection seems to be progressing in spite of this therapy, miconazole (1%) may be introduced hourly. Candida, which is a yeast, is treated with flucytosine combined with natamycin, nystatin, or miconazole. Sensitivity studies should be performed.

Sterile corneal ulceration

Peripheral corneal ulceration with little evidence of infectious aetiology occurs in association with connective tissue disorders, or, rarely, alone, when it is known as Mooren's ulcer. These conditions are rare and may lead to perforation. Hence they require emergency treatment.

The ulceration is probably an auto-immune process and is associated with the following inflammatory diseases:

- Diffuse or necrotising scleritis
- Postoperative cataract extraction, following use of silk sutures for the limbal wound
- Rheumatoid arthritis (*Figs. 5.30 & 5.31*)
- Polyarteritis nodosa
- Wegener's granulomatosis (*Figs. 5.32 & 5.33*)

5.30

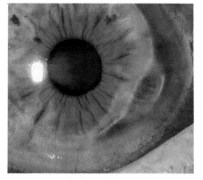

Fig. 5.30 Peripheral corneal ulceration in a patient with severe rheumatoid arthritis

5.31

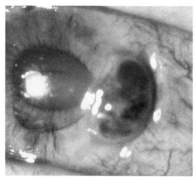

Fig. 5.31 Corneal perforation in a patient with rheumatoid arthritis

5.32

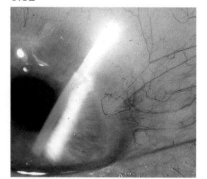

Fig. 5.32 Marginal corneal thinning in a patient with Wegener's granulomatosis

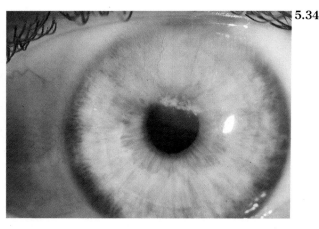

Fig. 5.33 Collapse of the bridge of the nose in a patient with peripheral keratitis, and Wegener's granulomatosis

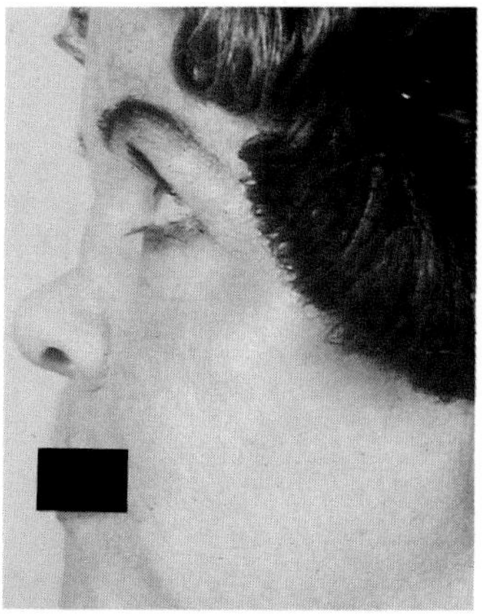

Fig. 5.34 Terrien's marginal ulcer, which must be differentiated from other forms of peripheral corneal ulceration

Symptoms: Persistent pain, redness, photophobia and watering.

Signs:

- Local limbal hyperaemia
- Conjunctival elevation alongside the peripheral furrow
- Severe peripheral corneal thinning, with sharply defined inner border
- Occasional cellular infiltration and vascularisation
- Descemetocele
- Perforation and iris prolapse
- Terrien's ulcer is unilateral, occurs in younger patients, and is associated with peripheral corneal thinning and lipid deposition (*Fig. 5.34*).

Management: The condition is serious and requires ⓢ consultant care.

- Topical antibiotic. Topical corticosteroid must be used cautiously, but can be beneficial
- Tear substitutes as many patients have concurrent KCS
- Systemic immunosuppression can be effective when the condition is bilateral and blindness is threatened
- Surgical procedures, such as annular corneal graft, conjunctival flap and limbectomy, may be tried with varying degrees of response

Tear deficiency

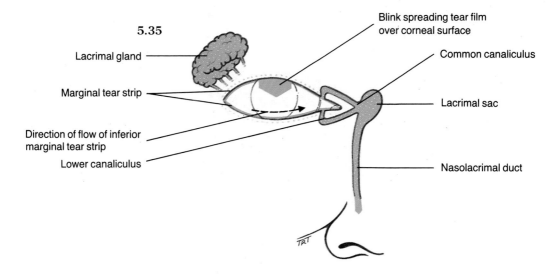

5.35

Lacrimal gland

Marginal tear strip

Direction of flow of inferior marginal tear strip

Lower canaliculus

Blink spreading tear film over corneal surface

Common canaliculus

Lacrimal sac

Nasolacrimal duct

Fig. 5.35 Illustration of tear film production, movement across the marginal tear film strip and blinking action, with drainage into nasolacrimal duct

The aqueous portion of tears is produced by the lacrimal gland, a tubulo-acinar exocrine gland in the upper and outer portion of the orbit, close to the margin. Its secretions reach the conjunctival sac via a series of 12 ducts into the upper fornix. There is an orbital portion, which is the major part, separated from a palpebral portion by the aponeurosis of the levator tendon. Tears are also secreted by the accessory lacrimal glands of Krause, found in the upper and lower conjunctival fornices. Some lacrimal secretion is produced by the glands of Wolfring, located in the supratarsal conjunctiva of the upper lid.

The functions of the tear film are:

- to maintain an optically smooth surface of the tear film

- mechanically to remove foreign matter from the cornea and conjunctival sac by lubrication of the surface

- to supply the nutritional requirements to the corneal epithelium

- to maintain an antibacterial function.

It is composed of three layers:

- A superficial lipid layer, secreted by the Meibomian glands, which prevents evaporation

- An aqueous layer, which is the largest

- An inner mucous layer produced by conjunctival goblet cells, responsible for the stability of the film by ensuring a uniform spread of the aqueous layer across the corneal epithelium

The tear film forms the marginal strip at its junction with the upper and lower lid margins, where the oily surface prevents spillage of the tear fluid over the lid margin. The tears are drained from the lacus lacrimalis via two puncta to the upper and lower canaliculi, then to a common canaliculus, which leads into the nasolacrimal sac, and finally down the nasolacrimal duct to the inferior meatus in the nose (*Fig. 5.35*).

Examination of the tear film

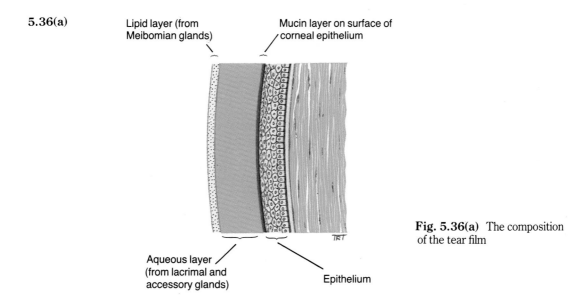

Lipid layer (from Meibomian glands)

Mucin layer on surface of corneal epithelium

Aqueous layer (from lacrimal and accessory glands)

Epithelium

Fig. 5.36(a) The composition of the tear film

The tear film is examined with a slit lamp (*Fig. 5.36(a)*). The marginal strip must be examined and an assessment made of its magnitude. In tear deficiency it will be reduced and may be barely discernible.

The instillation of a small amount of fluorescein will demonstrate the film when examined with the slit lamp. The patient is asked to refrain from blinking for about 30–40 seconds while the film is examined. The break-up time is the period elapsing before the film ruptures to leave an obvious area where the fluorescein layer is breached. A normal break-up time is considered to be at least 10 seconds.

Staining patterns of the conjunctiva and cornea, using fluorescein or rose bengal, preferably the latter, are useful in identifying patients with tear deficiency. Rose bengal drops, although the most instructive, cause severe stinging in some patients. They should be washed out with saline drops and only used infrequently. The typical staining pattern in the dry eye is punctate, involving the lower part of the cornea and spreading onto the adjoining conjunctiva. The tear film in the dry eye characteristically contains debris of mucous threads and clumps of epithelial cells.

Filaments attached to the corneal epithelium, usually in the upper half, are formed by disrupted epithelial cells, remaining attached at one point, together with a mucous coat. They stain brightly with rose bengal.

Schirmer's test is used to determine the presence of tear deficiency (*Fig. 5.36(b)*). It is measured with a strip of filter paper 5 mm in width, the folded tip of which is held in place by the lower lid. The strip is held in position for five minutes and the spread of tear fluid along the strip is measured. Normal levels are in the region of 10 mm and deficiency is generally thought to be at a level below 5 mm.

Lysozyme content of tears represents an accurate test in keratoconjunctivitis sicca. However, this measurement is not commonly available as a routine test.

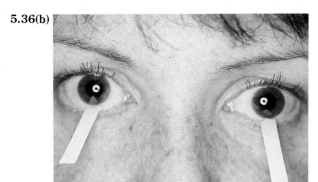

Fig. 5.36(b) Schirmer's test

Tear film abnormalities

These occur in the three layers of the tear film, lipid, aqueous and mucous, and in addition the surface epithelium of the cornea, conjunctiva and the tarsal plates.

Dry Eyes

Dry eyes are caused by a deficiency in any of the areas responsible for tear production.

Keratoconjunctivitis sicca (KCS) occurs as a result of reduction in the aqueous component of the film. It is due to atrophy of the lacrimal tissue, often idiopathic, occurring commonly in middle-aged women, sometimes in association with inflammatory disorders, e.g. sarcoid, or with auto-immune disorders as in Sjögren's disease.

5.37(a)

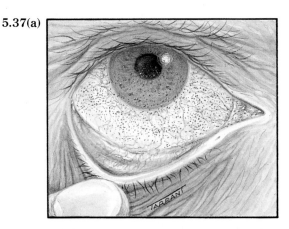

Fig. 5.37(a) Artist's impression of the typical staining pattern with Rose bengal drops in a patient with keratoconjunctivitis sicca

5.37(b)

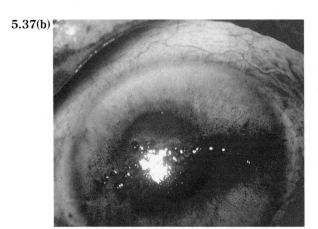

Fig. 5.37(b) Staining of the cornea and conjunctiva with Rose bengal drops in keratoconjunctivitis sicca

5.37(c)

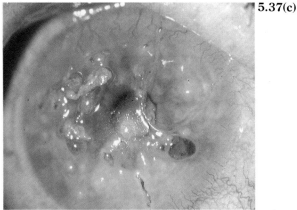

Fig. 5.37(c) Mucous plaque keratitis in a patient with keratoconjunctivitis sicca

Symptoms: Irritation, soreness and redness, particularly in smoky environments. Because the tear film is important in forming a perfect refractive surface, disruption leads to visual blurring.

Signs: Slight hyperaemia, reduced marginal strip, mucous strands and debris in the tear film, punctate staining with rose bengal and an abnormally low Schirmer test (*Figs. 5.37(a)–(c)*).
N.B. Rose bengal stain stings on application, especially in dry eyes, so it is kinder to instil local anaesthetic drops beforehand and essential to wash the excess stain out with sterile saline immediately after application.

KCS occurs in:

• Elderly menopausal females

• Sjögren's syndrome, when it is associated with a dry mouth and rheumatoid arthritis (with positive rheumatoid factor and anti-nuclear antibody)

• Mucous membrane pemphigoid

• Inactive trachoma

• Late Stevens-Johnson syndrome

• Following caustic burns

• Connective tissue disorders such as systemic lupus erythematosus and Wegener's granulomatosis

• Sarcoidosis

In the dry eye syndromes there is loss of the protective function of the normal tear film due to absence of lysozyme, IgA and other substances. Hence, patients are at greater risk of suffering from infections of the anterior segment. It is therefore unwise to use contact lenses for therapeutic or optical reasons.

Deficits in the mucous layer occur as a secondary phenomenon resulting from damage to the mucous-secreting goblet cells. This occurs in vitamin A deficiency. Areas of non-wettability occur on the surface as occurs for xerophthalmia, more commonly seen in developing countries. Secondary deficiency occurs in conditions that cause a loss of natural structure of the conjunctiva including:

• Mucous membrane pemphigoid
• Stevens-Johnson syndrome
• Severe trachoma
• Chemical burns

Mucous deficiency is characterised by an abnormally short tear break-up time.

Deficits in the lipid layer follow chronic, lid-margin disease, such as blepharitis or meibomitis, and are associated with the production of an altered lipid that does not form a stable, oily layer. Rarely, there may be congenital absence of the Meibomian glands which causes an incapacitating punctate epitheliopathy with severe photophobia.

Abnormality of surface epithelium may occur and induce staining patterns reminiscent of those seen in KCS, itself resulting in tear film abnormality. The epithelial cells possess microvilli which project finger-like receptors to which the mucous layer adheres. This structure is easily disturbed, altering the tear film and leading to persistent deficits.

Corneal irregularities and corneal anaesthesia are associated with breakdown in the epithelium. Failure of lid-closure reflex, as in nocturnal lagophthalmos, in which lid closure at night is incomplete, can induce epithelial drying and multiple erosions. Failure of lid-closure and blinking reflex is also seen in seventh nerve palsies with a poor Bell's phenomenon; that is inadequate upgaze when the eyes are closed, such as during sleep, and is associated with loss of epithelium and punctate staining of the lower third of the cornea.

Irregularities in the surface induced by elevation of the limbal conjunctiva, e.g. following certain forms of surgery, cause poor contact between tarsal conjunctiva of the upper lid and the ocular surface. Drying causes dehydration of the stroma and thinning, together with the formation of a shelving pit known as a dellen.

• Treatment depends on tear replacement using tear substitutes which depend upon the addition of absorptive polymers in their formulation.

Preparations for tear deficiency include:

a. Hypromellose

• Hypromellose Eye Drops
• Isopto Alkaline
• Isopto Plain
• Tears Naturale

b. Polyvinyl alcohol

• Hypotears
• Liquifilm tears
• Sno tears

These preparations have differences in their formulation and patients may show best responses to a particular formulation. It is therefore worth altering the prescription if the patient remains symptomatic. In severe KCS, drops must be instilled frequently, say hourly or even half-hourly.

• Lubricating ointments at night can be useful. Lacri Lube containing liquid paraffin is effective.

• Preservation of the existing tears using plugs, such (S) as the Freeman punctal plug, to obliterate the puncta can be helpful.

• Antiinflammatory therapy is not beneficial.

• Bandage contact lenses must be avoided because of the added risk of infection.

Rosacea keratitis

Rosacea keratitis is an uncommon and potentially serious condition, associated with the classical telangiectatic skin condition. Both conditions undergo remission and exacerbation, but not always in concert.

Signs:

• Scaly blepharitis and recurrent conjunctival hyperaemia

• Corneal lesions occur in the lower third with punctate epithelial keratitis at the limbus leading to greyish superficial stromal opacity

• Vascularisation

• Stromal thinning (*Fig. 5.38*)

• Lipid deposits at the inner edge

• Perforation can occur

(S) *Management:*

• Since inflammatory, lid-margin disease is common it must be controlled with hygienic measures, together with antibiotics.

• Topical antibiotics and corticosteroid can be used where there is active inflammation. Corticosteroid, although hastening resolution of the inflammatory response in the conjunctiva and corneal stroma, may increase stromal thinning and induce corneal perforation. Dilute corticosteroid drops must be used in the first instance.

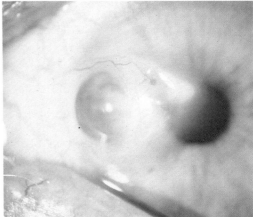

5.38

Fig. 5.38 Corneal thinning and threatened perforation in a patient with rosacea keratitis

• Systemic tetracycline is useful where chronic blepharitis is associated. This can be beneficial in the treatment of the cutaneous inflammation. The dosage is 250 mg, three times daily, for up to six weeks.

• Penetrating keratoplasty is necessary for perforation. This is usually eccentric, greatly adding to the technical difficulties and increasing the risk of allograft rejection.

Neurotrophic keratitis

Neurotrophic keratitis occurs when the sensory nerve supply to the cornea is compromised. Causes are surgery involving the trigeminal nerve, multiple sclerosis, tumours such as neurofibroma, meningioma in the posterior fossa and acoustic neuroma, aneurysm, cerebro-vascular accident causing the mid-pontine syndrome, herpes zoster and herpes simplex infection and radiation. The maintenance of normal corneal structure depends upon intact sensory innervation. Axoplasmic flow affords protective substances, although the mediators of this trophic influence are unknown.

Signs:

● Punctate epithelial erosions

● Generalised stromal infiltration with inflammatory cells

● Persistent erosion with an elevated or rolled edge

● Superficial and deep vascularisation

● Permanent opacification (*Fig. 5.39*)

Where there is damage to the fifth and the seventh nerve the risk of corneal damage is increased.

Ⓢ *Management:*

● Prophylactic antibiotics are necessary in the early stages, preceded by conjunctival bacterial culture.

● Corticosteroid therapy must be used with care and requires frequent monitoring for beneficial or adverse responses.

Facial nerve palsy

Facial nerve palsy or paralysis induces poor lid closure which can result in exposure keratitis. This is not always necessarily the case, as where there is a good Bell's phenomenon (elevation of the eyes on closure of the lids) the cornea is well protected during sleep since it is not exposed (*Fig. 5.40*).

The clinical consequence of facial nerve paralysis is desiccation of the corneal epithelium and occasional damage to the basement membrane, with eventual cell death. Multiple erosions in the lower cornea are an early sign. Stromal ulceration occurs in severe cases. The risk of superimposed infection must be excluded on clinical examination.

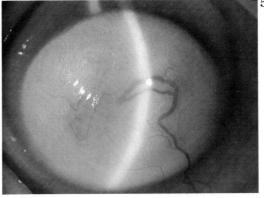

Fig. 5.39 Severe lipid deposition following infective keratitis in a patient with a completely anaesthetic cornea

● A moist chamber, in which a Cartella shield is fitted closely to the orbit and the holes occluded with tape, can be beneficial.

● Treatment of a large corneal erosion is beset with pitfalls. Strapping of the lids with a horizontal band of tape can result in improvement. Bandage contact lenses must be avoided because they are dangerous. Permanent tarsorrhaphy is occasionally necessary, particularly when associated with facial nerve palsy, such as follows operative treatment of an acoustic neuroma.

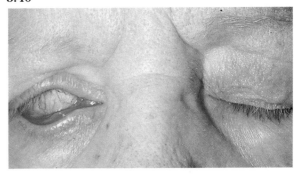

Fig. 5.40 A positive Bell's phenomenon in a patient with a right seventh nerve palsy

Management: Where the Bell's phenomenon is weak, treatment is necessary in the long term.

- Prophylactic antibiotic treatment is necessary in ointment form at night.

- Patients must be warned about signs of infection and advised to attend as an emergency if necessary.

- Good coverage of the corneal surface can be achieved by the application of a horizontal piece of tape either at night only, or day and night where surface damage is advancing. Temporary tarsorrhaphy using botulinum toxin infected into the levator may be an effective short-term measure.

- Permanent, central tarsorrhaphy remains a valuable Ⓢ treatment mode, but it is rarely necessary.

Corneal dystrophies

Corneal hereditary dystrophies are distinctive, chronic alterations in one of the three principle layers, leading to loss of vision and other symptoms occasionally resulting in presentation of the patient in the emergency department. It is therefore useful to describe briefly the most common of the dystrophies.

Epithelial dystrophies

The corneal epithelium, the basement membrane, or Bowman's layer is affected.

Recurrent erosion syndrome – This is characterised by a sudden attack of sharp, needle-like pain in the eye on waking in the morning. There is often a history of a corneal abrasion caused by objects such as paper, fingernails or twigs. Recurrence is in the originally affected area. Examination demonstrates the epithelial deficit using fluorescein drops. Subtle epithelial changes, such as microcysts, fingerprint lines and bleb- and net-like changes, may be seen in affected patients and help in reaching a diagnosis.

Management: The erosion is treated with antibiotic Ⓢ and a firm pad and bandage for 24 hours. Chloramphenicol ointment or Lacri Lube must be given q.i.d. for one week. Local anaesthetic drops must be avoided if possible as they delay healing.

Prophylactic measures must be taken. The affected eye can be strapped closed during sleep with micropore, following instillation of Lacri Lube.

Occasionally, prophylactic treatment with a bandage contact lens is effective.

Reis-Buckler dystrophy – This autosomal, dominant dystrophy primarily affects the basement membrane and Bowman's layer. Progressive and diffuse scarring occurs, which does not involve the stroma, with ring-like opacities which appear to form irregular projections into the epithelium. Recurrent erosion is a troublesome feature.

Meesman's dominant dystrophy – There are fleck-like opacities within the epithelial layer, only visible with the slit lamp microscope.

Stromal dystrophies

Two out of the three main examples can present as emergencies with recurrent abrasions.

Granular dystrophy – This is dominantly inherited, with superficial stromal discoid or nodular opacities which remain discrete in the anterior stromal layers of axial stroma (*Fig. 5.41*). A peripheral, clear zone remains. Spontaneous corneal erosion can occur, necessitating immediate care.

Lattice dystrophy – This demonstrates double-contoured, branching filaments forming a latticework, amongst which fine dots, eventually producing diffuse opacification, appear (*Fig. 5.42*). Recurrent erosions and significant loss of vision occur, the latter in middle age.

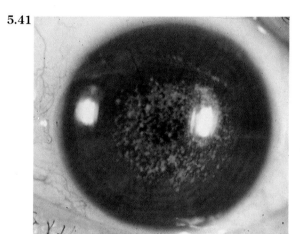

Fig. 5.41 Granular dystrophy

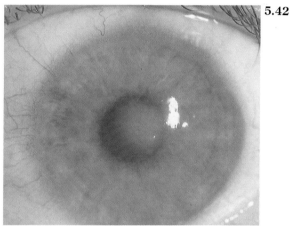

Fig. 5.42 Lattice dystrophy

Macular dystrophy – This recessive dystrophy is characterised by central cloudiness in the superficial layers (*Fig. 5.43*). The clouding eventually involves the entire thickness and extends to the periphery.

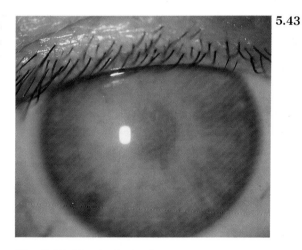

Fig. 5.43 Macular dystrophy

Endothelial dystrophies

These dystrophies can present as emergencies since decompensation and corneal oedema with epithelial bullae may provide painful symptoms if they rupture.

Cornea guttata – These are elevations in Descemet's membrane induced by stressed endothelial cells, sometimes associated in advanced cases with a beaten metal appearance. They may represent the early stages of Fuchs' endothelial dystrophy.

Fuchs' endothelial dystrophy – This is due to apparently spontaneous endothelial decompensation, with stromal and eventually epithelial oedema (*Fig. 5.44*). Rupture of bullae causes pain, and a gradual decline in visual acuity may indicate a penetrating keratoplasty.

Ⓢ *Management:*

• Hypertonic agents, such as 5% sodium chloride drops or ointment, help to dehydrate the epithelium and improve the visual acuity.

• Soft bandage contact lenses can be used for treatment of ruptured bullae, particularly when the pain is severe. There is a continuing risk of bacterial infection in these patients and so careful monitoring is needed.

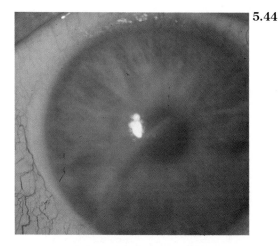

Fig. 5.44 Endothelial decompensation in a patient with Fuchs' dystrophy

Keratoconus

This is often bilateral and is due to central thinning which leads to coning of the cornea producing visual loss (*Fig. 5.45*). The early stages are treatable with gas-permeable contact lenses, but when the cone becomes pronounced, the lens cannot be retained and penetrating keratoplasty becomes necessary.

The condition can lead to severe corneal oedema (*Fig. 5.46*) because of ruptures in Descemet's membrane, and for this reason may present as an emergency.

Management: The patient can be reassured that the Ⓢ oedema spontaneously clears. It may be treated with patching and hypertonic saline drops or ointment. The patient must be referred to an ophthalmologist.

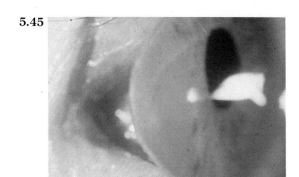

Fig. 5.45 Keratoconus

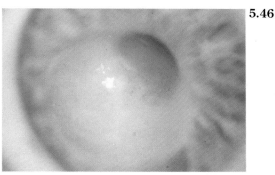

Fig. 5.46 Corneal oedema in a patient with severe keratoconus

6 Uveal tract – iris, ciliary body and choroid

Normal anatomy

6.1

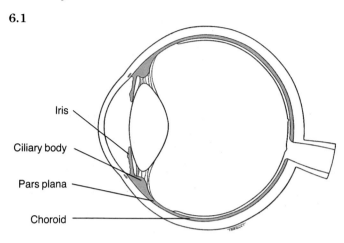

Iris

Ciliary body

Pars plana

Choroid

Fig. 6.1 Normal anatomy of the uvea

The uveal tract is the middle vascular layer of the eye. It is divided into three portions: iris, ciliary body and choroid (*Fig. 6.1*).

The iris is a pigmented structure that extends forwards from the ciliary body, dividing the aqueous compartment into anterior and posterior chambers. The pupil acts as a variable aperture to control the amount of light that enters the eye. The sphincter pupillae and dilator pupillae are smooth muscles of the iris which control pupil diameter. The sphincter pupillae is supplied by the parasympathetic nervous system via the short ciliary branches of the oculomotor nerve (see p. 192), while the dilator pupillae is supplied by the sympathetic nervous system via the long ciliary nerves (see p. 187). The level of pigmentation in the iris stroma determines the colour of the iris – the brown iris being the most heavily pigmented and the blue iris the least. This pigmentation is acquired in the first few months, or even years, after birth.

The ciliary body has two main functions:

● **Production of aqueous fluid from the ciliary epithelium** – Aqueous fluid produced from the ciliary body nourishes the avascular cornea and lens. It cir-culates through the posterior chamber, around the pupillary margin into the anterior chamber and drains via the trabecular meshwork and canal of Schlemm in the angle. The angle structures can be viewed by gonioscopy (see below).

● **Control of accommodation by the ciliary muscle** – Contraction of the muscle which circum-ferentially surrounds the lens, relaxes the tension on the zonular fibres supporting the lens and allows the lens to adopt a more spherical configuration. This increases the refractive power of the lens to allow accommodation for close targets.

The choroid runs posteriorly from the ciliary body to the optic nerve. It is highly vascular and nourishes the outer layers of the retina. It is pigmented due to the presence of uveal melanocytes and this is responsible for the background colour of the fundus. In highly pigmented individuals the colour is very dark red, masking any details of the choroid. In albinos there is no pigment present and all the blood vessels of the choroid are easily visualised.

Uveitis

Uveitis is inflammation of the uveal tract. It is divided into:

- anterior (iritis) (*Fig. 6.2*)
- intermediate (cyclitis – inflammation of the ciliary body)
- posterior (choroiditis, retinitis)
- panuveitis

In practice, the groups overlap. In about one third of cases no cause or related condition for the uveitis is found. The most common related conditions are:

- **Seronegative arthritides**, e.g. ankylosing spondylitis, juvenile chronic arthritis, Reiter's syndrome, Behçet's disease

- **Inflammatory bowel disease**

- **Chronic granulomatous conditions**, e.g. sarcoidosis, tuberculosis

- **Sexually transmitted diseases**, e.g. syphilis, gonorrhoea

- **Local infections**, e.g. *Herpes zoster* (see pp. 85–87) (chickenpox and shingles), *Herpes simplex* (see pp. 36, 63, 83), measles, influenza, cytomegalovirus, toxoplasmosis, toxocariasis, onchocerciasis, presumed ocular histoplasmosis syndrome, candidiasis

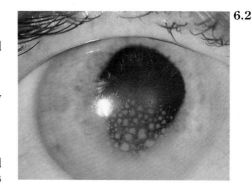

6.2

Fig. 6.2 Right iritis

- **Ocular syndromes**, e.g. Fuchs' heterochromic cyclitis, sympathetic ophthalmitis, Posner-Schlossman syndrome

- **Lens-induced uveitis**, e.g. a cataractous lens may leak proteins, giving rise to an anterior uveitis; an intraocular lens implant may cause a low-grade uveitis, especially iris-clip or anterior chamber lens

- **Masquerade syndromes**, that is tumours that masquerade as uveitis e.g. reticulum cell sarcoma, retinoblastoma, malignant melanoma, leukaemia, lymphoma

Anterior uveitis

Anterior uveitis may be acute or chronic. The acute form often presents to the general practitioner as an acute red eye to be differentiated from conjunctivitis or acute glaucoma.

Symptoms: Acute anterior uveitis presents with deep and throbbing ocular pain, photophobia and blurred vision. Chronic uveitis may be painless with slight blurring of vision. There may be a history of previous episodes, often undiagnosed, and associated disease, e.g. low back pain from sacroileitis, symptoms from inflammatory bowel disease, aching joints from peripheral arthritis, e.g. in Reiter's syndrome, and chronic cough or dyspnoea in sarcoidosis (*Fig. 6.3*), all of which may flare-up simultaneously.

6.3

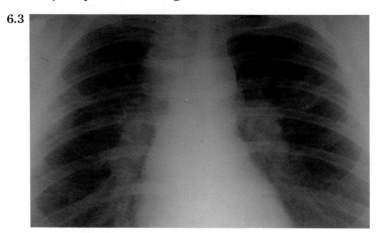

Fig. 6.3 Chest radiograph – acute sarcoidosis

Signs: Acute anterior uveitis (*Figs. 6.4(a)–(d), 6.5, 6.6*):

• **Limbal injection**, ranging from a faint pink blush to intense redness spreading out from the limbus due to dilatation of the blood vessels. This is graded from 0 to ++++.

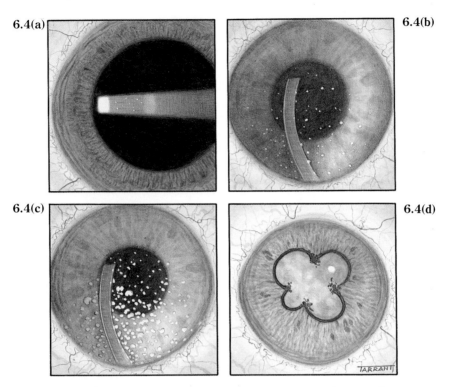

Fig. 6.4(a)–(d) Composite diagram of acute anterior uveitis. **(a)** Slit-lamp beam showing cells and flare in anterior chamber, **(b)** Small keratic precipitates, **(c)** Large (mutton fat) keratic precipitates, **(d)** Posterior synechiae and cataract formation

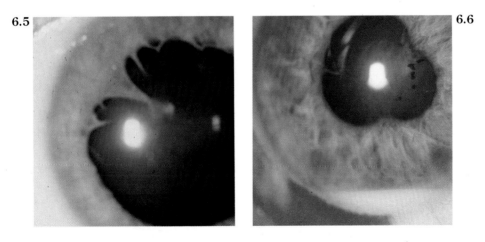

Fig. 6.5 Posterior synechiae

Fig. 6.6 Hypopyon and posterior synechiae in acute anterior uveitis

Ⓡ ● **Keratic precipitates** (KPs) are deposits of inflammatory cells on the corneal endothelium. They may form a fine dusting on the endothelial surface or they may form medium-sized or large-sized aggregates. The large, yellow deposits, known as mutton-fat KPs, are often associated with sarcoidosis. New KPs are white and round; old KPs are pigmented. The KPs are usually situated on the lower half of the cornea in an inverted cone distribution, except in Fuchs' heterochromic cyclitis when they are centrally distributed, or disciform keratitis (see p. 83), when they are situated posterior to the site of corneal involvement. The number of the KPs is recorded to monitor severity and progress. KPs cannot be seen by inexperienced observers without proper equipment such as a slit lamp microscope.

Ⓡ ● **Flare and cells** in the anterior chamber. To view these the slit lamp beam is shone obliquely across the anterior chamber so that the aqueous is viewed in front of the black contrast of the pupil. Maximum magnification and light intensity are used. Flare is due to protein exudation from leaky iris blood vessels. The cells are white, round and inflammatory. If large numbers are present, they can be seen to circulate with convection currents in the aqueous. They are distinguished from pigment cells and red cells by colour and size. Flare and cells are graded by using a beam of 1 mm width and 3 mm height. Flare is graded from 0 to ++++:

    0 - nil present
    + - faint
    ++ - moderate
    +++ - marked – iris and lens details hazy
    ++++ - gelatinous exudate in anterior chamber

Cellular activity is graded from 0 to ++++ according to the number of cells seen in the field of the beam:

    0 - no cells seen
    +/− - 0–5 cells
    + - 5–10 cells
    ++ - 10–20 cells
    +++ - 20–50 cells
    ++++ - >50 cells

● **Posterior synechiae** are adhesions of the iris pupillary border to the anterior surface of the lens. The pupil is small and irregular because of this. If there are 360° of posterior synechiae (seclusio pupillae), aqueous flow may be obstructed, causing the iris to billow forwards and the pressure to rise owing to angle obstruction. This is called iris bombé. There may also be pigment deposited on the anterior surface of the lens – remnants of previous broken-down posterior synechiae.

● **Intraocular pressure** may be normal, subnormal (owing to paralysis of ciliary body function), or raised (owing to inadequate aqueous drainage). If raised, there may be fine corneal epithelial oedema. Some patients, so-called 'steroid responders', have raised intraocular pressure as a result of steroid treatment. In this instance the dose of steroid is reduced if possible or the patient is changed to a type of steroid that is less likely to induce a pressure rise.

Chronic uveitis is more insidious in onset and there may be a complete absence of limbal injection, although slit lamp examination reveals the anterior chamber activity. The uveitis associated with juvenile chronic arthritis is often of this type (see pp. 230–31). Chronic uveitis is more commonly associated with posterior uveitis. The following features are seen in addition to those listed above:

● **Anterior vitreous inflammation**, which is seen if the beam is angled through the pupil and focused behind the lens. The cells seen are larger than anterior chamber cells and may be graded similarly. They may only become apparent once the anterior chamber activity has settled to allow a clearer view.

● **Lens opacities**, which tend to start as a posterior, subcapsular opacification and are associated with chronic uveitis (especially if uncontrolled) as well as with steroid treatment.

● **Iris atrophy**, which is seen in all chronic uveitis, but especially in Fuchs' heterochromic cyclitis. Dilatation of iris blood vessels is commonly seen in uveitis.

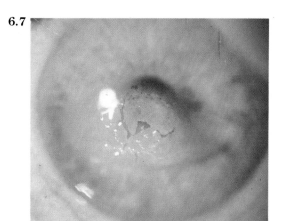

6.7

• **Band keratopathy** (*Fig. 6.7*) which is a band-shaped deposition of calcium in deeper corneal epithelium and adjacent to Bowman's membrane. It starts to form at 3 o'clock and 9 o'clock and spreads slowly inwards. It is often seen with chronic uveitis in children, associated with juvenile chronic arthritis.

Fig. 6.7 Band-shaped keratopathy

A full fundal examination is carried out in all cases of anterior uveitis, looking for associated posterior uveitis – chorioretinitis, pars planitis, and also retinal detachment and the 'masquerade' syndromes. If the visual acuity is decreased, the macula is examined with a contact lens or a Hruby lens to detect cystoid macular oedema.

Ⓡ *Management of acute anterior uveitis:* Cases of uveitis detected by the general practitioner should be referred immediately to an ophthalmologist. The immediate management is carried out by the eye casualty officer, but complicated cases are referred to the consultant eye specialist.

• Intensive pupillary dilatation using, if necessary, several instillations of cyclopentolate 1%, phenylephrine 10% to break the posterior synechiae.

• If unsuccessful, further different types of dilating drops are used, e.g. adrenaline 1/1000 and cocaine 4%, and a heated pad (Maddox) is applied.

• If still unsuccessful, and the posterior synechiae are known not to be longstanding, a subconjunctival injection of Mydricaine (a mixture of atropine, adrenaline and procaine) is given (see below). The Mydricaine is often combined with betamethasone (about 2 mg) to act as a depot injection of steroids in severe cases.

For the administration of subconjunctival injection (*Fig. 6.8*):

a. The patient should be lying on a couch. Amethocaine and cocaine 4% drops are instilled to anaesthetise the conjunctiva.
b. The patient is instructed to look up as far as possible.

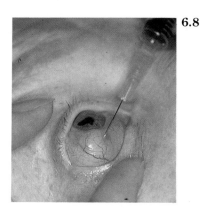

6.8

Fig. 6.8 Administration of subconjunctival injection

c. The syringe containing the drugs to be injected is fitted with a 25-gauge needle. The tip of the needle is inserted gently under the bulbar conjunctiva and Tenon's capsule at a point well away from the limbus, with the needle almost parallel to the eye and the bevel pointing upwards. A subconjunctival bleb is raised as the syringe contents are expelled. The maximum amount that can be injected is about 2 mls.
d. The eye is closed and lightly padded for a few hours.

- A Collagen shield is a relatively new method of controlled drug delivery

- Further treatment – The mainstay of treatment is topical steroids to reduce inflammation and mydriatics (with cycloplegic action) to relieve spasm of the ciliary muscle and prevent posterior synechiae formation. The severity of attack determines the strength of steroid and cycloplegic required.
N.B. Steroids should be used with caution if the suspected aetiology is *Herpes simplex* virus or bacterial.

Ⓡ Ⓢ **Severe attacks**: Dexamethasone 0.1% drops hourly for 24–48 hours or until a good response to treatment is seen, then decreased to two hourly for the next 24–48 hours and then further decreased to q.d.s. This is maintained until the eye is quiet after which it may be tailed off slowly, e.g. t.d.s. for 3 days, then b.d. for 3 days, then o.d. for 3 days, then stop. It may be necessary to tail off more slowly in some cases, using alternate day dexamethasone or a weaker preparation for a period of weeks to prevent relapse.

Atropine drops 1% b.d. or t.d.s. or homatropine drops 2% t.d.s. until the inflammation has settled, after which it may be tailed off.

Betamethasone ointment is used at night.

Moderate attacks: Betamethasone drops q.d.s. with **cyclopentolate 1%** t.d.s. with or without betamethasone ointment at night depending on severity. The treatment is tailed off as outlined above.

Mild attacks: Prednisolone 0.5% drops are used q.d.s. together with **cyclopentolate 1%** drops t.d.s., tailing off as above.

In steroid responders, when there is a rise in intraocular pressure in response to steroid treatment, fluoromethalone (FML) drops are substituted as the steroid, although they have a less powerful anti-inflammatory action. If the pressure rises over 28 mm Hg it may be controlled with Timolol drops 0.5% b.d. (if there are no contra-indications) in the short term until the inflammation is settled, after which it can be stopped. The pressure should be rechecked later when the patient is off treatment.

Investigations: It is not essential to investigate patients with their first attack of acute anterior uveitis if there is no apparent systemic association. If the uveitis is recurrent, bilateral, associated with systemic symptoms, e.g. arthralgia, in an only eye or associated with posterior uveitis, it is investigated. Routine tests performed include full blood count, viscosity, VDRL and, if indicated, chest radiograph (to exclude sarcoidosis) and radiograph of the sacroiliac joints (to exclude sacroileitis). Further investigations may include auto-immune profile and the tests outlined in the section on posterior uveitis (see below).

Posterior uveitis

Posterior uveitis has an insidious onset. The most common causes are toxoplasmosis, sarcoidosis, histoplasmosis (in the USA), syphilis, toxocariasis, tuberculosis, auto-immune disease and Behçet's disease.

Symptoms: The main symptoms are blurring of vision and floaters. The floaters are abundant in pars planitis (peripheral posterior uveitis). The vision may be especially decreased in posterior pole chorioretinitis.

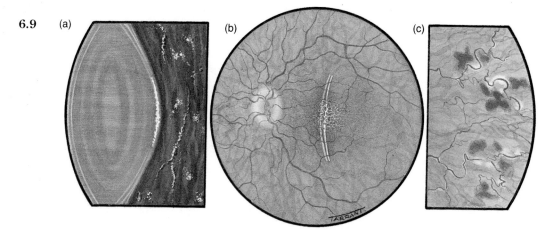

Fig. 6.9(a)–(c) Composite diagram of posterior uveitis. **(a)** Slit-lamp view showing posterior subscapular cataract and anterior vitreous opacities, **(b)** Disc swelling and cystoid macular oedema, **(c)** Vasculitis: exudates and haemorrhage around inflamed blood vessels

Signs: The main features of posterior uveitis (*Fig. 6.9(a)–(c)*) are:

- **Vitreous opacities**, which are seen in the anterior vitreous by shining the beam through the pupil and focusing behind the lens, and in the posterior vitreous by direct and indirect ophthalmoscopy. Fine opacities are individual inflammatory cells. Large peripheral opacities ('snowball' opacities), which may progress to form a plaque inferiorly ('snowbanking'), are seen in pars planitis. Large opacities may also be seen in sarcoidosis. Vitreous opacities may be graded from 0 to ++++:

> 0 - no vitreous opacities
> + - few opacities, clear retinal view
> ++ - moderate numbers of opacities with slight obscuration of retina
> +++ - large numbers of opacities with marked blurring of retinal view
> ++++ - dense opacities with no fundal view

- **Choroiditis**, which appears as white or yellow lesions with a fluffy border due to retinitis, which may be contiguous with previous inactive lesions as in toxoplasmosis. The inactive lesions appear as pale areas of chorioretinal atrophy, surrounded by a well-defined, pigmented border.

- **Retinitis**, which is often associated with choroiditis, causes a greyish, ill-defined appearance to the retina.

- **Cystoid macular oedema**, which is a fine microcystic change at the macula associated with chronic uveitis.

- **Disc swelling**, which is seen in chronic uveitis.

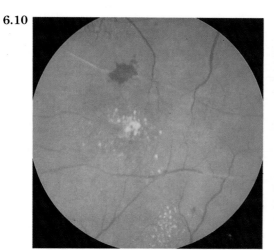

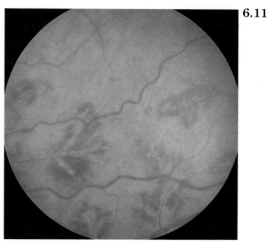

Fig. 6.10 Vasculitis in systemic lupus erythematosus

Fig. 6.11 Vasculitis in Behçet's syndrome

- **Vasculitis** (*Figs. 6.10 & 6.11*)

- **Neovascularisation**, which may occur anywhere in the retina. In histoplasmosis it occurs at the macula as a subretinal neovascular membrane, causing central visual loss.

Ⓡ Ⓢ *Management of posterior uveitis:* This is carried out at a specialist eye centre.

- **Treatment of underlying disease**, e.g. tuberculosis, syphilis, sarcoidosis.

- **Treatment of anterior uveitis** with topical steroids and mydriatics (v.s.).

- **Treatment of posterior uveitis.** Drops or ointments are not adequate if the uveitis is posterior to the iris–lens diaphragm because of lack of penetration. Peribulbar injections of steroids are used.

- **Indications for systemic steroids** include chorioretinal inflammation, which is close to the posterior pole and thus sight-threatening, cystoid macular oedema and persistent uveitis (anterior or posterior) failing to respond to topical treatment.

The dose used depends on the severity of the lesion and the cause. If sight is threatened, doses of up to 60–100 mg prednisolone daily are used. If the indication is for a persistent uveitis, doses of around 30 mg daily are used. Inpatient treatment is necessary if high dose steroids are used. If children are treated with any dose of systemic steroids, they should be under the care of a paediatrician.

Patients with chronic uveitis on long-term steroids may develop posterior subcapsular lens opacity.

Specific conditions

A few conditions that deserve special mention are discussed in the next few pages.

Ankylosing spondylitis

The uveitis associated with this seronegative arthritis is usually **acute, anterior** and **recurrent**. It accounts for about 15% of all cases of **acute** anterior uveitis. The disease typically affects young, adult males – >90% are HLA-B27 positive.

There is initially a sacroiliitis (*Fig. 6.12*), followed by involvement of the lumbar spine and cervical spine, leading eventually to bony ankylosis in severe cases, with the typical 'bamboo spine' appearance. The disease can also affect children, in whom it starts as an inflammation of peripheral joints, especially the knees.

The sacroiliitis is often subclinical and therefore young, male patients with anterior uveitis are screened for this condition. To avoid unnecessary pelvic irradiation, females are only screened if they have symptoms of low back pain.

The sacroiliitis, which often flares up at the same time as the anterior uveitis, is treated with non-steroidal anti-inflammatory drugs. The anterior uveitis is treated with topical steroids and mydriatics in the usual way. Episodes usually resolve within two months and few permanent sequelae result.

6.12

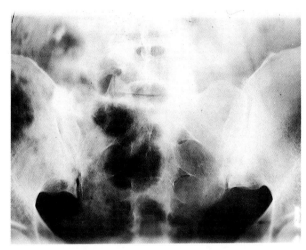

Fig. 6.12 Sacroiliitis of the left sacroiliac joint in a patient with ankylosing spondylitis (Courtesy of Dr. W.D. Jeans)

Reiter's syndrome

The classical triad of Reiter's syndrome is **arthritis**, (usually knees and ankles, but also hands, sacroiliac joints, wrists, and calcaneal spur formation), **urethritis**, and **conjunctivitis** or **uveitis** (or occasionally punctate keratitis). It typically affects young, adult males, a high proportion of whom are HLA-B27 positive. The aetiology remains unknown; many of the adult males have an onset of urethritis two weeks post-intercourse, other males and some females may have a post-dysentery form and some have arthritis as the presenting feature. Chlamydia has been implicated in the venereal form.

Management: The anterior uveitis is treated with Ⓢ topical steroids and mydriatics in the usual way. In suspected Chlamydia cases a 10-day course of tetra-cycline, 250 mg q.d.s. orally, is prescribed.

Toxoplasmosis

This is due to an infection with the protozoa *Toxoplasma gondii* and causes a retinochoroiditis (*Fig. 6.13*). It may be acquired *in utero* by the transplacental route or as an adult. Ocular toxoplasmosis is almost always acquired *in utero*.

T. gondii lives in the intestines of cats and the eggs are shed in cat faeces. Flies transfer the eggs onto food which is ingested by man. It may also infect cows and other herbivores, passing to man through ingestion of inadequately cooked meat. Adult toxoplasmosis is usually a subclinical infection, or occasionally a glandular fever-type illness. It is dangerous when acquired during pregnancy as it may lead to death of the foetus or congenital toxoplasmosis.

The features of the latter are systemic illness including fever and jaundice at birth, congenital abnormalities, convulsions and mental retardation. Intracranial calcification is seen on the skull radiograph. Ocular manifestations include congenital cataracts, microphthalmos and chorioretinitis. The healed scars of chorioretinitis may be the only evidence of past infection seen in milder cases and it is these old lesions that become reactivated in adult life, giving rise to retinochoroiditis and posterior uveitis.

Signs: Typically there is a posterior uveitis, which is often more active over the site of the lesion, with a mild anterior uveitis. Active retinochoroiditis is seen as a fresh white, fluffy area on the edge of an old chorioretinal scar. Occasionally, the posterior uveitis may be florid and accompanied by tractional retinal detachment. Rarely, the optic nerve may become inflamed.

Investigations: ELISA (Enzyme Linked Immunosorbent Assay) serology or fluorescent antibody test confirms past infection, but gives no indication as to whether the disease is current.

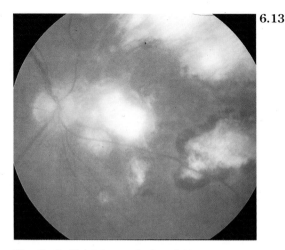

Fig. 6.13 Toxoplasma chorioretinitis

Differential diagnosis: Toxocariasis (v.i.).

Management: Treatment is used if the condition is sight-threatening, e.g. if there is a macular lesion, optic nerve involvement or a florid vitritis. Various regimes are used such as Prednisolone 30–50 mg daily initially, tailing off as clinical response is seen, or Clindamycin 300 mg q.d.s. for four weeks, which is being used more commonly now. It may lead to diarrhoea, in which case the treatment should be stopped. In a small proportion of cases the diarrhoea is due to pseudomembranous colitis, which is serious and requires urgent hospitalisation. Sigmoidoscopy and stool examination for *Clostridium difficile* infection is carried out. Pseudomembranous colitis is treated with oral vancomycin.

Sulphonamides and pyrimethamine (which needs to be used with folinic acid to prevent thrombocytopenia and leucopenia) are further treatment options.

Toxocariasis

Toxocariasis (*Fig. 6.14(a)–(d)*) is a roundworm infestation of dogs and cats that can accidentally infect humans, usually children. *Toxocara canis* and *Toxocara catis* are the two species which respectively infest dogs and cats. The *catis* variety is probably not important in man.

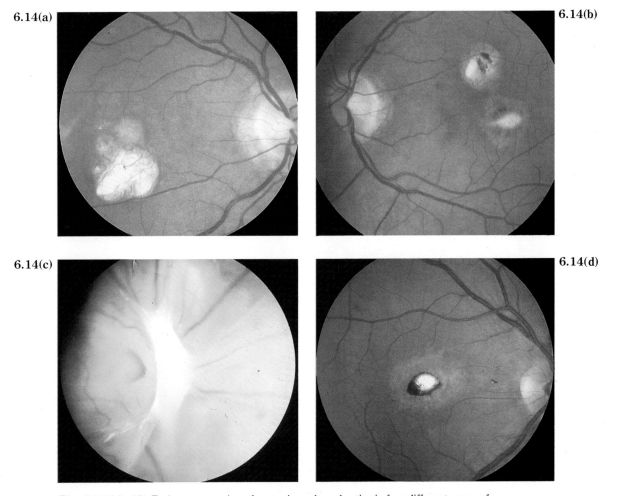

6.14(a)

6.14(b)

6.14(c)

6.14(d)

Fig. 6.14(a)–(d) End-stage scarring of posterior pole and retina in four different cases of toxocariasis

T. canis infects pregnant bitches and is passed transplacentally to the puppies. Infection is acquired by ingestion of embryonated eggs from soil or the dog's fur. It is mainly a disease of children. Infection can lead to visceral larval migrans syndrome as the larvae migrate from the intestine through the tissues, giving rise to fever, eosinophilia, hepatomegaly, asthma and seizures, but no ocular manifestations. Ocular involvement occurs with subclinical infection and may manifest as the following:

• Localized posterior pole granulomata (age 6–14 years)

• Peripheral granulomata, which may cause dragging of the disc similar to that seen in retrolental fibroplasia (age 6–40 years)

• Chronic destructive endophthalmitis, which may give rise to exudative lesions and tractional retinal detachment (age 2–9 years). This is one of the differential diagnoses in leukocoria (see pp. 231–36), but, unlike 75% of cases of retinoblastoma, it does not calcify.

Investigations: ELISA test for antibodies to *Toxocara*, which is positive at 1 in 8, but may be significant at even lower dilutions.

Management: Preventative measures include periodic ⓢ worming of dogs with piperazine and health education to reduce contact of children with dog faeces. Visceral larval migrans is treated with thiobendazole. Ocular inflammatory lesions are treated with systemic steroids. Pars plana vitrectomy may be necessary when vision is threatened by impending tractional retinal detachment.

Tuberculosis

This may cause an acute iritis, a recurring iritis, a chronic iritis associated with cataract formation and glaucoma, or tubercle formation. Choroidal tubercles, which appear in miliary tuberculosis, are white–yellow nodules with ill-defined borders, and are associated with systemic symptoms. They need to be differentiated from 'histo spots' in presumed ocular histoplasmosis.

Fuchs' heterochromic cyclitis

This easily missed diagnosis (*Fig. 6.15(a)*) accounts for about 2% of anterior uveitis. Onset is typically in young adulthood.

Symptoms: Blurred vision, which is due to either the development of a posterior subcapsular cataract or vitreous opacities.

Signs: Early signs include heterochromia iridis (*Fig. 6.15(b)*) (in unilateral cases) as the iris stroma becomes atrophic. A brown iris will look paler and a blue iris will look bluer when compared with the other side. The iris has a moth-eaten appearance easily demonstrated on transillumination. Posterior synechiae do not develop. The keratic precipitates are medium-sized and star-shaped. They are distributed over the entire posterior surface of the cornea rather than being confined to the inferior part. The anterior chamber activity is mild. Later complications include secondary glaucoma and posterior subcapsular cataract formation. Anterior vitreous activity may be present.

● Heterochromia iridis may also be inherited, idiopathic or due to other causes, e.g. siderosis, congenital Horner's syndrome or melanoma.

Management: Topical steroids may be used in the short term if they are beneficial in controlling the inflammation, but not otherwise. Mydriatics are not necessary. Cataract extraction with an intraocular lens implant may be performed.

6.15(a)

6.15(b)

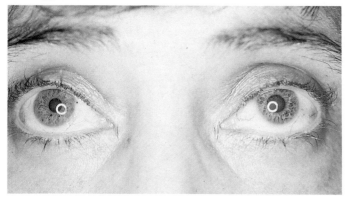

Fig. 6.15(a) Heterochromia iridis

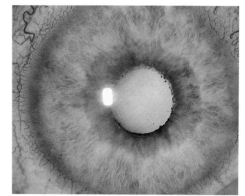

Fig. 6.15(b) Fuchs' heterochromic cyclitis

Posner-Schlossman syndrome — acute glaucomatocyclitic crisis

This is a rare syndrome of unknown aetiology affecting young adults. It causes intermittent attacks of acute pressure rise, associated with mild anterior uveitis, affecting one eye only. The attacks usually last a few hours, occasionally longer.

Symptoms: Blurring of vision associated with corneal oedema due to the acute rise in intraocular pressure.

Signs: Corneal oedema, a few keratic precipitates and mild anterior uveitis with minimal conjunctival injection. The pupil is usually dilated and there is no posterior synechiae formation. The intraocular pressure is 40 to 60 mmHg. Mild heterochromia may develop in the long-term.

Investigations: Gonioscopy should be performed to exclude attacks of acute, intermittent, angle-closure glaucoma.

Management: Reduction of pressure is achieved by Ⓢ Ⓡ using Timolol drops 0.5% b.d. and Adrenaline drops 1% b.d. and Acetazolamide 250 mg q.d.s. Topical steroids are not necessary.

Behçet's disease

This is an immune occlusive vasculitis which affects young adults, especially from the eastern Mediterranean region and Japan (*Figs. 6.16 & 6.17*). It is characterised by recurrent painful aphthous ulcers, genital ulcers, uveitis, synovitis, cutaneous vasculitis (giving rise to pustular eruptions), and meningoencephalitis.

Ocular manifestations occur mainly in males and may start in the late teens. They consist of a recurrent anterior uveitis, sometimes with hypopyon formation, posterior uveitis with retinal exudation, vasculitis, leading to venous occlusion, disc swelling, cystoid macular oedema and diffuse retinal oedema. There is usually marked vitreous activity. The usual pattern is of recurrent episodes, becoming less frequent as time goes on, but often with progressive loss of vision.

Investigations: The diagnosis is made on clinical criteria since there are no definitive tests to date. There is an increased prevalence of HLA-B5 in Behçet's disease. A tuberculin-type response occurs upon accidental needle-stick injury, but this is not advocated as a diagnostic test.

Management: The initial treatment is with topical Ⓢ steroids. In severe cases systemic steroids are necessary, but frequently do not prevent the relentless progression of the ocular inflammation, which often leads to blindness within three years of onset. Immunosuppressive drugs, e.g. chlorambucil and cyclosporin A, are used in extreme cases, in consultation with a haematologist and nephrologist to monitor treatment.

6.16

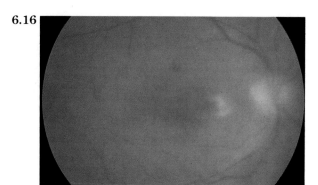

Fig. 6.16 Behçet's disease – posterior uveitis and retinal inflammation

6.17

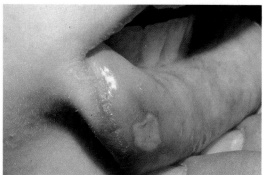

Fig. 6.17 Mouth ulcers in Behçet's disease

Sympathetic ophthalmitis

This is a bilateral panuveitis which follows a penetrating injury or intraocular surgery (usually with associated uveal tissue prolapse) to one eye. It is now rare, following improvement in operative techniques and less delay in the repair of penetrating wounds. The most common time of onset is 4–8 weeks after injury, although the earliest time is nine days after injury and the latest is 50 years. The aetiology may be an auto-immune reaction to pigment epithelium to which the body has become sensitised through the injury.

Symptoms and signs: The eye which received the initial trauma, the 'exciting' eye, develops a panuveitis. The other eye, the 'sympathising' eye, develops photophobia and blurring as inflammation in the ciliary body occurs. Either an anterior uveitis ensues with large keratic precipitates, iris nodules and extensive posterior synechiae, or, sometimes, a posterior uveitis develops with disseminated, yellow–white, retinal spots (Dalen-Fuchs nodules), subretinal oedema and papillitis. Eventually, it evolves into a florid panuveitis. In the initial stages the eye often shows no external signs of inflammation.

Management: If performed within nine days of injury, Ⓢ the condition is prevented by enucleation of the injured eye. In the presence of sympathetic ophthalmitis, the exciting eye should be enucleated if there is no potential for visual recovery as it may aggravate the sympathetic ophthalmitis in the other eye. Topical steroids and high dose steroids orally are used to treat the condition. If there is no response, immuno-suppressive drugs may be required.
N.B. After a penetrating injury or intraocular surgery, especially if complicated by iris prolapse, the other eye should always be examined for signs of sympathetic ophthalmitis. A fundal examination is mandatory.

Endophthalmitis

This is a catastrophic condition which consists of widespread inflammation of intraocular tissues, usually as a result of infection, but sometimes due to foreign body reaction (e.g. starch within the eye). Often the infection arises by direct entry into the eye, e.g. during surgery or penetrating injury, and usually manifests in the first two days postoperatively.

Sometimes the infection occurs weeks, months or years later via a persistent portal of entry into the eye, e.g. drainage bleb or vitreous wick syndrome (where vitreous appears at the wound and prevents the two edges healing), or after removal of intraocular sutures. Occasionally, the infection arises from haematogenous spread from septic foci, e.g. indwelling catheters or intravenous lines, or in intravenous drug abusers. The most common infecting organisms are *Staph. epidermidis, Staph. aureus,* gram-negative bacilli and pneumococci.

Symptoms: Acute bacterial endophthalmitis manifests as a sudden onset of increased pain and decreased vision. Fungal endophthalmitis has a slower onset of decreasing vision and less pain. Sterile endophthalmitis, e.g. due to starch on surgeons' gloves, presents 2–8 days postoperatively with similar symptoms of pain and decreasing visual acuity, but is less florid than bacterial endophthalmitis.

Signs: In bacterial endophthalmitis there is loss of visual acuity, lid swelling, lid spasm, chemosis, purulent discharge, hypopyon and poor fundal view. In fungal endophthalmitis, there is a transient hypopyon, followed by vitreous 'fluff-ball' lesions and satellite lesions. Sterile endophthalmitis has an appearance intermediate between the two other forms.

Ⓡ Ⓢ *Management of bacterial endophthalmitis:* Suspected cases require immediate admission to a specialist eye centre.

Investigations: N.B. Microbial identification is of vital importance.

• Swabs of conjunctiva and any other infected site, e.g. discharging stye, skin lesion, indwelling catheter, are taken for culture. Blood cultures are taken if indicated, e.g. systemic disturbance, drug addiction and so on.

• Anterior chamber paracentesis (*Fig. 6.18*) is carried out, using a 25-gauge needle through a small, peripheral, corneal stab to withdraw 0.1–0.2ml of aqueous.

• Vitreous sampling (*Fig. 6.19*) is performed using a 23-gauge needle through a pars plana incision to withdraw 0.3ml of vitreous. Through the same incision, 200µg of gentamicin in 0.1ml and 2.0mg of cephazolin in 0.1ml are administered. Smears for Gram stain and cultures are carried out using bacteriological and fungal culture media. Vitreous sampling has a bacteriological yield of up to 50% positive cultures compared with 30% for anterior chamber sampling.

6.18

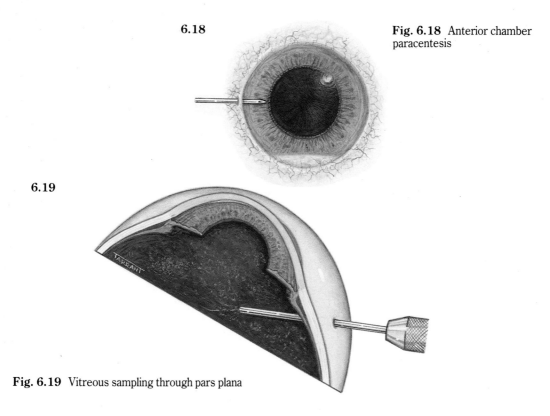

Fig. 6.18 Anterior chamber paracentesis

6.19

Fig. 6.19 Vitreous sampling through pars plana

Treatment: In many centres the results of the microbiological investigations will be ready within half an hour, when appropriate treatment is begun. If microbiological results are not available immediately or are negative, blind therapy is carried out, but the treatment is re-evaluated once culture results are available.

The initial treatment regime prior to Gram stain or negative culture results is:

• topical gentamicin forte drops every 15 to 30 minutes

• atropine 1% drops t.d.s.
• subconjunctival methicillin 150mg, gentamicin 20mg
• intravenous gentamicin 1 mg/kg every 8 hours and cephazolin 1g every 6 hours (or cephaloridine 1g every 6 hours)
• oral steroids (after the first 24 hours), but not if fungal infection is suspected.

Once the culture results are available the antibiotics are modified accordingly:

- **Streptococcus** – Intravitreal cephazolin, subconjunctival methicillin with 0.1 mg dexamethasone, topical penicillin drops half-hourly and systemic benzyl penicillin.
- **Strep. pneumoniae** – as for *streptococcus*, but no subconjunctival steroids.
- **Staphylococcus** – Intravitreal cephazolin, subconjunctival methicillin with dexamethasone 0.1 mg, topical chloramphenicol and gentamicin, systemic cephazolin 1 g every 6 hours (vancomycin, tetracycline and erythromycin are alternatives).
- **E. Coli** – Intravitreal gentamicin, subconjunctival gentamicin, topical fortified gentamicin drops and chloramphenicol drops alternating half-hourly, topical cycloplegics, subconjunctival steroid injection, systemic antibiotics depending on sensitivity of the organism.

Ⓡ Ⓢ *Management of fungal endophthalmitis (Fig. 6.20(a) & (b))*: Cases are treated with systemic antifungal therapy and steroids (after 48 hours of antifungal treatment alone). In known posterior chamber infection, vitrectomy, followed by intravitreal antifungal agents, e.g. amphotericin B, is used.

6.20(a)

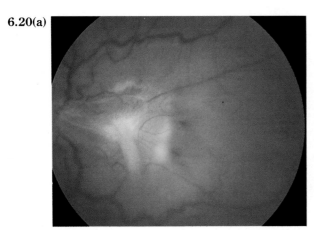

6.20(b)

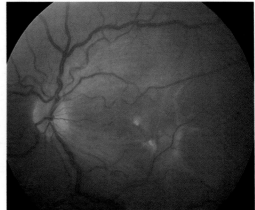

Fig. 6.20(a) Candida endophthalmitis before treatment

Fig. 6.20(b) Candida endophthalmitis after treatment

Ⓡ Ⓢ *Management of sterile endophthalmitis:* This is treated with subconjunctival and topical steroids. It has a slightly better prognosis.

Glaucoma

Glaucoma is categorised according to whether it is acute or chronic, open or closed angle and primary or secondary. The angle referred to is the drainage angle of the eye where the trabecular meshwork is situated. The angle structures can be viewed by gonioscopy (*Fig. 6.21(a) & (b)*).

A contact lens, with an angled mirror and slit-lamp examination, is used to view the angle structures. This overcomes the problem of total internal reflection at the cornea, which normally prohibits viewing of the angle. Several layers are seen in the gonioscope mirror, corresponding to the angle structures.

Working from anterior to posterior, **Schwalbe's line** is seen first. This is the junction between Descemet's membrane, the innermost layer of the cornea and the trabeculum. It appears as an opaque line. Next is the **trabecular meshwork** which is mostly pigmented. Sometimes a deeper pigmented line is seen, which represents the **canal of Schlemm**. The next, whiter area is the **scleral spur**, the most anterior part of the sclera and the site of attachment of the longitudinal ciliary muscle. A darker, grey band, representing the **ciliary body**, is the next structure to be seen. Finally, there is an angle recess and occasionally the **iris processes** may be seen (usually only in childhood). In open angles most of these structures may be seen, but in narrow angles only Schwalbe's line, with or without part of the trabecular meshwork, is seen. With a closed angle none of the angle structures are seen. Peripheral anterior synechiae, which are adhesions of the peripheral iris across the angle, may sometimes be seen.

For the purposes of this book, it is convenient to divide glaucoma into acute and chronic glaucoma.

6.21(a)

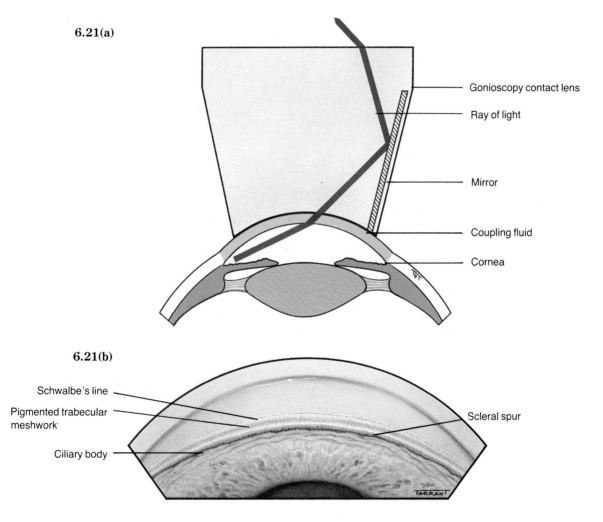

Gonioscopy contact lens

Ray of light

Mirror

Coupling fluid

Cornea

6.21(b)

Schwalbe's line

Pigmented trabecular meshwork

Ciliary body

Scleral spur

Fig. 6.21(a) & (b) Gonioscopy appearances – **(a)** Passage of a ray of light from drainage angle of eye to viewer, **(b)** View of angle structures

Acute glaucoma

There are three main types of acute glaucoma:

Primary angle-closure glaucoma

This is a cause of a painful, red eye (*Fig. 6.22*). It occurs mainly in the elderly, more commonly in females and hypermetropic individuals. It has a familial tendency. The pressure increase is due to episodes of pupil block, when the pupil margin is in close apposition to the lens in a semi-dilated position. This prevents the aqueous from draining from the posterior to the anterior chamber and the relative pressure builds up behind the iris, causing it to bow forwards when the peripheral part of the iris occludes the angle. This leads to failure of drainage of aqueous and acute pressure rise. Factors leading to its occurrence include a shallow anterior chamber with narrow angle, which is more likely with age, due to enlargement of the lens, and a semi-dilated pupil as occurs in the evening or with dilating drops.

Symptoms: Pain, often in association with headache, abdominal pain, nausea and vomiting, blurred vision and perception of coloured haloes around lights (due to corneal oedema). There may have been previous 'warning' attacks when the eye became red and painful and haloes were seen. These usually occur in the evening, and spontaneously resolve with miosis due to sleep or brighter illumination.

Signs: Reduced visual acuity, ciliary injection, diffuse haziness of the cornea due to corneal epithelial oedema, and a fixed, oval, semi-dilated pupil. Slit lamp examination reveals a shallow anterior chamber (less than 2.5mm), which is also seen on the unaffected side, with raised intraocular pressure, as measured by applanation tonometry, of around 50–65 mmHg. Intensive treatment with glycerine drops is used to draw oedema out of the cornea, allowing a clearer anterior chamber view. Spiralling of the iris fibres (*Fig. 6.23*) with mild anterior chamber activity is seen. Gonioscopy shows a closed angle on the affected side and usually a narrow or very narrow angle on the other side. The optic discs are often swollen.

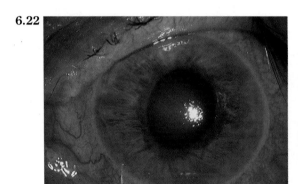

Fig. 6.22 Acute angle-closure glaucoma

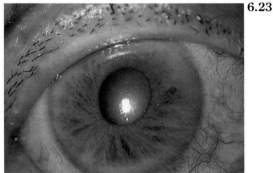

Fig. 6.23 Iris spiralling following acute angle-closure glaucoma

Differential diagnosis:

• Glaucoma secondary to anterior uveitis, when there is marked anterior chamber activity, an open angle and the intraocular pressure is generally not as high, e.g. 35–45 mmHg.

• Acute anterior uveitis, when the cornea may appear hazy to the naked eye, but this is due to keratic precipitates, the pupil is small and posterior synechiae are present, together with marked anterior chamber activity.

• Neovascular glaucoma, when there is a history of diabetes, or central retinal vein occlusion. Rubeosis, with blood vessels in the angle, is seen on examination.

• Phakolytic glaucoma, when there is a mature cataractous lens and proteins cause a uveitic glaucoma. Treatment is to lower pressure and then perform cataract extraction.

• Phakomorphic glaucoma, when a swollen, cataractous lens causes pupil block and angle-closure glaucoma. Treatment is prompt cataract extraction.

Ⓡ *Management:* Emergency treatment is required as the optic nerve may become compromised by the high intraocular pressure within a few hours.

• The patient is referred as an emergency and admitted.

• Immediate treatment (preferably in the casualty department) with a slow, intravenous injection of acetazolamide 500 mg to reduce the pressure. The patient should be lying down as he may feel faint following this.

• Timolol 0.5% drops b.d. are begun to decrease aqueous production.

• Pilocarpine 4% drops are begun and given every 15 minutes. This acts to miose the pupil and draw the iris out of the angle. Initially, when the pressures are high, the iris is ischaemic and the pilocarpine may not be effective. Prophylactic pilocarpine 1% q.d.s. is given to the other eye.

• If intraocular pressure remains high, osmotic agents are used, e.g. glycerol 1.0–1.5 g/kg p.o. or mannitol 1.0–2.0 g/kg i.v.

• Betamethasone drops q.d.s. are begun to decrease secondary uveitis.

• Analgesics and anti-emetics are given as necessary.

• Once the pressure has been reduced, repeat Ⓢ gonioscopy is performed to assess the angle damage and anterior synechiae formation. If there is extensive angle damage or if the pressure fails to be controlled on pilocarpine, a drainage procedure, e.g. trabeculectomy, is required. If the pressure is down to normal, a laser iridotomy or surgical peripheral iridectomy (*Fig. 6.24*) is performed on the affected eye. A prophylactic laser iridotomy (or peripheral iridectomy) is performed on the other eye a few days later.

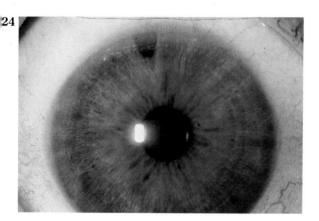

24

Fig. 6.24 Peripheral iridectomy

Neovascular glaucoma

This develops when new vessels grow in the drainage angle and a fibrotic "zipping-up" of the angle occurs (*Figs. 6.25, 6.26*). This happens in diabetes, or after central retinal vein occlusion, and is associated with neovascularisation elsewhere, e.g. disc and iris.

Symptoms: Painful, blind eye.

Signs: Ciliary injection, corneal oedema, rubeosis iridis, mild anterior uveitis and raised intraocular pressure.

(S) *Management:* The best management is prevention by treating early neovascularisation with panretinal photocoagulation to induce natural regression of the new vessels.

Medical management of neovascular glaucoma consists of dexamethasone 0.1% drops q.d.s. and atropine drops 1% t.d.s. If this fails to control symptoms, techniques such as cyclocryotherapy, to stop ciliary body production of aqueous fluid, or insertion of a Molteno tube, which drains aqueous to the subconjunctival space, are tried. The interested reader is referred to textbooks of surgery for further information on these techniques.

6.25

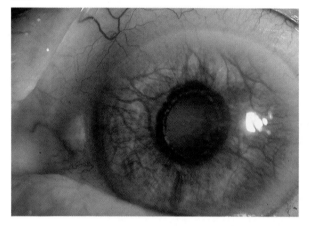

Fig. 6.25 Neovascular glaucoma showing iris new vessels

6.26

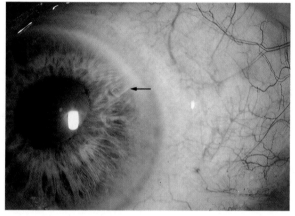

Fig. 6.26 Neovascular glaucoma showing Molteno tube (arrow)

Uveitic glaucoma

This is a raised intraocular pressure associated with uveitis.

Symptoms & Signs: As for acute anterior uveitis (see pp. 104–8) with the addition of pain, reduced visual acuity, corneal oedema and raised intraocular pressure. There may also be seclusio pupillae with consequent iris bombé.

(R) *Management:*

● Admission may be necessary if the pressure is over 40 mmHg or the uveitis is severe.

● Intravenous acetazolamide 500 mg if the pressure is over 40 mmHg followed by acetazolamide 250 mg q.d.s.

● Intensive dilatation and steroid drops as described in the section on uveitis.

● Timolol 0.5% b.d.

● *Herpes zoster ophthalmicus* and *Herpes simplex* are two of the most common causes. In the latter, steroid drops should be used with caution.

Chronic glaucoma

Primary open-angle glaucoma

Primary open-angle glaucoma (or chronic simple glaucoma) is the most common form of glaucoma in the community, affecting over 1 in 200 of the population over 40 years of age. It consists of progressive loss of field due to optic nerve damage through raised intraocular pressure. It is insidious in onset and entirely asymptomatic until pronounced field loss is evident in the end stages. It is usually bilateral and there is a strong familial tendency. In order to make the diagnosis four factors are important:

1. Raised intraocular pressure (>21 mmHg): This is most accurately assessed using applanation tonometry (see p. 26). In a few cases there may be all the other factors present, but in the presence of a normal intraocular pressure. This is referred to as 'low tension glaucoma'. If raised pressure is present in the absence of field loss or optic nerve cupping this is referred to as 'ocular hypertension'

2. Open angle on gonioscopy (by definition) (see *Fig. 6.21*)

3. Cupping of the optic disc (*Fig. 6.27(a)–(d)*): This is due to a loss in the number of nerve fibres passing through the disc. Because of a variation in size of the discs, the size of the cup is recorded as a cup:disc ratio in the **vertical** direction (as glaucomatous cups are often oval in shape with the greatest extension superiorly and inferiorly). The edge of the cup is taken as the position where the small blood vessels curve over the central indent in the surface of the disc, not to be confused with the limit of disc pallor. Suspicious factors include a cup:disc ratio >0.6 *per se*, or a cup:disc ratio >0.3 in the presence of other factors, e.g. glaucomatous field loss, any asymmetrical extension of the cup or difference in cupping between the two eyes. The discs are best assessed using a Hruby lens, 90 D lens or fundus contact lens.

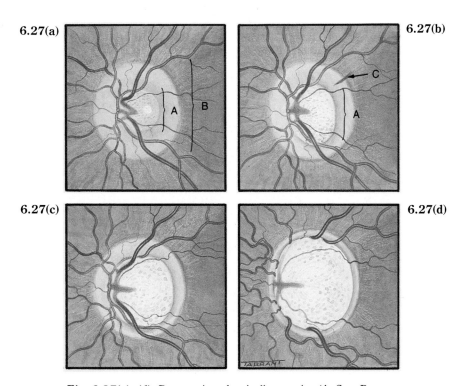

Fig. 6.27(a)–(d) Progression of optic disc cupping (A–Cup, B–Disc, C–Flame-shaped haemorrhage). **(a)** Normal optic disc and cup, **(b)** Early superior and inferior extension of cup, **(c)** Further extension of optic disc cupping, **(d)** Advanced optic disc cupping

4. Glaucomatous field loss: Early field loss includes arcuate (*Fig. 11.31*) or paracentral scotomata (sometimes reversible on commencing treatment). Later peripheral field loss leads to a nasal step or temporal wedge. Altitudinal defects and loss of the entire peripheral field then occur, with the central island remaining. The central island may finally be lost altogether.

(S) *Management:* Referral is urgent if there is extensive field loss or cupping of the disc, or an intraocular pressure over 30mmHg.

The mainstay of treatment is using drops to reduce intraocular pressure. The principal ones used are:

• Beta-blockers, e.g. Timolol drops, which reduce aqueous secretion. They are usually tried in the lower strength 0.25% b.d. initially and increased to 0.5% b.d. if not effective. They are contra-indicated in patients with obstructive airways disease, heart block or bradycardia.

• Cholinergic agonists, e.g. pilocarpine, which increases aqueous outflow. Pilocarpine is usually tried in the lower strength of 1% q.d.s., increasing to 2% or 4% q.d.s. if lower strengths are not effective. It mioses the pupil, which has the advantage of acting as a pinhole for refractive errors, but the disadvantage of reducing light entry in low lighting conditions and visual fields. This is especially difficult if there are developing axial lens opacities. It also reduces accommodation in young patients and may cause a frontal headache initially (which usually improves). The pupil should be dilated at least annually for fundal examination in a person on long-term miotics.

• Alpha adrenergic agonists, which increase aqueous outflow. Adrenaline, although a mixed agonist, is used in this respect. It can be used in the 0.5% strength b.d., increasing to 1% or 2% as necessary. It leads to conjunctival hyperaemia, nasolacrimal blockage and, in the long-term, to harmless brown–black, sub-conjunctival, 'adrenochrome' deposits which may be mistaken for foreign bodies. Side-effects include precipitation of angle-closure glaucoma, cystoid macular oedema in the aphakic and tachyarrhythmias. Systemic absorption should be reduced by punctal occlusion upon instilling the drops.

• Carbonic anhydrase inhibitors, e.g. acetazolamide 250mg o.d. to q.d.s. p.o., are used to reduce aqueous secretion. They may be used as a short-term measure in addition to all the drops to control pressure, e.g. before trabeculectomy is arranged.

Surgical treatment consists of trabeculectomy, which creates an artificial drainage channel from the posterior chamber to the subconjunctival space via a filtering bleb, or laser trabeculoplasty, which opens up the trabecular meshwork to facilitate drainage. These procedures tend to be used when medical management has failed to control the intraocular pressure and further field loss has occurred or when medical management is not tolerated. There is increasing debate among ophthalmologists concerning the earlier place of trabeculectomy in glaucoma management. The risks of trabeculectomy include a further loss of visual field and early or late endophthalmitis due to entry of organisms via the filtering bleb.

Chronic primary angle-closure glaucoma

This occurs when the angle becomes progressively closed, usually superiorly to inferiorly. The field loss and optic disc cupping is similar to that seen in chronic open-angle glaucoma. The treatment is surgical: peripheral iridectomy or filtration surgery, depending on the amount of permanent anterior synechiae formation.

Pseudoexfoliation syndrome

This condition (*Fig. 6.28*) is commonly seen in Scandinavian countries, but there is marked geographical variation in prevalence. Flakes of basement membrane-like substance from the lens become deposited on the anterior lens capsule, the pupillary margin and, most importantly, in the trabecular meshwork. This gives rise to chronic open-angle glaucoma in about 60% of affected eyes, and often in the unaffected eye as well. Gonioscopy demonstrates dandruff-like deposits overlying the trabecular meshwork, which is hyperpigmented. Treatment is as for primary open-angle glaucoma.

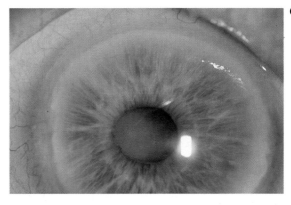

Fig. 6.28 Pseudoexfoliation (seen just inside pupillary margin)

Pigment dispersion syndrome

Pigment lost from the iris is deposited in a vertical, spindle-shaped pattern on the corneal endothelium ('Krukenberg's spindles'), and within the trabeculum, giving rise to a raised intraocular pressure and a hyperpigmented band on gonioscopy (*Fig. 6.29(a) & (b)*). The iris looks atrophic which is well demonstrated on transillumination. Treatment is as for primary open-angle glaucoma.

6.29(a) 6.29(b)

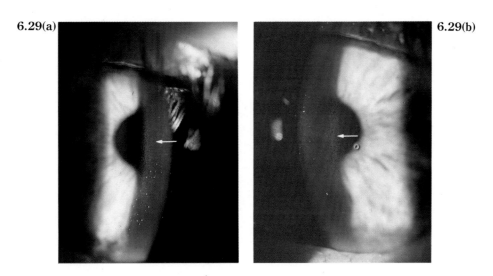

Fig. 6.29(a) & (b) Slit lamp views of pigment dispersion syndrome – Krukenberg's spindles (arrows)

Glaucoma secondary to trauma

The initial injury is usually blunt trauma which leads to a hyphaema. Gonioscopy is usually carried out after the hyphaema has settled and may show some angle recession. If there is greater than 180° of angle recession, there is a high risk of developing glaucoma in later life and this should be screened for, using annual pressure checks.

Glaucoma secondary to developmental anomalies

The example shown here (*Fig. 6.30*) is a patient with Rieger's syndrome, which includes iris and angle anomalies together with facial and dental abnormalities.

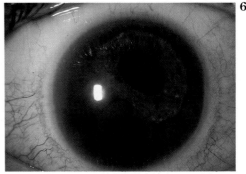

Fig. 6.30 Reiger's syndrome

Iris tumours

Iris naevi

These are brown, flat or slightly elevated swellings on the anterior iris surface (*Fig. 6.31*). Found most commonly on paler irides, they have little or no malignant potential. In neurofibromatosis there may be multiple iris naevi called Lisch nodules, but these are often less pigmented than the common iris naevi.

6.31

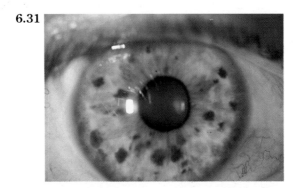

Fig. 6.31 Iris naevi

Juvenile xanthogranuloma

This is a yellow, raised, fairly vascular swelling that arises over the iris (*see Fig. 13.19*). It most commonly occurs in the first year of life, but occasionally occurs in adults. It may be associated with yellowish skin lesions. In the eye it produces spontaneous hyphaemas and secondary glaucoma.

Iris melanoma

This appears as an elevated swelling over the iris (*Fig. 6.32(a) & (b)*). It usually occurs in the fourth or fifth decade. It may be pigmented or non-pigmented (amelanotic melanoma). It often distorts the iris architecture giving rise to ectropion uveae, pupillary distortion, neovascularisation and unilateral glaucoma. It may also be associated with a localised lens opacity adjacent to the lesion. Iris melanomas account for 5–10% of uveal tract melanomas and have fewer malignant features on pathological examination and a much better prognosis than do ciliary body melanomas. It may be observed initially, but if there is any sign of spread to the angle, it is treated (s) by local excision or enucleation. Differential diagnosis includes iris cyst (*Fig. 6.33*), leiomyoma, naevi and metastases.

6.32(a)

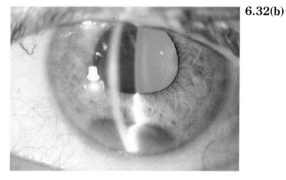

6.32(b)

Fig. 6.32(a) Iris melanoma

Fig. 6.32(b) Iris melanoma

6.33

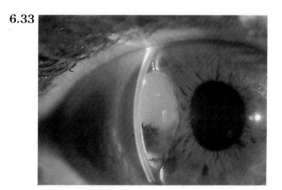

Fig. 6.33 Iris cyst (Courtesy of Institute of Ophthalmology)

Ciliary body melanoma

This tumour is more common than an iris melanoma and has a worse prognosis because of later detection and more aggressive histology (*Figs. 6.34, 6.35(a) & (b)*). It presents as a late onset astigmatism due to pressure exerted on the lens, or as a pigmented lesion seen on the bulbar conjunctiva, or, in advanced cases, as a mass in the anterior chamber. The findings are a pigmented lesion appearing through the sclera near the limbus with dilated episcleral blood vessels coursing towards it. After pupillary dilatation a localised lens opacity near the tumour is sometimes seen, with a pigmented mass arising from behind the iris and occasionally a retinal detachment due to posterior extension. Gonioscopy reveals a pigmented lesion invading the angle. Further investigations (S) include ultrasonography, transillumination, ^{32}P uptake and nuclear magnetic resonance imaging. Treatment is iridocyclectomy for small, localised tumours and enucleation for large tumours.

6.34

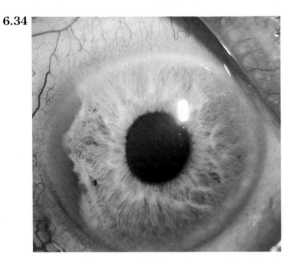

Fig. 6.34 Ciliary body melanoma
Fig. 6.35(a) & (b) Ciliary body melanoma
(Courtesy of Institute of Ophthalmology)

6.35(a)

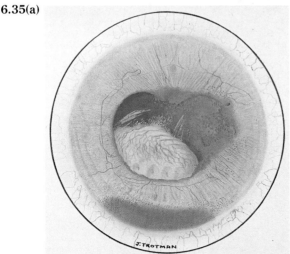

6.35(b)

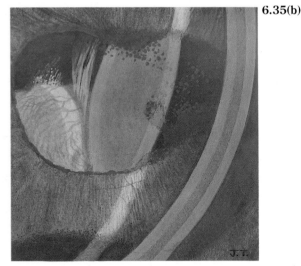

Choroidal melanoma

This is the most common intraocular tumour in adults (*Fig. 6.36*). It usually occurs after the fifth decade and is rare in blacks. It may arise *de novo* or from an existing naevus. Small lesions may be difficult to distinguish from benign naevi. Naevi appear as flat, grey lesions with an ill-defined edge, usually less than three optic disc diameters in size, but occasionally larger and often with drüsen on their surface. They are frequently present at birth and may enlarge throughout childhood. However, they tend to stop growing after puberty.

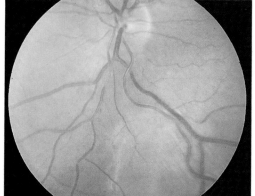

Fig. 6.36 Choroidal malignant melanoma

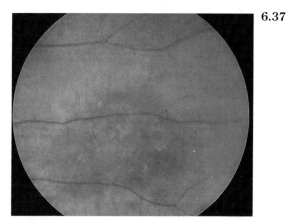

Fig. 6.37 Benign choroidal naevus

Features suggestive of a small melanoma include photopsia, an elevated lesion, an increase in size (best documented by fundal photography), visual field loss (although this can occur in benign lesions), serous detachment over the lesion (although this can also occur occasionally in posterior pole naevi), and the presence of orange lipofuscin pigment on the surface. Larger melanomas may present as a solid retinal detachment, often as a 'collar stud' lesion which is waisted where it breaks through Bruch's membrane and then balloons out into the vitreous cavity. It is usually pigmented, but sometimes is amelanotic. It may be complicated by vitreous haemorrhage, retinal haemorrhage, chronic uveitis and glaucoma. The differential diagnosis of a solid, grey, elevated lesion includes choroidal haematoma, choroidal effusion, choroidal metastasis and choroidal haemangioma.

To distinguish a benign naevus from a small malignant melanoma: If any doubt exists, the patient should be referred for ophthalmic opinion. The clinical criteria listed above are used. Indirect ophthalmoscopy is extremely useful for detecting if elevation is present as it gives a three-dimensional view. Normal visual fields imply a benign lesion (*Fig. 6.37*). Fluorescein angiography is often helpful. A baseline fundal photograph is taken and the patient is followed up to observe any change in size.

To investigate a large solid retinal detachment: Most malignant melanomas can be diagnosed on indirect ophthalmoscopy appearances (*Fig. 6.38*). In the presence of lens opacities, ultrasound may be helpful. Transillumination, where a light probe is placed on the sclera whilst viewing through the indirect ophthalmoscope (without its light source), helps to differentiate a choroidal haemangioma and effusion, which transilluminate, and a melanoma, which does not. General examination is carried out to exclude any secondary metastasis (commonly to the liver or lung) or any other primary (most commonly bronchus or breast) if a choroidal metastasis is suspected. Examination of the other eye is essential to exclude mimicking conditions since melanomas are unilateral. Further investigations include chest radiograph, full blood count and viscosity, liver function tests, liver ultrasound and orbital computerised tomography to detect orbital extension. In the future, nuclear magnetic resonance imaging may prove useful.

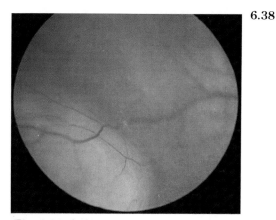

Fig. 6.38 Solid retinal detachment – malignant melanoma (Courtesy of Mr. R. Humphry)

(S) *Management of choroidal melanoma:* This is controversial and depends on size, location, rate of growth, extension into the orbit and presence of metastases. Enucleation is currently used for eyes that have lost vision due to a large melanoma that has not metastasised (as the prognosis for life expectancy is less than one year if this has occurred). Observation is more appropriate in elderly or chronically ill individuals with slow-growing tumours. Some believe that enucleation may actually lead to dissemination of tumour cells at the time of removal and certainly care should be taken to ensure the least traumatic removal. After enucleation some surgeons use a silastic implant to provide a good base for a prosthesis, but others disagree as it makes the detection of orbit recurrences very difficult. A temporary shell is fitted initially and then after a few weeks a permanent prosthesis is made for the patient. In the case of large tumours in frail, elderly individuals, or in metastatic disease, palliative radiotherapy or chemotherapy is given.

Small choroidal melanomas (less than 10mm diameter and 3mm depth) in eyes with normal visual acuity are usually observed in the first instance as they are often very slow-growing with little tendency to metastasise. Other possibilities include laser photocoagulation, cryotherapy, localised radioactive plaques, e.g. ^{106}Ru plaques, and the newest technique of charged particle beam irradiation.

Prognosis depends on size, extension, histological type, presence of pigment (amelanotic melanoma has a better prognosis), extension through Bruch's membrane and age of patient (older patients have a poorer prognosis).

Choroidal metastases

These occur most commonly from bronchus or breast primaries. They are often multiple and bilateral and present with blurring of vision (*Fig. 6.39*).

Signs: Single or multiple, ill-defined, pale, slightly elevated lesions in one or both fundi. Fluorescein characteristics are not dissimilar to choroidal melanoma.

(S) *Management:* Although life expectancy is often short owing to disseminated disease, it is of great value to the patient to treat these lesions to restore vision. Choroidal metastases tend to respond dramatically to radiotherapy.

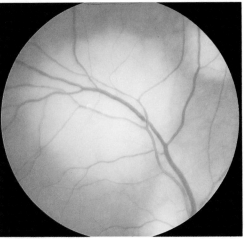

6.39

Fig. 6.39 Choroidal metastases from carcinoma of the breast (Courtesy of Mr. C. Dean Hart)

7 Lens

The lens is made up of layers like an onion. The central part, the nucleus, is formed first as an embryo and surrounding layers are added throughout life. The outer layers are called the cortex, and the 'skin' surrounding the entire lens is called the capsule, which is divided into anterior and posterior parts.

Cataract

A cataract is a lens opacity that causes loss of vision (*Figs. 7.1(a)–(c), 7.2(a)–(c), 7.3, 7.4 & 7.5(a) & (b)*). It is usually classified on the basis of aetiology and anatomical site within the lens, although the mode of treatment is not affected by these factors.

7.1(a)

7.1(b)

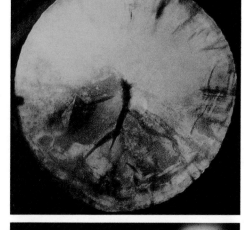

7.1(c)

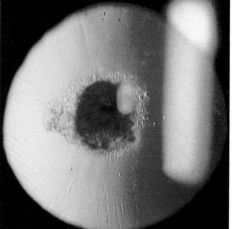

Fig. 7.1(a) Optical section of nuclear sclerosis demonstrating a brunescent nuclear change (Courtesy of Mr. N. Brown)
Fig. 7.1(b) Cortical spoke cataracts demonstrated against the red reflex (Courtesy of Mr. N. Brown)
Fig. 7.1(c) Posterior subscapular cataract against the red reflex (Courtesy of Mr. N. Brown)

Senile cataract

This is the most common type of cataract and appears to be a natural ageing process. No aetiological factors are known, but there is a hereditary component. There are three types of senile cataract that often coexist:

● **Nuclear sclerosis** (*Fig. 7.1(a)*), which is a yellow ageing of the central part of the lens, causing an altered colour perception (objects appear duller and more yellow in colour), and myopia owing to an increased refractivity of the lens. This often leads to a renewed ability to read without reading spectacles, a so-called 'second sight'.

● **Cortical cataract** (*Fig. 7.1(b)*), which is often seen as radiating 'spoke-like' opacities, progressing to complete white opacification.

● **Subcapsular cataract** (*Fig. 7.1(c)*), which may consist of anterior or posterior opacities situated directly under the capsule. These are more subtle in appearance, but may cause loss in visual acuity, if axial, especially on reading. Alternatively, they may be quite disabling owing to glare from sunlight or car headlights at night.

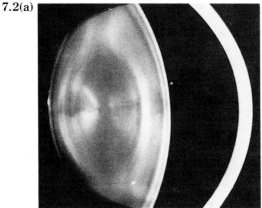

7.2(a)

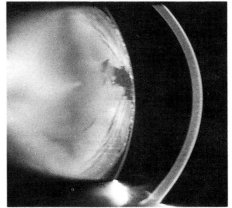

7.2(b)

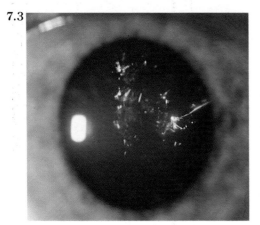

7.2(c)

Fig. 7.2(a)–(c) Slit-lamp views of
(a) normal lens, **(b)** nuclear sclerosis and
(c) cortical cataract (Courtesy of
Mr. N. Brown)
Fig. 7.3 'Christmas Tree' cataract
(Courtesy of Mr. N. Brown)
Fig. 7.4 Cortical lens opacities against a red
reflex (Courtesy of Mr. N. Brown)

7.3

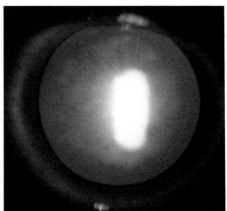

7.4

Symptoms: Gradual onset of blurring of vision and difficulty in reading fine print, threading a needle, recognising faces from a distance, or night driving. Often there is glare (v.s.) and yellowing of colours. There may be monocular diplopia, that is double vision from one eye only, which adds to the visual difficulty.

Occasionally patients may describe a sudden loss of vision in one eye, owing to the fact that they have suddenly covered over the other eye and only then become aware that there is poor vision in that eye, even though it may have been there for some time.

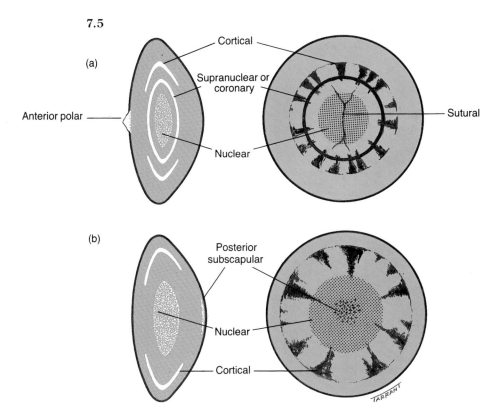

7.5

(a)

Cortical

Supranuclear or coronary

Anterior polar

Nuclear

Sutural

(b)

Posterior subscapular

Nuclear

Cortical

TARRANT

Fig. 7.5 Cross-sectional and anterior-posterior views of (**a**) a congenital type cataract and (**b**) an adult type cataract

Signs: Reduced visual acuity: distance and near visual acuity should both be tested as some patients' difficulty in reading with a posterior subcapsular cataract is only demonstrated with a near vision test. The cataract may be easily outlined in black against a red reflex when viewing through the direct ophthalmoscope set on a +10 lens about 10 cm away. A nuclear cataract appears as a black smaller 'lens within a lens', whereas cortical lens opacities may be seen as radiating, black spokes. Often the cataract is less well defined. Slit-lamp examination allows a detailed characterisation of the cataract. Very dense cataracts appear as leukocoria (white pupillary reflex).

Ⓢ *Management:* Surgical removal of the cataractous lens is the only treatment. No medical treatment is known to be of benefit. Ocular assessment includes visual acuity, lid inspection, anterior segment inflammation, intraocular pressure, severity of lens opacities and retinal pathology. Pupil responses are completely normal in cataracts and any abnormality may imply optic nerve or retinal pathology. Cataract surgery may be carried out under local anaesthetic using retrobulbar or peribulbar anaesthetic injection. The lens is either extracted extracapsularly, that is leaving the posterior capsule behind to separate the vitreous from the anterior compartment of the eye, or intracapsularly, when the entire lens plus capsule is taken. The first technique has a lower long-term complication rate, for example retinal detachment or macular oedema. It allows the insertion of a posterior chamber lens implant, which is the most successful type of lens, but is a relatively new approach. Intracapsular surgery requires less sophisticated equipment and is still the most widely used technique world-wide. Anterior chamber intraocular lenses may be inserted, but often the aphakic refractive error is corrected using a contact lens or aphakic spectacles. With aphakic spectacles, and to a lesser extent with contact lenses, there is a difference in image size between the two eyes until the other eye is also operated on.

Criteria for cataract surgery:

• Interference in lifestyle owing to the presence of cataracts. In a younger patient this may be inability to drive if the visual acuity falls below the legal limit of 6/12. In the older patient, inability to read or to thread a needle may take away the pleasures of life. In some elderly patients no difficulty is noticed until the visual acuity is 6/36 or less, at which point simple household duties become hampered. In many instances a new refraction will improve visual acuity significantly before deciding whether or not to operate.

• Attitude of the patient. This may seem obvious, but the patient must actively want something done.

• Absence of retinal pathology and especially amblyopia. Sometimes with macular lesions, cataract extraction may be indicated purely to provide field of vision, even though acuity may not be greatly improved.

• Ability to cope with postoperative care. Many elderly patients find it hard to manage a contact lens and an intraocular lens implant is more successful in these circumstances. If this is not possible and aphakic spectacles are needed, the surgery should be delayed until the other eye also has poor sight so that image disparity is not a problem.

• Complications of cataracts remaining in the eye. These include phacomorphic glaucoma, in which an intumescent cataractous lens causes a narrow angle and induces angle-closure glaucoma, and phacolytic glaucoma, in which a mature cataract leaks lens protein into the anterior chamber. This induces production of large numbers of macrophages which block the trabecular meshwork. Prompt cataract extraction is required in both cases.

• After a successful first eye operation, the second eye is operated on if the patient is young and/or good binocular vision is required, or if the patient is greatly troubled by using only one eye. Financial constraints may intervene here.

Other causes of cataract:

• **Metabolic**, e.g. diabetes mellitus, when white, spot-like opacities appear in the lens, or there may be premature development of senile cataract. Hypoglycaemia may induce cataract formation owing to osmotic swelling of the lens. Advanced rubeosis is often associated with cataract formation (*Fig. 7.6*). Hypocalcaemia, galactosaemia (see section on congenital cataracts pp. 232–33), Lowe's syndrome and other inherited metabolic diseases may give rise to congenital cataracts.

• **Ocular conditions** including chronic anterior uveitis, high myopia and hereditary and retinal pigmentary disorders, for example retinitis pigmentosa.

• **Trauma** to the eye including penetrating or blunt ocular injury, irradiation, for example therapeutic irradiation for ocular tumours, and electric shock.

• **Drug-induced**, for example topical corticosteroids in high concentrations or over a prolonged period of time, miotics, e.g. pilocarpine, or systemic corticosteroids may lead to cataract formation. Chlorpromazine therapy leads to deposition of brown crystals in the anterior lens cortex, but rarely causes visual loss (*see Fig. 16.4*).

• **Congenital** (*Figs. 7.7(a) & (b), 7.8*) (see Chapter 13) e.g. due to rubella, toxoplasmosis, cytomegalovirus.

• **Other associated conditions** e.g. myotonic dystrophy, Down's syndrome, atopic eczema.

7.6

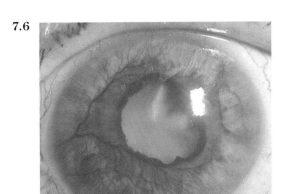

Fig. 7.6 Dense lens opacity in rubeosis
iridis

7.7(a)

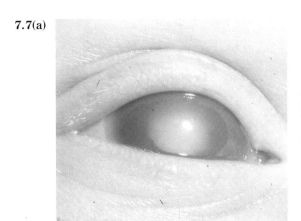

Fig. 7.7(a) Cataract in congenital rubella
(Courtesy of Institute of Child Health)

7.7(b)

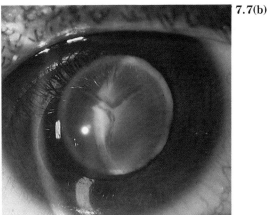

Fig. 7.7(b) Congenital cataract

7.8

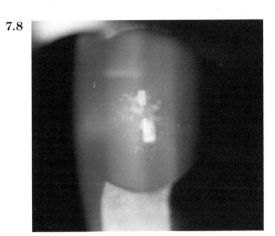

Fig. 7.8 Congenital cataract – blue dot
opacities

Dislocated lenses

Congenital disorders

• *Marfan's syndrome*

This is a dominantly-inherited disorder of connective tissue, characterised by arachnodactyly, long limbs, joint laxity, chest deformities, high arched palate, cardiovascular abnormalities, including aortic valve abnormalities, and aortic aneurysm, which is often the cause of death. The ocular abnormalities include lens dislocation (upwards), myopia, glaucoma due to angle anomalies, iris hypoplasia and retinal detachment.

• *Homocystinuria*

This is a recessively-inherited disorder caused by a deficiency of cystathione synthetase. The body habitus is similar to that of Marfan's, but there is often mental deficiency, osteoporosis, fractures and vascular thrombosis. The lens often subluxates (*Fig. 7.9*), but, in contrast to Marfan's, it is usually downwards. There is associated glaucoma.

(Dislocated lenses are also seen in Weill-Marchesani syndrome and hyperlysinaemia.)

7.9

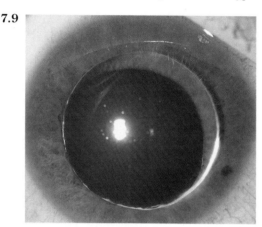

Fig. 7.9 Complete anterior dislocation of the lens in homocystinuria

Acquired causes

- Trauma
- Hypermature cataract
- Large eye, e.g. buphthalmos
- Ciliary body melanomas

(S) *Management:* If the lens is acutely dislocated anteriorly into the anterior chamber, corneal endothelial damage may occur due to friction by the lens and there may be secondary, acute glaucoma. The patient should lie down flat on his back and then the pupil be intensively dilated using g cyclopentolate 1% and g phenylephrine 10%. In some cases the lens will relocate. The pupil should then be constricted using carbachol 3% drops or pilocarpine 2% and once it is safe the patient may be allowed home. The patient is started on g beta-methasone drops q.d.s. to reduce inflammation and regular miotic drops are continued. If indicated the lens is extracted.

Chronically dislocated lenses (usually posterior dislocations) are removed if there is intractable uveitis, monocular diplopia or secondary glaucoma. This involves vitreous surgery techniques.

8 Fundus

Normal anatomy of the retina

8.1

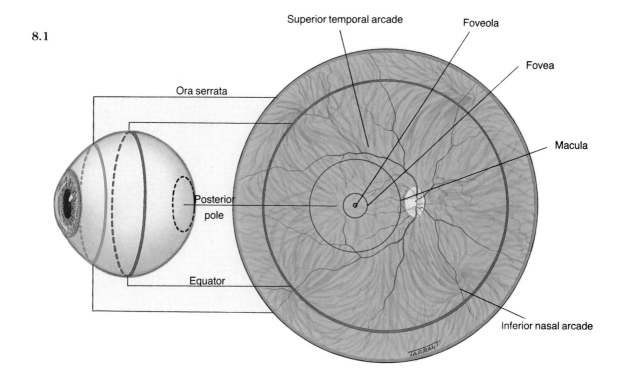

Fig. 8.1 Normal anatomy of the retina and corresponding picture on globe

The retina is the innermost layer of the eye (*Fig. 8.1*). The anterior limit of the retina is at the ora serrata where it merges with the ciliary epithelium. The 'equator' is an imaginary line dividing the anterior half of the eye from the posterior half. Continuing the analogy with the globe, the posterior pole is the area at the back of the eye and it encompasses the macula region between the retinal blood vessel arcades.

The retina consists of two layers both derived from the neuroectoderm which becomes invaginated to form the optic cup. The outer layer forms the retinal pigment epithelium, a single sheet of hexagonal-shaped cells which support the photoreceptors, while the inner layer forms the neurosensory retina. The neurosensory retina is made up of layers of cells and their connections and is concerned with the conversion of light into electrical signals to the brain.

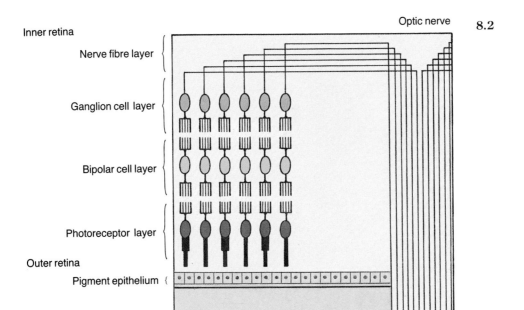

Fig. 8.2 Neuronal pathways in retina

There is essentially a two-neuron pathway (*Fig. 8.2*) in the retina from the receptors to the optic nerve. Outermost are the photoreceptors, the rods and the cones, which are not, in fact, neurons. These synapse with the middle layer, the bipolar cells, which in turn synapse with the inner ganglion cells. Nerve fibres from the ganglion cells form the innermost layer of the retina, bar an internal limiting lamina. As well as this vertical, two-neuron connection, numerous horizontal connections exist, namely the horizontal and amacrine cells, which modify the outgoing signal to increase its definition. The inner retina is supplied by the retinal arteries and the outer retina by the choriocapillaris, a capillary network in the choroid.

The macula region is the area concerned with precise, central vision. It is here that most of the cones for colour vision are concentrated. The macula is a circular area approximately 4.5mm (three optic disc diameters) in diameter, the centre of which is the fovea (1.5mm in diameter), which lies 3mm temporal to the disc and 0.5mm inferior to it. At the fovea the retina is adapted to maximise visual acuity. There are no blood vessels running in front of the retina and the innermost retinal layers are swept outwards from the centremost pit, the foveola, to allow direct access of light to the photoreceptors.

The clear, vitreous jelly fills the posterior cavity of the eye and has a supportive and metabolic role. It is made up of a collagen framework filled with a gel-like substance, which is composed of hyaluronic acid. It is normally attached to the retina around the optic disc, at the ora serrata and at the macula zone, to the blood vessels of the arcade, and the fovea.

Optic disc

The optic disc is about 1.5 mm in diameter and is the exit point of approximately 1.2 million retinal nerve fibres in each optic nerve. These fibres pass along the optic nerves to the chiasm where the fibres subserving the nasal half of the retina cross over, whilst those subserving the temporal half of the retina continue posteriorly on the same side. Thus, field defects due to lesions anterior to the chiasm are uniocular and may cross the vertical midline, but posterior to the chiasm they are binocular and do not. The one exception to this is a lesion at the junction of the optic nerve and chiasm, where the inferonasal fibres from one eye sweep forwards at the chiasm into the other optic nerve. Thus, a prechiasmal lesion will produce an ipsilateral, central scotoma and a contralateral, upper temporal quadrantanopia (or more usually just a step). The fibres synapse in the lateral, geniculate bodies and thereafter form the optic radiations to the cortex. The macula is bilaterally represented in the cortex. The papillomacular bundle, which subserves the macula and thus the central field of vision, is the most important group of fibres. It consists of small, delicate nerves which occupy the centre of the optic nerve and are most vulnerable to compressive lesions of that optic nerve, e.g. optic glioma. The typical field losses seen in optic nerve disease are:

• Central scotoma, e.g. optic neuritis (see Chapter 11), compressive lesions, ischaemic lesions.

• Arcuate scotoma. This is a comma-shaped defect, typically arising from or pointing towards the blind spot with a sharp border on the horizontal meridian. This is seen in chronic glaucoma, ischaemic optic neuropathy and optic atrophy secondary to glaucoma.

• Altitudinal field defects, that is loss of upper or lower half of field, e.g. anterior ischaemic optic neuropathy or coloboma of optic nerve.

• Centrocaecal scotoma. This is caused by damage to the macula fibres in the central core of the optic nerve (central scotoma) and to the fibres around the optic disc (enlarged blind spot). The classical example is toxic optic neuropathy, but it may also occur in demyelinating disease, infiltrations and compressive lesions.

• Junctional scotoma as seen in prechiasmal lesions.

Normal optic disc appearance

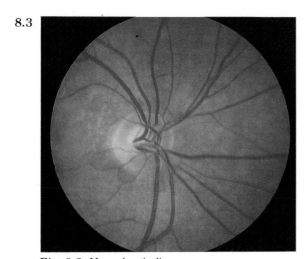

8.3

8.4

Fig. 8.3 Normal optic disc

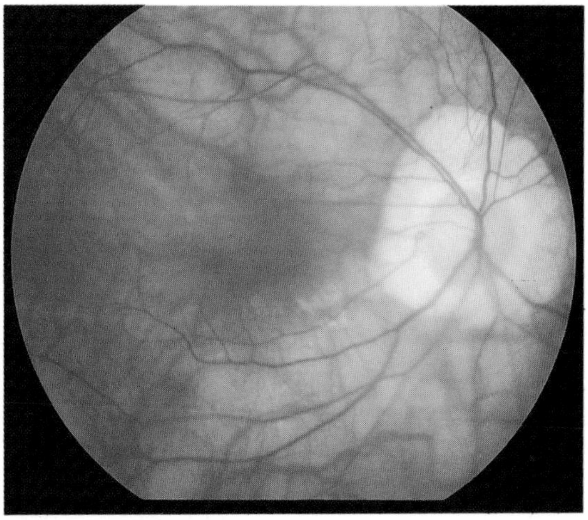

Fig. 8.4 Myopic disc

There is quite a variation in normal disc appearances (*Fig. 8.3*). **Hypermetropic discs** tend to look small and crowded with an ill-defined disc margin, in some cases pronounced enough to confuse with papilloedema. In contrast, the **myopic disc** (*Fig. 8.4*) is larger and often has a crescent of chorioretinal degeneration around it. It may enlarge to form an area of peripapillary atrophy and there may be associated areas of chorioretinal degeneration elsewhere in the retina.

The central cup is a depression in the base of the disc. Blood vessels course over the rim, an effect which may be barely noticeable or very pronounced (physiological cupping; see p. 123, for cup:disc ratio). Deep physiological cupping is differentiated from pathological cupping by the symmetry of the two discs, the circular rather than oval shape of the cup, the good pink rim of healthy neural tissue around the cup together with the absence of field defects and raised intraocular pressure.

Hypoplastic discs are small discs which appear crowded and often have a disparity between the scleral and retinal openings. They may be unilateral or bilateral and are associated with poor vision. They may be associated with midline abnormalities, e.g. absent septum pellucidum (septo-optic dysplasia of de Morsier), pituitary abnormalities (especially growth hormone deficiency), hypoglycaemia in the neonatal period and testicular hypoplasia.

Optic nerve pits (*Fig. 8.6*) are greyish excavations, usually found on the temporal side of the optic disc. From the second decade onwards they may be complicated by the development of serous retinal detachments of the macula region due to leakage of fluid from the pit. Occasionally laser photocoagulation, aimed at the pit or disc edge, is helpful.

Tilted discs (*Fig. 8.5*) are caused by oblique entry of the optic nerve into the globe and failure of correct symmetrical development of the disc. They are usually small bilateral, optic discs which are tilted obliquely such that the upper temporal margin lies anterior to the lower part. The inferonasal retina is often hypopigmented and there are upper bitemporal field defects which may be confused with bitemporal hemianopia except that they cross the midline. There is often associated astigmatism.

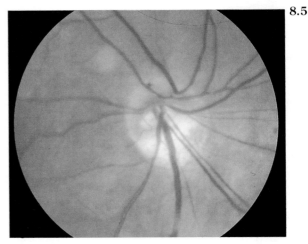

8.5

Fig. 8.5 Tilted disc

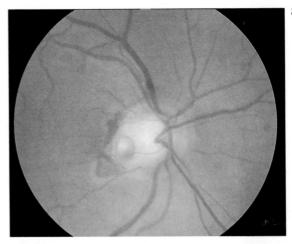

8.6

Fig. 8.6 Optic nerve pit with sub-retinal fluid over macula region

Optic disc colobomata are one of a group of colobomata caused by a failure of the foetal cleft to close. They vary in appearance from an area of hypoplasia of the disc inferiorly to a large excavation of the disc, which may be associated with a coloboma of the retina, choroid, lens or iris. The defects are almost always inferior, often bilateral and sometimes dominantly inherited. They are associated with superior visual field defects which cross the midline. The 'morning glory' disc is a variant whereby a large central mass of glial tissue overlies the optic disc and the blood vessels radiate outwards from this. The vision is poor and there may be associated abnormalities, e.g. basal encephalocoeles, accessory facial nodules, hypertelorism and palatal abnormalities.

Optic disc drüsen (*Fig. 8.7*) are pearly excrescences on or in the optic disc and are caused by degenerated glial material. The disc appears full with anomalous branching, e.g. trifurcation of retinal vessels over it. They are dominantly inherited with incomplete penetration. In childhood the drüsen are not visible and the appearances may be confused with papilloedema. The visual acuity is usually normal, but there may be an enlarged blind spot, an arcuate or paracentral scotoma, or a narrowing of the lower nasal field. Complications may occur from the third decade onwards and include peripapillary haemorrhage which may extend to the macula.

Myelinated nerve fibres (*Figs. 8.8 & 8.9*) are seen when the nerve fibres acquire myelin sheaths in the retina. Usually they are only myelinated posterior to the lamina cribrosa. The optic disc is surrounded by a burst of radiating, white fibres. Sometimes white, feathery patches of myelination are seen elsewhere in the retina. There is usually no loss of visual acuity, but there may be an enlarged blind spot. It is seen more commonly in neurofibromatosis.

Bergmeister's papilla is a glial remnant of primary vitreous tissue. Persistent hyaloid artery is another embryonic remnant.

For papilloedema, papillitis, anterior ischaemic optic neuropathy and optic atrophy see Chapter 11.

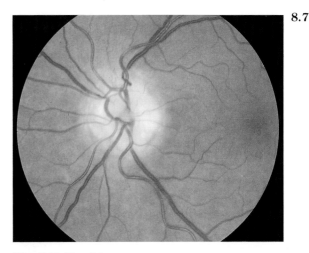

8.7

Fig. 8.7 Disc drüsen

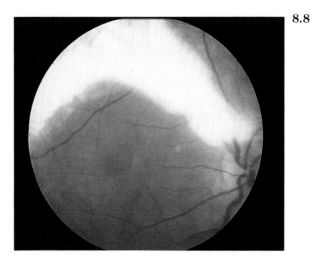

8.8

Figs. 8.8 & 8.9 Myelinated nerve fibres

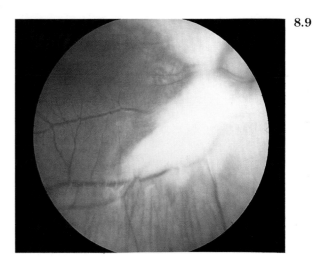

8.9

Retina

Common retinal signs

- **Dot haemorrhages** are small, intraretinal haemorrhages occurring from microvascular abnormalities, e.g. microaneurysms, commonly seen in background diabetic retinopathy (*Fig. 8.10*).

- **Blot haemorrhages** are larger and represent haemorrhagic infarcts in the nerve fibre layer (also visible in *Fig. 8.10*).

- **Flame-shaped haemorrhages** (*Fig. 8.11*) occur in the nerve fibre layer and are from larger retinal vessels.

8.10

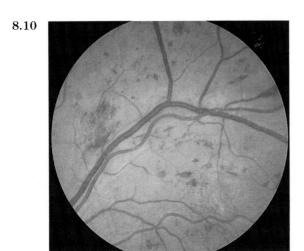

Fig. 8.10 Diabetic retinopathy demonstrating dot and blot haemorrhages

8.11

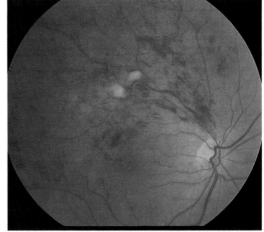

Fig. 8.11 Superior temporal branch vein occlusion demonstrating flame-shaped haemorrhages and cotton wool spots

- **Cotton wool spots** (*Fig. 8.12*) (a more appropriate term than soft exudates) are pale, fluffy areas caused by a build-up of axoplasmic contents after an infarct in the retinal nerve fibre layer. They indicate retinal ischaemia as seen in diabetes, hypertension, vein occlusions and vasculitis.

- **Hard exudates** (*Fig. 8.13*) are well-circumscribed, bright yellow deposits of lipid and lipoprotein which have leaked from retinal or subretinal vasculature. They sometimes form a circular pattern around a leakage point and are then referred to as a circinate exudate. They may also be arranged radially around the macula – a macular star.

- **Deep intraretinal haemorrhages** (*Fig. 8.14*) appear as pink, more diffuse areas of haemorrhage and may surround a subretinal haemorrhage.

- **Subretinal haemorrhages** (visible on *Fig. 8.14* also) are very dark red or even brown if they are deep to the pigment epithelium. They are often due to bleeding from subretinal neovascular membranes as in disciform macular degeneration.

- **Preretinal or retrohyaloid (subhyaloid) haemorrhages** (*Fig. 8.15*), e.g. those occurring from new disc vessels, occupy the space between the retina and the posterior vitreous face where it has detached. They have a crescentic border inferiorly, which is the limit of the posterior vitreous detachment, and a fluid level superiorly where the blood has settled. These haemorrhages may extend into the vitreous where they appear as a diffuse, red area obscuring fundus detail – an **intragel haemorrhage**.

- **Blood vessel sheathing and emboli** are seen in *Fig. 8.16*.

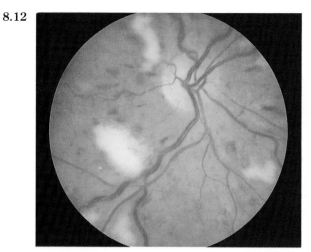

Fig. 8.12 Detail of cotton wool spots

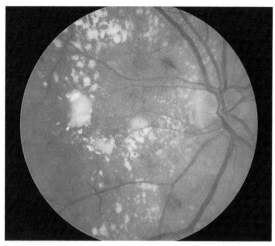

Fig. 8.13 Hard exudates forming circinate ring

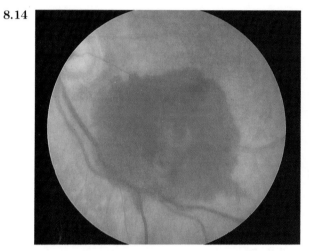

Fig. 8.14 Subretinal haemorrhage surrounded by deep intraretinal haemorrhage

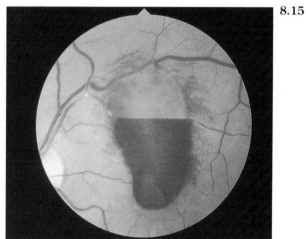

Fig. 8.15 Retrohyaloid haemorrhage

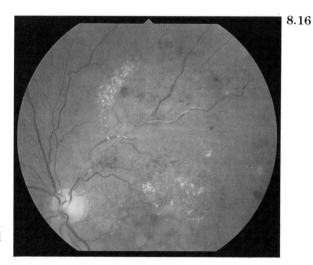

Fig. 8.16 Branch vein occlusion demonstrating blood vessel sheathing, emboli, drüsen

Macula

The macula (*Fig. 8.17*) is the most important area of the retina and is used for central vision. Over 90% of the visual field is contributed by the macula. It is an area at the posterior pole, just over three optic discs in size and situated just under three optic disc diameters (ODDs) temporal to and 1/2 ODD below the optic disc. The fovea is an area approximately the size of the optic disc in the centre. A small depression in the centre is the foveola. Healthy foveolas show a light reflex from their central pit as a torch is shone in. This is called the foveola reflex (sometimes the 'macular reflex') and is lost if the macula is diseased. To facilitate accurate image perception in the centre of the fovea, the neurosensory retinal parts are displaced laterally and there is an avascular zone.

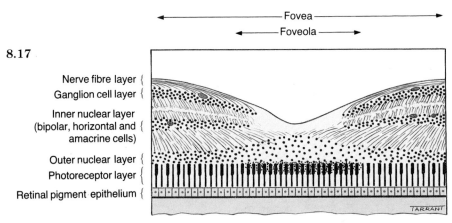

8.17

Fovea
Foveola

Nerve fibre layer {
Ganglion cell layer {
Inner nuclear layer (bipolar, horizontal and { amacrine cells)
Outer nuclear layer {
Photoreceptor layer {
Retinal pigment epithelium {

TARRANT

Fig. 8.17 Macula showing details of the layers of the retina

Symptoms of macular disease: A variety of pathological processes may affect the macula, but a common collection of symptoms results:

● **Decreased visual acuity**, often first noticed as difficulty in reading fine print or threading a needle.

● **Positive scotoma**, in which a small part of the vision is blocked out. (This is in contrast to optic nerve 'relative' scotomas where a part of the vision is 'missing' or ill-defined.)

● **Distortion of vision – metamorphopsia**. This usually takes the form of straight lines, e.g. window frames, appearing bent, or printed words having distorted letters, parts missing or straight horizontal lines appearing wavy. **Micropsia** and **macropsia**, which are alterations in image size due to distortion of the cone receptor configuration, may occur.

Signs of macular disease:

● Decreased visual acuity as seen on the Snellen chart. Sometimes, the near vision tests are a more sensitive indicator of macular disease.

● An Amsler grid, which is a 10 cm × 10 cm square divided up into 5 mm squares with a central fixation spot, whereby each square subtends 1° at 0.33 m, is an extremely useful way of mapping out macular disease. The patient is asked to fixate on the central spot with one eye only, covering the other, and to map out any irregularities, distortion or parts missing. It becomes immediately evident whether the lesion is located at the fovea, or to one side of it. Note that the fundal lesion, with relation to the fovea, will be diametrically opposite its position relative to the central fixation spot on the Amsler grid.

• The photostress test demonstrates a decreased ability of the macula to regenerate visual pigments after a bright light stimulus. The lowest line on the Snellen chart which is accurately read is recorded for one eye. The patient then fixates on a pen-torch shone at that eye from a few centimetres away for 10 seconds. The time taken to reread three letters from the same Snellen chart line as before the test is the photostress recovery time. Normally this is under 50 seconds, but it is prolonged in macular disease.

• An initial view with the direct ophthalmoscope will often provide the diagnosis of macular disease (*Fig. 8.18*). However, greater definition and a three-dimensional picture are seen with a Hruby lens, a 90 D lens or a fundus contact lens.

• If there is low visual acuity with opacities in the media, e.g. cataract such that the macula cannot be viewed, the Purkinje entopic test is performed. Here the patient gently rubs the illuminated end of a pen-torch over the closed eye. The patient will then be able to describe a vascular pattern, seen if the macula is healthy.

• Unlike optic nerve disease, the pupil reactions are normal (except in severe maculopathy), colour desaturation is less common (in formal colour testing there is a red–green colour deficit in optic nerve disease and a blue–yellow colour deficit in macular disease) and usually there is no dimming of vision in macular disease.

8.18

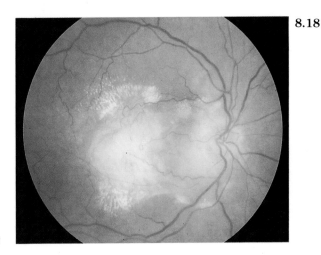

Fig. 8.18 Macula degeneration – disciform scar

Age-related macular degeneration

Age-related (senile) macular degeneration (ARMD) is the most common cause of registered blindness in the Caucasian population. It is far less common in other races. It occurs bilaterally, with the average age of onset of blindness in one eye being 65 years. The other eye is often affected by the age of 70. It leads to loss of central vision, but does not affect the periphery, so these patients retain navigational vision.

The macular degeneration occurs in two forms: wet and dry. This refers to the presence or absence of subretinal fluid at the macula. Dry macular degeneration is a pure degeneration of the retina and is untreatable, but often only slowly progressive. Wet ARMD occurs in several forms, but the most important to recognise is **disciform macular degeneration**. This is caused initially by dry macular degeneration, followed by the formation of a subretinal neovascular membrane (SRNVM) which may lead to haemorrhage and sudden visual loss at the macula. If the SRNVM is outside the fovea, it is potentially treatable with laser therapy. The results are only favourable in a small percentage of cases (about 20%) at present, but this is the only chance for these patients. If left untreated, it will lead to total loss of central vision in most cases.

Dry, age-related macular degeneration

Symptoms: Slow, progressive loss of central vision, noticed especially because of difficulty reading or sewing.

Signs: Decreased visual acuity, especially for near vision. Discrete, yellow–white deposits of lipofuscinoid material called drüsen, or colloid bodies associated with focal pigment deposits and atrophy, are seen at the macula. Soft drüsen are seen at the macula in *Fig. 8.19*, whereas hard drüsen are seen in the rest of the fundus on *Fig. 8.20*.

Management: There is no active treatment. If the ⓢ visual acuity is markedly reduced, magnifying lenses and good illumination are extremely useful. The patient is told that there is degeneration at the back of the eye which may progress, but that they will never go blind as they will maintain good peripheral vision. This is extremely important for the patient to know. At an appropriate level of decreased visual acuity they may be registered partially sighted or blind and thus be entitled to certain welfare benefits.

8.19

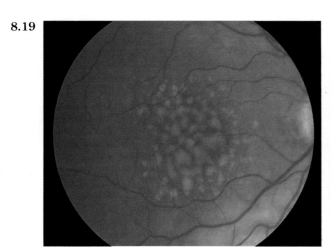

Fig. 8.19 Soft drüsen at the macula

8.20

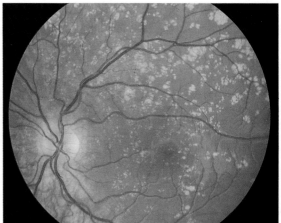

Fig. 8.20 Hard drüsen

Disciform macular degeneration

Symptoms: The patient may have noticed some steady deterioration in central vision, as in dry ARMD. The patient then notices blurring and distortion of vision, e.g. window frames look bent. This is due to subretinal fluid (*Figs. 8.21(a) & (b)*). Following this there may be a sudden deterioration of vision or development of a positive scotoma (due to a macular haemorrhage from the SRNVM) (*Fig. 8.22*).

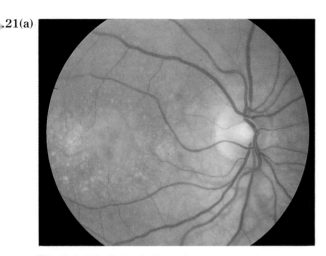

Fig. 8.21(a) Right disciform degeneration

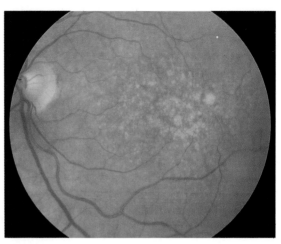

Fig. 8.21(b) Left macula drüsen (Same patient as Fig. 8.21(a)

Signs: The visual acuity is decreased. In early disciforms it may be 6/12, but in late disciforms it may be a case of counting fingers or hand movements. The Amsler grid demonstrates distortion or scotomas (ensure that reading spectacles are worn otherwise blurring due to refractive error may be interpreted as being 'distortion'). Normal pupil responses. The signs at the macula include drüsen, subretinal fluid and haemorrhages, sometimes at the edge of a greyish lesion – the SRNVM. A late disciform is seen as a pale, fibrous scar at the macula.

N.B. Because of the difficulty of accurately identifying early macular disciforms without sophisticated slit-lamp examination, it is crucial that all patients with a new history of distorted vision are seen **the same day** by an ophthalmologist for early assessment and possible treatment.

Management: After specialist assessment, if the disciform is deemed to be early and potentially treatable, the patient has a fluorescein angiogram without delay. If there is an SRNVM and it is outside the foveal avascular zone, it is treated with argon laser therapy.

Other conditions in which disciform degeneration occurs include high myopia (*Fig. 8.23*), angioid streaks (see p. 161), traumatic choroidal ruptures (see p. 217), presumed ocular histoplasmosis (see p. 162), optic nerve head drüsen (see p. 141), choroidal naevus (see pp. 128–29), melanoma or haemangioma and Best's disease.

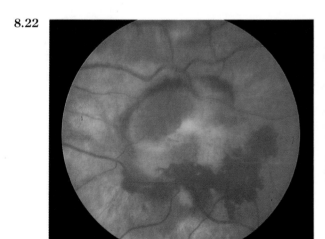

Fig. 8.22 Extensive disciform degeneration – left macula

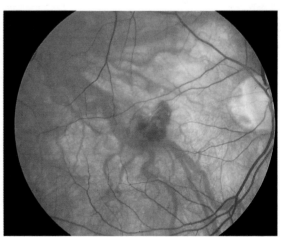

Fig. 8.23 Disciform degeneration in a myope showing haemorrhage

Central serous choroidopathy (central serous retinopathy)

This is a condition of unknown aetiology which usually affects adult males between 20 and 45 years of age (*Fig. 8.24*). A defect in the pigment epithelium allows serous fluid to pass from the choriocapillaris in between the pigment epithelium and photoreceptors, causing a localised, small, serous retinal detachment at the macula.

Symptoms: Sudden onset of a blurring of central vision, distortion, micropsia and positive scotoma.

Signs: Visual acuity is usually slightly reduced to 6/9 or 6/12. Characteristically, the visual acuity may be improved with a +1 lens which will focus on the elevated area of macula. The abnormal area may be plotted on the Amsler chart. There is a prolonged photostress recovery time. Direct ophthalmoscopy shows a loss of foveal light reflex and general definition of the macula. Hruby or fundus contact lens reveals a thin, blister-like elevation at the macula, often away from the fovea.

Management: The vision usually recovers spontaneously to normal or near normal over the succeeding few months. If there is doubt about the diagnosis, a fluorescein angiogram is performed which demonstrates the fluid leak at the macula (smoke-stack appearance). Laser photocoagulation is performed to expedite visual recovery in those patients who require excellent vision in both eyes for their occupation, have poor vision in the other eye, have suffered a loss of vision through previous attacks or have persistent symptoms after four months.

8.24

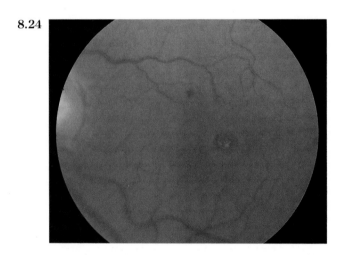

Fig. 8.24 Central serous choroidopathy (Courtesy of Mr. C. Dean Hart)

Pigment epithelial detachment

This is a localised detachment at the macula, between the pigment epithelium and underlying Bruch's membrane, i.e. deeper than a serous retinal detachment (*Fig. 8.25*). It occurs in two age-groups: 20–40 years, when it may be part of the central serous choroidopathy group, and in the elderly as a degenerative disorder.

Symptoms: Decreased visual acuity (more than central serous choroidopathy), with distortion, positive scotoma and positive photostress test.

Signs: A well-defined elevation at the macula region, thicker in appearance than central serous retinopathy. Fluorescein angiography demonstrates an area of leakage of dye, followed by pooling under the pigment epithelial detachment.

(s) *Management:* In both populations the best course is no treatment. The younger group has a good prognosis for visual recovery. The older group has a worse prognosis, but there is no evidence that laser treatment improves the outcome.

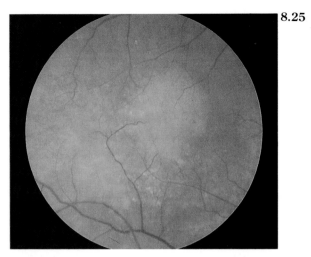

Fig. 8.25 Pigment epithelial detachment (Courtesy of Mr. R. Grey)

Cystoid macular oedema

This collection of fluid-filled cysts develops within the neuroretina, centred around the fovea (*Fig. 8.26*). There are several causes including retinal vein occlusion, severe or chronic anterior uveitis, a complication of cataract surgery (most often intracapsular), topical adrenaline in aphakic patients and diabetic maculopathy.

Symptoms: Decreased visual acuity.

Signs: Usually the anterior chamber or posterior chamber signs are not sufficient to explain the drop in visual acuity. Direct ophthalmoscopy may show a slightly enlarged, yellowish zone at the fovea with loss of the foveal reflex. Examination using the Hruby lens or fundus contact lens demonstrates a slightly elevated, cystic area at the fovea.

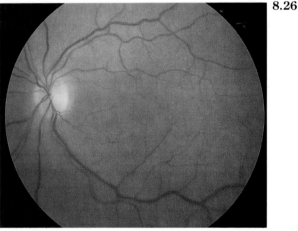

Fig. 8.26 Cystoid macular oedema (Courtesy of Mr. R. Grey); see also **Fig. 6.9(b)**

(s) *Management:* In most cases there is no treatment of proven benefit. In severe posterior uveitis, systemic steroids and acetazolamide 250 mg three times daily orally may help. In diabetic maculopathy, grid laser has been evaluated with fairly good results. In most cases the condition settles spontaneously within a few weeks or months, leaving good vision. However, it may be complicated by lamellar hole formation or macular degeneration. Indomethacin 25 mg t.d.s. orally in the early stages post-cataract extraction may be preventive.

Macular hole

There are two types of hole that occur at the macula (*Fig. 8.27(a) & (b)*), usually directly over the fovea:

• **True macular hole**. This is a full-thickness lesion, i.e. through retina down to choroid. The vision is moderately to severely impaired (6/18 or less). It has a punched-out appearance, with yellow pigment in the base of the hole and a greyish halo around the hole caused by localised subretinal fluid. The main causes are senile (when about 10% are bilateral), myopic and traumatic. Retinal detachment is a rare complication and occurs only in the myopic types.

• **Lamellar hole**. Here the hole is partially through the neuroretina and the pigment epithelium is not affected. The vision is mildly to moderately impaired. It usually arises as a complication of cystoid macular oedema, when the fluid-filled cysts coalesce and the roof of the cyst breaks down. It appears as a shallower defect with no yellow pigment in the base.

Management: There is no treatment for lamellar holes (s) or for most true macular holes. Macular holes associated with detachment are treated with detachment surgery and vitrectomy, with laser treatment around the hole.

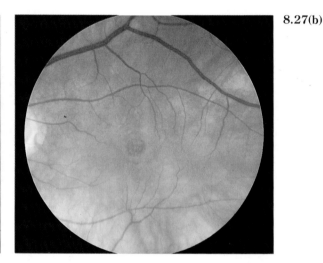

8.27(a) 8.27(b)

Fig. 8.27(a) & (b) Macular hole

Solar retinopathy (foveomacular retinitis)

This is a discrete foveal burn which usually occurs in individuals who stare at the sun during a solar eclipse or during religious experiences (*Fig. 8.28*). Soon after it has happened the patient notices a central scotoma and distorted vision with decreased visual acuity. The fovea becomes oedematous and often there is a yellow exudate in the foveola. The condition settles and may resolve completely over the ensuing months, but often a lamellar hole forms.

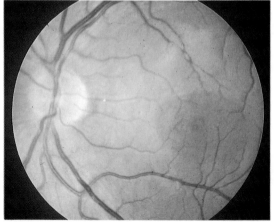

8.28

Fig. 8.28 Solar retinopathy (Courtesy of Mr. C. Dean Hart)

Macular dystrophies

There are a number of rare, inherited macular dystrophies, e.g. Stargardt's maculopathy (which is associated with pale flecks on the retina), cone dystrophy (which is an abnormality of cone receptors associated with loss of colour vision and central vision and with pigment epithelial degeneration at the macula), and Best's vitelliform dystrophy (which is an 'egg-yolk'-like degeneration at the macula). In each case a careful drug history must be taken since many drugs, e.g. antimalarials and major tranquilizers, may lead to a toxic maculopathy (see p. 263). Macular dystrophies are generally investigated by carrying out colour (s) vision testing, fluorescein angiography and electro-diagnostic testing.

Central retinal artery occlusion

This is an acute blockage of the central retinal artery, caused by embolism (*Fig. 8.29*). It occurs mainly in the elderly, when the main aetiological factors are hypertension, embolism from carotid artery disease, mural thrombus following myocardial infarction or associated with atrial fibrillation, calcified aortic valves, infective endocarditis, temporal arteritis and diabetes. Other rarer causes include atrial myxoma, syphilis, increased orbital pressure, e.g. retrobulbar haemorrhage, and, in younger patients, systemic lupus erythematosus, polyarteritis nodosa, dermatomyositis or infected emboli in intravenous drug abuse. Occasionally raised intraocular pressure, e.g. in acute angle closure glaucoma, gives rise to central retinal artery occlusion.

Symptoms: Sudden, painless loss of vision in one eye, sometimes not noticed immediately by the elderly.

Signs: The visual acuity is decreased to perception of light or hand movements unless there is a continued blood supply to part or all of the macular zone by a cilioretinal artery (present in about one in five cases), in which case central vision may be preserved. There is an afferent pupillary defect. In the acute stages (first 24–48 hours), the retina appears white and swollen due to infarction of retinal tissues. The arteries are attenuated with dark red blood owing to stagnation. At the fovea there is little retina to infarct and the red choroid shows through the thin retina as the characteristic 'cherry-red spot'. Other causes of 'cherry-red spot' include inherited gangliosidoses, such as Tay–Sachs disease, Niemann–Pick disease and sialidosis.

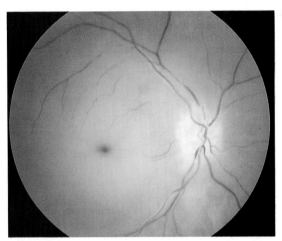

8.29

Fig. 8.29 Central retinal artery occlusion

Here deposition of lipid in the neural tissues causes a general pallor of the retina, sparing the fovea where the choroid shows through as a 'cherry-red spot'. The disc often appears swollen owing to build up of axoplasm at the nerve head. Over the following few days to weeks the retinal appearance often returns to normal, except that the arteries remain thin and the disc is pale. The intra-ocular pressure is measured prior to dilation to check for glaucoma.

Investigations: Blood pressure measurement, urine for glycosuria, full blood count and erythrocyte sedimentation rate (and plasma viscosity) to exclude temporal arteritis and connective tissue disease, carotid doppler studies, echocardiography and investigation of other sources of emboli as appropriate.

Management: If the history is less than 12 hours, it is reasonable to attempt to reverse the retinal artery blockage. The patient lies flat and ocular massage is applied for 15 minutes to reduce the intraocular pressure. In addition 500mg acetazolamide is given intravenously. Anterior chamber paracentesis and inhaling a mixture of 5% CO_2 and 95% O_2 may also be attempted, but these and the other measures described above to reduce intraocular pressure are rarely suc-cessful in alleviating the artery occlusion.

A central retinal artery occlusion may be a warning of impending cerebrovascular accident; therefore after the source of embolus is determined, appropriate treatment, e.g. carotid endarterectomy, aortic valvu-loplasty etc., is carried out. If the patient is not fit enough for this, therapy with antiplatelet drugs, e.g aspirin enteric coated 300mg daily, may be used.

Branch artery occlusion

This is usually caused by an embolus, commonly from the carotid artery or calcified aortic valve, blocking one of the retinal arteries (*Fig. 8.30*). Loss of vision in the territory supplied by that branch occurs, e.g. upper or lower half of field or a quadrant of field loss. Occasionally a cilioretinal artery occlusion may occur, causing loss of central vision.

Symptoms: Sudden loss of a part of the visual field of one eye only.

Signs: An area of pale, infarcted retina in the early stages, often with an embolus seen at the site of occlusion. Later, the retinal appearances return to normal, but the field loss is permanent. Carotid bruits or aortic murmurs may be heard.

ⓇⓈ *Management:* The source of emboli is identified and treated if possible. Again, low dose aspirin may be used if carotid endarterectomy is too hazardous.

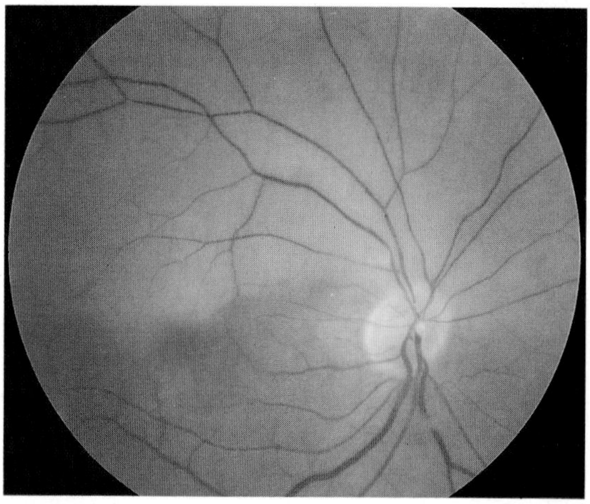

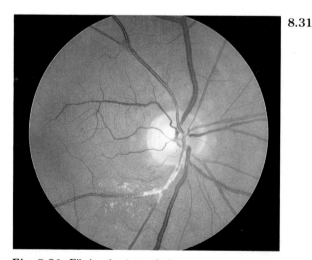

Fig. 8.30 Branch retinal artery occlusion

Types of emboli

- **Cholesterol emboli** (*Fig. 8.16*) appear as multiple, tiny, round, highly refractile crystals that rarely impede blood flow in the retinal arterioles. Also known as Hollenhorst plaques.

- **Fibrinoplatelet emboli** (*Fig. 8.31*) are larger and appear as whitish sludge blocking the arteriole. They are usually symptomatic and lead to episodes of amaurosis fugax (see below).

- **Calcific emboli** are the most dangerous as they cause permanent occlusion of major retinal arteries. They are usually single, large, non-refractile and white, and are located near the disc often at branch points.

Fig. 8.31 Fibrinoplatelet emboli

Amaurosis fugax

This is a fleeting loss of vision which is caused by an embolus occluding the central retinal artery, or a branch of it, and then passing on.

Symptoms: Typically, the patient describes a curtain or shutter coming over their vision either from the top downwards or the bottom upwards. It is **uniocular**. The vision is blacked out for a period of seconds to minutes, occasionally longer, and then reappears in a similar way. Sometimes the visual symptoms may be blurring rather than blacking-out and if this occurs in both eyes, it may be due to a transient ischaemic attack affecting the cortical visual pathways.

Signs: During an attack there may be an afferent pupillary defect and retinal oedema. Occasionally emboli, which are most likely to be the fibrinoplatelet type, are seen.

Management: Investigation of sources of emboli and (S) aspirin (enteric coated) 300mg daily. (The actual (P) dosage remains controversial; some sources say 75mg daily is adequate.) Advise to stop smoking.

Transient ischaemic attacks

Vertebro-basilar ischaemia and carotid ischaemia both give rise to visual symptoms. The causes include emboli, generalised arteriosclerotic disease or, in the case of vertebro-basilar ischaemia, compression from cervical vertebrae.

Symptoms: Sudden onset of blurring of vision, affecting both eyes and sometimes hemianopic. Each episode lasts minutes to hours and can be associated with dizziness, tingling around the mouth, diplopia and hearing and speech disturbances in brain stem ischaemia, and hemiparesis in cortical ischaemia.

Signs: Examination of the eyes is normal. Visual field disturbance may be present.

Investigations: General medical examination and investigations to exclude cardiovascular abnormalities, e.g. hypertension, emboli, carotid artery studies and cervical spine radiography if appropriate.

Management: Advise to stop smoking. Aspirin therapy. (P) Referral to vascular specialist if appropriate.

Migraine

Migraine is associated with a number of symptoms that may cause the sufferer to attend an eye casualty department. A classical attack of migraine may be preceded or associated with visual symptoms. There is usually a past history of migraine.

Sometimes the visual symptoms may dominate the clinical picture, with only minimal, if any, headache or nausea. The visual symptoms are typically bilateral, although unilateral cases have been described. In the case of sudden unilateral visual loss a local ocular cause should be sought first, for example central retinal artery or vein occlusion. Other forms of migraine that may occur include ophthalmoplegic migraine, more commonly affecting the younger age groups and atypical migraine, giving rise to facial or ocular pain (v.i.).

Symptoms
• **visual phenomena**, such as zig-zag lines, or shapes, that may have the appearance of fortifications on a castle (fortification spectra), with tiny, bright, coloured flashing lights filling the visual field

• **loss of visual field** which may be hemianopic, or occasionally all the visual field or sometimes constriction of the field.

Atypical Migraine

This may give rise to various types of orbital or facial pain. **Cluster headaches** are seen in middle-aged men, often with no past history of migraine. There is a pattern of nightly attacks of excruciating pain around the eye that wakes the patient up. There is often injection and chemosis of the conjunctiva of the eye on the affected side, associated with watering. The attacks usually last from 30 minutes to 2 hours. The series of attacks may last up to 3 months.

Orbital migraine gives rise to a deep boring pain behind the eye with occasional exacerbations of sharp, stabbing pain in the eye. It may be associated with other migrainous symptoms and an attack may last several days.

Management: Simple analgesics or, in severe attacks, (S)(P) ergotamine preparations.

8.32

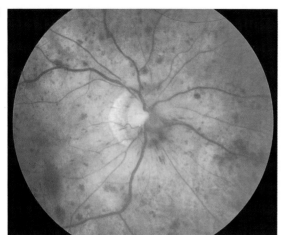

8.33

Fig. 8.32 Central retinal vein occlusion – few haemorrhages

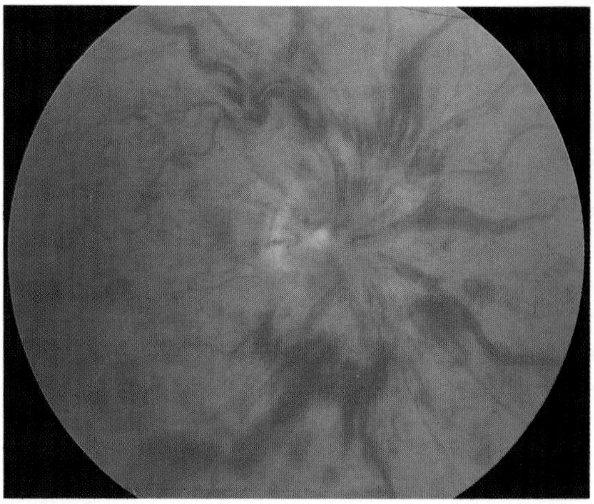

Fig. 8.33 Central retinal vein occlusion – haemorrhagic

8.34

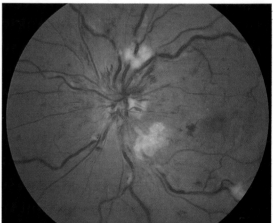

Fig. 8.34 Central retinal vein occlusion – ischaemic

Occlusion of the central retinal vein (*Figs. 8.32, 8.33, 8.34*) produces a range of clinical pictures, depending on the amount of occlusion present. It is more common in diabetes mellitus, hypertension and chronic glaucoma. It may be related to generalised arteriosclerosis, causing thickening of the central retinal artery that shares a sheath with the central retinal vein and which may cause compression. In young patients a similar, although less severe, picture is seen and may be related to a vasculitis, e.g. sarcoidosis. In severe cases, where there is extensive retinal ischaemia (as demonstrated by cotton wool spots, blot haemorrhages and capillary drop-out on fluorescein angiography), there is a 30–50% chance of developing neovascular glaucoma, known as '90-day glaucoma' because it can develop within three months after the initial event. It is a devastating complication which may be prevented by prophylactic, panretinal photocoagulation.

Symptoms: Vary from mild blurring to severe painless loss of vision. It is often noticed upon waking, with normal vision the night before.

Signs: In mild cases there are a few haemorrhages radiating from the disc to the periphery. In more severe cases there is venous dilatation and multiple flame-shaped and blot haemorrhages and cotton wool

spots extending from the disc, where they are the most dense, to the equator. The disc is often swollen and there may be subretinal fluid at the macular region. The intraocular pressure may be normal in the affected eye, even in the presence of glaucoma, since the pressure may be lowered acutely in central retinal vein occlusion. The other eye may then be found to have an elevated pressure owing to chronic glaucoma. In neovascular glaucoma, rubeosis iridis is seen, but rarely disc or retinal new vessels. Shunt vessels often develop on the disc as new routes of drainage of retinal blood are opened up.

Differential diagnosis: Stage III or IV hypertensive retinopathy (see p. 179) is bilateral and the haemorrhages do not extend as far peripherally. There is often a macular star of hard exudate. Hyperviscosity syndromes, e.g. macroglobulinaemia, polycythaemias etc., are bilateral and show venous dilatation and beading ('string of sausages' appearance), but few haemorrhages. Diabetic retinopathy is bilateral and the haemorrhages are more randomly placed, not radiating from the disc, which is not swollen.

Investigations: FBC and viscosity, urinalysis for glucose, and, in young patients, investigations for causes of vasculitis, e.g. sarcoid, auto-immune disease, Behçet's disease and so on, if appropriate.

Management: There is no treatment for the acute Ⓢ Ⓡ stages of central retinal vein occlusion. Glaucoma, if present, is treated in the usual way. In less severe cases the vision may show some improvement as the haemorrhages and the macular subretinal fluid clear. If retinal ischaemia is present clinically (cotton wool spots and blot haemorrhages) (*Fig. 8.35*), fluorescein angiography is performed to determine its extent. If severe, panretinal photocoagulation may be appropriate.

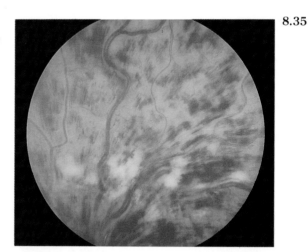

8.35

Fig. 8.35 Central retinal vein occlusion – detail of cotton wool spots and haemorrhages

Hyperviscosity syndrome

High plasma viscosity (*Fig. 8.36*) is caused by high protein states such as Waldenström's macroglobulinaemia, myeloma, or high cell states, e.g. leukaemia. It leads to a picture of venous stasis in the retina, similar to central retinal vein occlusion, but occurring bilaterally.

Initially the veins become dilated and beaded ('string of sausages' appearance) and then flame-shaped and blot haemorrhages appear, together with retinal oedema and disc swelling.

The management of the underlying condition is imperative.

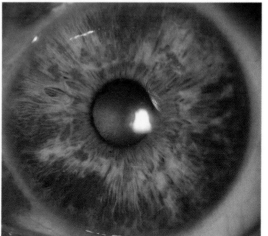

8.36

Fig. 8.36 Spontaneous haemorrhages into iris in patient with leukaemia and low platelet count

Branch retinal vein occlusion

Occlusion of a branch of the central retinal vein (*Figs. 8.37(a) & (b)*) occurs, often temporally, at a crossing point where artery and vein share a fascial sheath and an artery, enlarged owing to hypertension or arteriosclerosis, causes compression of the vein. Sometimes it occurs nasally, e.g. in diabetes. It may occur anywhere in periphlebitis. In glaucoma it may occur at the rim of a deeply-cupped, glaucomatous disc.

Symptoms: Blurring of central vision is noticed in a temporal branch vein occlusion which affects the macular zone. Nasal and peripheral branch vein occlusions are often asymptomatic.

Signs: Flame-shaped haemorrhages, with or without cotton wool spots, in the area served by the occluded vein with macular subretinal fluid if macular drainage is affected. Intraocular pressure is measured for glaucoma. Later complications include disc and retinal neovascularisation, often in the area between normal and ischaemic retina. This may lead to vitreous haemorrhage. Hard exudates may develop in the macular zone if there is chronic vascular leakage.

Investigations: Blood pressure measurement (hypertension is the most common aetiological factor), FBC and viscosity, urinalysis for glucose, vasculitis investigations as appropriate.

Management: There is no acute treatment. The vision often improves over a period of weeks to months as the haemorrhages clear and the macular oedema settles. Fluorescein angiography is performed to determine the side of leakage if retinal ischaemia or neovascularisation is suspected, or in the presence of macular hard exudates. In neovascularisation, retinal photocoagulation is performed in the affected quadrant. In chronic macular oedema, laser burns are placed over the points of leakage.

8.37(a)

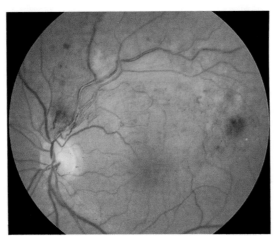

8.37

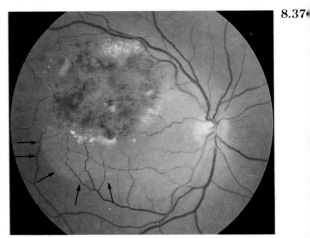

Fig. 8.37(a) Branch retinal vein occlusion – site of occlusion at crossing point on disc margin (Courtesy of Mr. C. Dean Hart)

Fig. 8.37(b) Branch retinal vein occlusion – involving macular region. Subretinal fluid (arrowed) seen inferior to the area of haemorrhage and exudate at the macula

Posterior vitreous detachment (PVD)

The vitreous gel is normally attached posteriorly around the optic disc (Weiss ring) at the posterior vitreous face and anteriorly at the vitreous base to the ora serrata and to the posterior lens capsule. As individuals age, the vitreous gel shrinks in volume and at a certain stage becomes too small to fill the cavity available to it. It then detaches at the posterior vitreous face, remaining attached anteriorly to the posterior lens capsule by a small rim around the equator. This may happen acutely over the age of 40 years.

Symptoms: Sudden onset of floaters (vitreous opacities) or mild blurring of vision, appearance of a ring-shaped object (the previous attachment of the vitreous around the optic nerve head), flashing lights or photopsia (often an intense, white streak of light at the temporal periphery experienced especially in low illumination and lasting a few seconds). Occasionally a dark streak is seen or blurring of vision is experienced when a vitreous haemorrhage occurs.

Signs: The pupil must be dilated. Direct ophthalmoscopy is often normal. Indirect ophthalmoscopy may reveal peripheral holes or tears, or vitreous haemorrhage. Examination with a three-mirror contact lens is essential to demonstrate any peripheral holes or tears. It also demonstrates the posterior vitreous face away from the retina, often with the Weiss ring clearly seen, which is diagnostic of a PVD.

Management: All patients with sudden onset of flashing (S)(R) lights or floaters should be seen within 1–2 days at an eye centre for a fundal examination to ensure that there are no retinal tears. If there is a vitreous haemorrhage, they may require admission. The majority of patients do not have any retinal holes and may be discharged with instructions to return promptly if their symptoms worsen or fail to settle, or if they have any symptoms of retinal detachment (v.i.). Those with peripheral tears are managed as outlined below.

Retinal detachment

The most common type of retinal detachment (*Fig. 8.38(a) & (b)*) is that caused by a retinal hole or tear, when fluid from the vitreous cavity accumulates under the neuroretina (the anterior part of the retina) and strips it off the pigment epithelium (the posterior part of the retina). This is a **rhegmatogenous** retinal detachment whioch occurs more commonly in highly myopic individuals and following acute posterior vitreous detachment. It also occurs after trauma (see below).

8.38(a)
8.38(b)

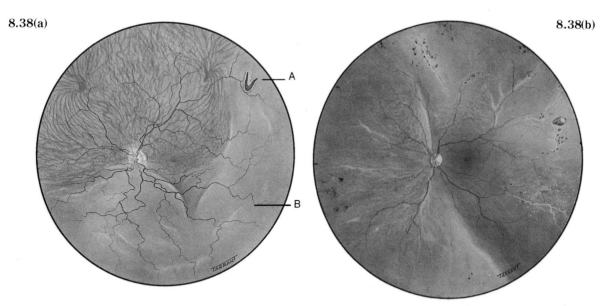

Fig. 8.38(a) Retinal detachment – showing superior temporal tear and bullous detachment. A – U-shaped tear, B – Bullous detachment

Fig. 8.38(b) Total retinal detachment (Courtesy of Institute of Ophthalmology)

A second type of retinal detachment is the **exudative** or **secondary** type, in which leakage of fluid from the choroid or retinal vessels causes elevation of the neurosensory retina. This is most commonly seen in malignant hypertension, especially toxaemia of pregnancy, renal disease, e.g. glomerulonephritis, and retinal vasculitis, retinal vein occlusion, retinal vascular anomalies and choroidal tumours. Treatment is directed at the underlying condition, which if corrected may lead to spontaneous resolution of the detachment. Detachment surgery is not appropriate.

A third type is a **tractional** retinal detachment. This occurs when inflammatory exudates or haemorrhages in the vitreous become organised into condensations of fibrous tissue or bands which then contract and pull on the retina, leading to a funnel-shaped retinal detachment. This occurs most commonly in proliferative diabetic retinopathy, but also in perforating injuries with intraocular foreign bodies, endophthalmitis, and as a complication of previous, complicated, detachment surgery. Highly specialised, closed, intraocular, microsurgical techniques to free the traction bands and flatten the retina are required.

These types of retinal detachment need to be differentiated from a solid choroidal detachment as a result

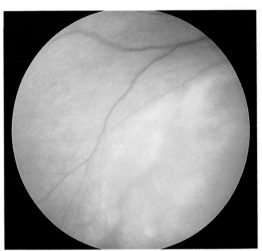

8.39

Fig. 8.39 Solid detachment due to malignant melanoma

of tumour (primary choroidal malignant melanoma (*Fig. 8.39*) or secondary deposits), a retinoschisis and a choroidal detachment following intraocular surgery.

Rhegmatogenous retinal detachment

This type commonly presents in primary health care or to an optician (*Fig. 8.40*). Peripheral retinal degeneration and/or vitreous traction (after acute posterior vitreous detachment) lead to retinal tear or hole formation which may progress to retinal detachment as vitreous fluid tracks under the neurosensory retina. Degenerations in the peripheral retina, which occur as an age-related process from the age of 40, and 20 years earlier in severe myopes, occur in several descriptive forms:

• Benign chorioretinal degeneration, including 'paving-stone', microcystoid, 'snowflake', drüsen and pigment clumping. Although any of these peripheral degenerations may be associated with hole formation if vitreous traction occurs, no prophylactic treatment is necessary when seen.

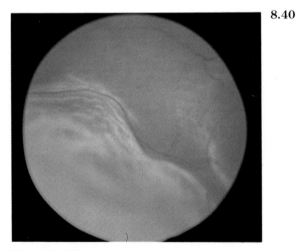

8.40

Fig. 8.40 Rhegmatogenous retinal detachment

• Degenerations predisposing to tear formation, including lattice and snail-track, require prophylactic treatment with laser or cryotherapy when seen (*Fig. 8.41*).

• Senile retinoschisis, when splitting occurs in the retina especially in the inferotemporal area, often bilaterally. If holes occur in both leaves of the schisis, a retinal detachment may occur (around 1% incidence). Most ophthalmologists would not treat retinoschisis alone unless the fellow eye had suffered a retinal detachment as a result.

Other predisposing factors include trauma, aphakia, positive family history, inherited connective tissue disorder, e.g. Marfan's syndrome.

Symptoms: The most common presentation is sudden onset of flashing lights (photopsia) and a shower of floaters which is associated with a posterior vitreous detachment. This initial occurrence may be ignored by the patient and is often followed by the development of a 'curtain' or 'cloud-like' obstruction to the vision. This is often described as a 'lid coming down over the vision' and it occurs as the retina detaches. In slowly progressive detachments the patient may not present until the macula has detached, at which point central vision is lost.

Signs: Visual acuity may be normal or reduced (if the macula is off). Reactive anterior uveitis may be present. The presence of 'tobacco dust', i.e. brownish specks in the anterior vitreous, is a fairly sensitive indicator of retinal detachment. A relative afferent pupillary defect may be seen in macula-off retinal detachment and the red reflex is lost in the area of the detachment. A bullous detachment appears as a ballooning of the retina, which is grey, owing to loss of red reflex from the choroid, and wrinkled, and the vascular markings are dark instead of red. There is a clear demarcation between the flat and detached retina and sometimes the detachment will be seen as a black shadow against the pupillary red reflex. It is seen most easily by indirect ophthalmoscopy, although direct ophthalmoscopy with a dilated pupil will reveal some detachments. Examination with a three-mirror contact lens is essential to delineate the detachment, determine if the macula is on or off, and to identify the position of the hole(s). A retinal detachment chart should be drawn. The shape of the retinal detachment is often a good guide as to the position of the hole since subretinal fluid tracks downwards from a hole and then fills up from below, so that in the absence of obvious holes attention can be concentrated at the predicted position. Thus, in an inferior retinal detachment the side with the highest fluid level will have the hole at the top. Superior retinal detachments progress far more rapidly than inferior ones.

8.41

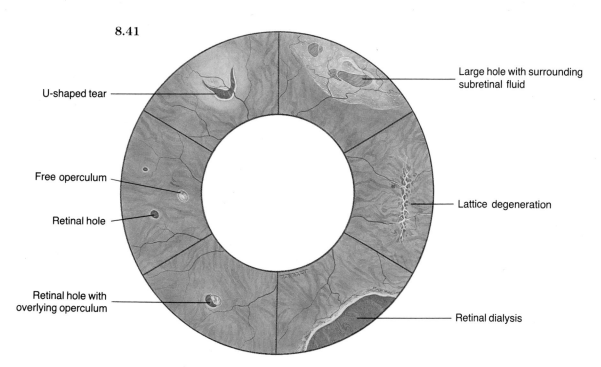

Fig. 8.41 Composite diagram of peripheral retinal degenerations that lead to retinal detachment

Management: All possible retinal detachments should be referred to a specialist eye centre for immediate assessment. If the macula is still attached, as indicated by good visual acuity, the potential for visual recovery is good and the detachment is repaired as soon as possible, preferably the same day. The patient should be kept fasting from the time of referral (if reasonable). If the macula is detached, there is less urgency, but the patient should be referred within a day. The principle of retinal detachment repair is to identify the holes or tears and to use laser or cryotherapy to induce adhesions between the retinal layers around the holes. The sclera is then indented using plombs (sponge-like material) or encircling bands to support the hole and relieve vitreous traction. It may be necessary to drain excessive quantities of subretinal fluid. If the scleral buckling is correctly positioned, the retina will usually go flat over the subsequent few days. If there is a retinal tear without a detachment or vitreous traction, laser or cryotherapy alone is the treatment of choice.

Prognosis: This depends on the length of the history and whether or not the macula is detached. Chronic retinal detachments have a worse prognosis since the photoreceptors may have degenerated as they are separated from their source of nutrients, the choriocapillaris, and the retinal folds may have become fixed. Giant retinal tears are exceptionally difficult to manage and require vitrectomy techniques. Detachment surgery requires expertise and the patient should be given a fairly guarded prognosis even in the better prognostic groups.

Retinal dialysis

This is a disinsertion of the retina from its attachment at the ora serrata (*Fig. 8.42*). It often occurs in younger age groups either spontaneously or as a result of trauma. It may progress to extensive retinal detachment and Ⓢ is treated by conventional detachment surgery.

8.42

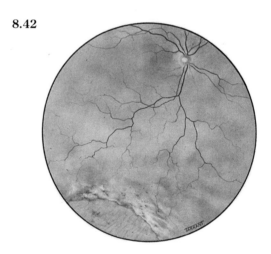

Fig. 8.42 Retinal dialysis (Courtesy of Institute of Ophthalmology)

Retinoschisis

This is a superficial splitting of the retina, occurring at or below the nerve ganglion layer. It appears as a thin, translucent veil over the retina with preservation of normal colour and the vascular pattern of the deeper layers of the retina underneath. There are two main groups of retinoschisis:

• **Congenital X-linked retinoschisis**. This is characterised by progressive visual deterioration with formation of peripheral retinoschises and microcysts at the macula. There is an increased risk of vitreous haemorrhage and retinal detachment. This may occur spontaneously or with minimal trauma and contact sports should be avoided. Electrodiagnostic tests show characteristic features.

• **Senile or acquired retinoschisis**. These cases are bilateral and usually inferotemporal. They are usually asymptomatic and picked up on routine examination. If holes occur in the anterior and posterior leaflets, a retinal detachment may develop (incidence about 1%). An absolute field defect is seen in the area of the schisis. No treatment is required for a schisis alone. The patients should be warned of the risk of retinal detachment and asked to reattend promptly if any worrying symptoms occur.

Angioid streaks

These are breaks in Bruch's membrane (the layer separating the pigment epithelium and choriocapillaris), which appear as dark cracks with serrated edges, wider than the blood vessels, radiating from the optic disc (*Fig. 8.43*). They may be associated with peripheral mottling of the retina and drüsen of the optic nerve head. If an angioid streak occurs at the fovea, central vision is impaired. Otherwise, visual problems arise from the formation of disciform macular degeneration and choroidal rupture. Minimal eye trauma may provoke visual loss from these complications. Patients with this condition should avoid contact sports. Only rarely are the disciform lesions treatable. Many patients with angioid streaks have associated systemic conditions, e.g. pseudoxanthoma elasticum (with characteristic yellow papules in the neck and axilla) (*Fig. 8.44*), Ehlers-Danlos syndrome, Paget's disease and sickle cell anaemia.

8.43

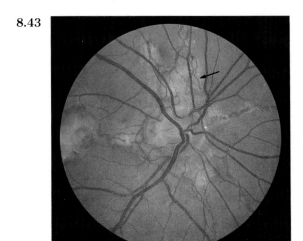

Fig. 8.43 Angioid streaks (one arrowed) in pseudoxanthoma elasticum

8.44

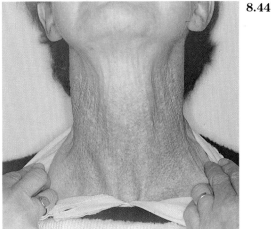

Fig. 8.44 Pseudoxanthoma elasticum showing skin changes

Asteroid hyalosis (or hyalitis)

This is a condition in which collections of minute, highly refractile, white bodies made of calcium lipid salts are seen in the vitreous. It is usually an incidental finding, present in normal individuals, and may be partly inherited. Usually no treatment is required.

Histoplasmosis or presumed ocular histoplasmosis syndrome

Histoplasmosis is a fungal infection, usually caused by *Histoplasma capsulatum*, which is endemic in the midwest of the USA, but does not occur in the UK (*Fig. 8.45*). The vast majority of histoplasmic infections are benign and asymptomatic. It is during childhood infections that the earliest ocular presentation, the 'histo spots', occur and lay down the foundations for the later manifestations. The identical ocular picture to histoplasmosis is found in certain parts of Europe, where the fungus does not occur, thus the condition is best called 'presumed ocular histoplasmosis syndrome'.

Ocular findings: Multifocal choroiditis with 0–70 histo spots in either eye, peripapillary and peripheral linear chorioretinal atrophy and haemorrhagic macular disci-

form degeneration, which is the major cause of loss of vision. The maculopathy typically occurs between the ages of 20 and 40 years. The vitreous is clear, which is a distinguishing feature of this condition.

Investigations: Histoplasma skin testing is positive in two-thirds of cases and there is an increased frequency of HLA-B7.

Management: There is no proven benefit from ⓢ treatment with corticosteroids or antifungal therapy. Occasionally the early macular disciform may be treated with laser to try to prevent severe visual loss, but even expert treatment may be disappointing.

8.45

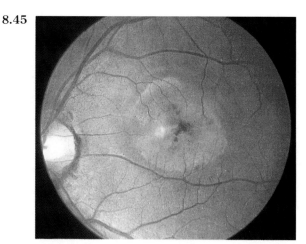

Fig. 8.45 Presumed ocular histoplasmosis syndrome showing macular lesion

Retinitis

Retinal infections usually occur in conjunction with endophthalmitis (see pp. 116–18) and chorioretinitis, e.g. toxoplasmosis (see p. 112). Rarer causes of isolated retinitis are seen in viral and fungal infections, of which the most important are discussed below.

Candida retinitis

This infection (*see Fig. 6.20(a) & (b)*) occurs in intravenous drug abusers, patients with longstanding, central intravenous lines and immunocompromised individuals. The patient notices initial blurring of vision due to a posterior uveitis, followed by loss of visual acuity due to focal areas of retinitis at the posterior pole. These appear as fluffy, 'snowball' opacities with thread-like extensions into the vitreous. There may be foci of candida infection elsewhere in the body, e.g. urinary tract infection. Treatment consists of vitrectomy to clear the bulk of the infection and injection of antifungal agents locally into the vitreous cavity, combined with systemic antifungal therapy.

Cytomegalovirus (CMV) retinitis

This is mainly seen in immunocompromised individuals (*Fig. 8.46(a)–(c)*) and, in recent years, in patients with AIDS (Acquired ImmunoDeficiency Syndrome). The main symptom is visual loss in one or both eyes. The appearance of the fundus is described as 'tomato sauce and cottage cheese', referring to the widespread haemorrhages and the retinitis, a whitish infiltration with vein occlusion. The organism is cultured from urine or eyes. Treatment is with antiviral agents – gancyclovir has been used recently.

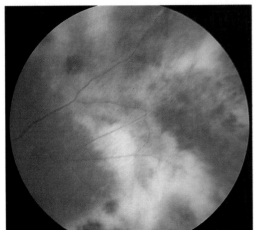

Fig. 8.46(a) Cytomegalovirus retinitis

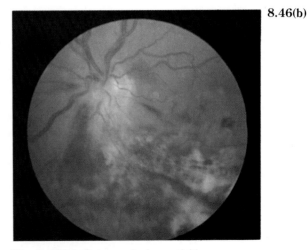

Fig. 8.46(b) Cytomegalovirus retinitis
(Courtesy of Mr. R. Humphry)

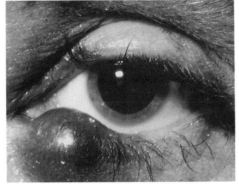

Fig. 8.46(c) Kaposi's sarcoma of lid
(Courtesy of Mr. R. Marsh)

Retinitis pigmentosa

This is a group of inherited conditions which leads to progressive visual loss (*Figs. 8.47, 8.48*). The severity is often linked with the mode of inheritance, thus autosomally recessive and X-linked recessive cases are more severely affected than autosomal dominant cases. Other features include night blindness, constriction of the visual fields, cataract, optic atrophy (waxy pallor), typical pigment spicule appearance, arteriolar attenuation, myopia and maculopathy. There are several systemic disorders associated with a pigmentary retinopathy including abetalipoproteinaemia, Refsum's disease, Usher's syndrome, Laurence-Moon-Biedl syndrome, Kearns-Sayre syndrome and Friedreich's ataxia.

8.47

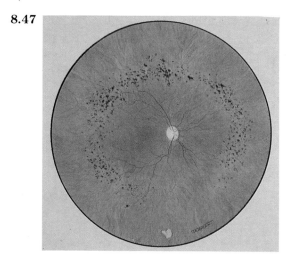

Fig. 8.47 Retinitis pigmentosa

8.48

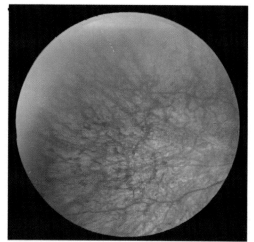

Fig. 8.48 Retinitis pigmentosa – detail showing bone spicule pigmentation (Courtesy of Mr. R. Humphry)

9 Orbit

Normal anatomy

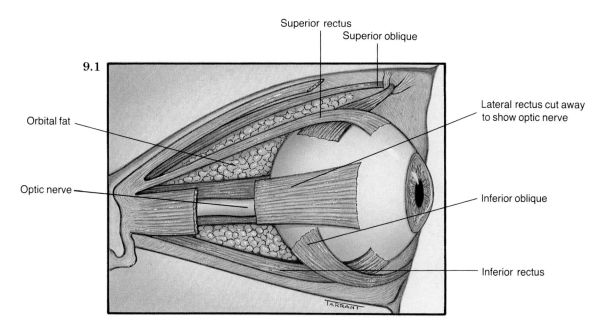

Superior rectus

Superior oblique

Lateral rectus cut away to show optic nerve

Orbital fat

Optic nerve

Inferior oblique

Inferior rectus

Fig. 9.1 Anatomy of the orbit

The orbit is the bony cavity that contains the eyeballs, extraocular muscles, vessels, nerves, fat and glands, including the lacrimal gland (*Fig. 9.1*). It is a four-sided pyramid with the apex posterior and the base anterior. The medial walls of the two orbits are parallel to each other and the lateral walls are at 90° to each other.

The **roof**, formed by the orbital plate of the frontal bone anteriorly and the lesser wing of the sphenoid bone posteriorly, separates the orbit from the anterior cranial fossa. The **floor**, which is formed by the maxilla medially and the zygoma laterally, separates the orbit from the maxillary sinus. Posteriorly lies the

inferior orbital fissure, through which the maxillary nerve and its zygomatic branch (from the pterygo-palatine fossa) and some communicating veins, pass. Anteriorly lies the canal of the infraorbital nerve.

From anterior to posterior, the **medial** wall is made up of the frontal process of the maxilla, the lacrimal bone, the orbital plate of the ethmoid and the body of the sphenoid. It separates the orbit from the nasal cavity and the ethmoid air sinuses. The naso-lacrimal duct runs down a canal at the inferomedial angle. The **lateral** wall, which separates the orbit from the temporal fossa, is formed by the zygomatic bone and the greater wing of the sphenoid.

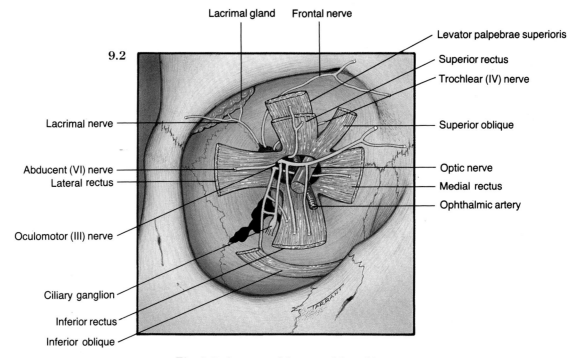

Lacrimal gland   Frontal nerve

9.2

Levator palpebrae superioris

Superior rectus

Trochlear (IV) nerve

Lacrimal nerve

Superior oblique

Abducent (VI) nerve

Lateral rectus

Optic nerve

Medial rectus

Ophthalmic artery

Oculomotor (III) nerve

Ciliary ganglion

Inferior rectus

Inferior oblique

Fig. 9.2 Anatomy of the apex of the orbit

The **superior orbital fissure** lies between the greater and lesser wings of the sphenoid bone and opens into the middle cranial fossa. The **optic canal** opens into the apex of the orbit (*Fig. 9.2*) and transmits the optic nerve and ophthalmic artery. A common tendinous ring, which surrounds the medial end of the superior orbital fissure and the optic canal, affords origin to the extraocular muscles, excluding the inferior oblique which arises from the anteromedial aspect of the floor of the orbit. The recti attach directly to the globe several millimetres behind the limbus in their respective locations: superiorly, inferiorly, medially and laterally.

The superior oblique passes through a pulley, the trochlea, situated in the anteromedial angle of the orbit, makes a sharp angle backwards and inserts onto the posterolateral quadrant of the superior aspect of the globe. The levator palpebrae superioris arises from just superior to the common tendinous ring. The superior orbital fissure above the common tendinous ring transmits the lacrimal and frontal branches of the trigeminal nerve and trochlear nerve. The part of the fissure enclosed by the ring transmits the oculomotor nerve (superior and inferior branches), nasociliary branch of the trigeminal nerve and the abducent nerve. The ophthalmic veins pass through the superior orbital fissure to the cavernous sinus.

The lacrimal gland sits in a fossa in the superolateral angle of the orbit behind the upper lid.

General features of orbital disease

The main disorders affecting the orbit are infection, tumours, pseudotumour, thyroid eye disease (see below) and trauma (see pp. 222–24). The main presenting features of orbital disease are displacement of the globe, sometimes pain (malignancy or inflammation), sometimes pulsation of the globe (sphenoid bone defects or arteriovenous shunts) or bruits (caroticocavernous fistula), decreased visual acuity (optic nerve compression) and diplopia (involvement of cranial nerves III, IV and VI and extraocular muscles). If there is a space-occupying lesion arising anterior in the orbit, the predominant symptom is proptosis, whereas a more posterior lesion causes optic nerve compression and minimal proptosis.

History includes details of duration of symptoms, rapidity of progression, history of systemic disease, e.g. thyroid, sinus disease, malignancy, diabetes, hypertension and vasculitis, as well as the features noted above.

Examination:

- **Visual acuity** – decreased acuity, e.g. due to optic nerve compression, when it is associated with an afferent nerve defect, field loss and disc swelling; exposure keratitis with proptosis and chorioretinal folds due to external compression of the posterior pole.

- **Proptosis**, which is forwards displacement of the globe in the direction of the visual axis (axial), is measured using an exophthalmometer (see p. 28). A difference of more than 2mm between the two sides is significant. A rough guide is obtained by comparing the patient's two eyes from above. Displacement of the globe may also be non-axial, that is superior, inferior, medial or lateral. This is due to an extraconal lesion, that is, one outside the muscle cone. It is important to differentiate proptosis from pseudo-proptosis, e.g due to facial asymmetry or a contra-lateral Horner's.

- **Eyelid retraction, lid lag, superior limbic keratoconjunctivitis** and **injection over horizontal recti insertions** are suggestive of thyroid disease.

- **Pulsation** from within the orbit (sphenoid bone defects, arteriovenous fistulae), **bruits** (carotico-cavernous fistulae), **alteration in size** of orbital mass (varices enlarge with Valsalva manoeuvre) (*see Fig. 9.11(b)*) .

- **Palpable masses** – the orbital margin is palpated.

- **Extraocular movements**, looking for muscle palsies or muscle restriction, including Hess chart if necessary.

- **Pupillary responses**, looking for a relative afferent pupillary defect.

- **Fundal examination**, looking for disc swelling, opticociliary shunt vessels (seen in optic nerve sheath meningioma) and chorioretinal folds.

- **Visual fields** – Goldmann perimetry to look for enlarged blind spot and other defects.

- **Cranial nerve abnormalities** are looked for, especially absent corneal reflexes.

Investigations include FBC, plasma viscosity, fasting blood glucose or urinalysis for glycosuria, thyroid function tests and skull and orbital radiography with computerised tomography if indicated.

Thyroid eye disease

The vast majority of unilateral and bilateral proptosis in the adult is caused by **dysthyroid eye disease**. Hyperthyroidism, e.g. due to Graves' disease, over-correction of hypothyroidism with thyroxine (T_4), toxic goitre and thyroiditis may give rise to lid retraction and lid lag, but only Graves' disease presents a serious ophthalmic problem and is discussed here.

Graves' disease is an auto-immune condition mainly affecting women aged 20–50 years. Release of thyroid-stimulating antibodies causes overaction of the gland, and a similar process can affect the muscles and tissues of the orbit. Some individuals with eye manifestations are hyperthyroid, showing raised T_3, +/− raised T_4 and low TSH. Others may be euthyroid and have so-called Ophthalmic Graves' disease. This has similar ocular manifestations to Graves' disease.

Ocular manifestations:

• **Lid retraction** (*Fig. 9.3*) – Normally the upper lid covers the top 2 mm of the cornea. In lid retraction the lid is either at or above the upper limbus exposing the sclera. Lid lag, in which the upper lid appears slowed in its descent on downgaze, is part of the same phenomenon. It is due to overstimulation of Müller's muscle (sympathetic part of levator palpebrae superioris). It is asymptomatic. Occasionally, for cosmetic (S) reasons, Müllers muscle may be recessed (loosened). Superior limbic keratoconjunctivitis is sometimes seen (*Fig. 9.4*).

• **Infiltrative eye disease** (*Fig. 9.5*) – A general increase in connective tissue of the orbit and muscle hypertrophy occurs as the result of stimulation by a humoral agent as yet unidentified. This leads to ocular discomfort and photophobia and can lead to visual impairment. The main features are:

(a) Proptosis – unilateral or bilateral – which is seen as an exposure of the sclera inferiorly and may be measured with an exophthalmometer. It may result in exposure keratitis. In mild to moderate cases, lubri- (S) cating ointment should be instilled at night, together with taping of the lids and the use of artificial tears during the day. In severe cases, lateral tarsorrhaphy may be required to protect the cornea.

(b) Hypertrophy of conjunctiva with chemosis, hyperaemia over the horizontal rectus muscle insertions and lid swelling. Artificial tears provide symptomatic (S) relief.

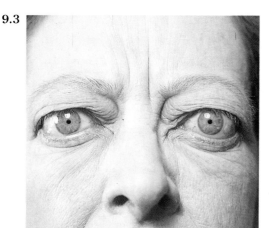

Fig. 9.3 Thyroid eye disease showing lid retraction and mild exophthalmos

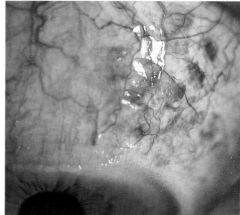

Fig. 9.4 Superior limbic keratoconjunctivitis

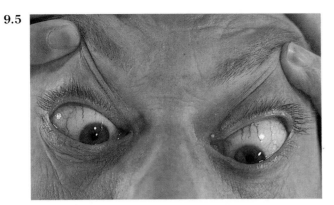

Fig. 9.5 Thyroid exophthalmos – moderate to severe. The patient should be observed from behind while looking down

(c) Optic neuropathy is caused by compression of the optic nerve and its blood supply by the swollen orbital tissues. There is often mildly raised intraocular pressure which may increase on elevation of the eyes. There is progressive impairment of central vision with a central or paracentral scotoma and arcuate defects on field testing. Fundoscopy reveals swelling of the optic disc with retinal folds and, later, optic atrophy is seen. Optic neuropathy is a serious complication referred to as 'malignant exophthalmos'. It requires Ⓢ urgent, inpatient management with high dose steroids (initial dose 80–100mg prednisolone daily) to reduce orbital tissues and proptosis. Alternative treatments are radiotherapy and orbital decompression.

(d) Restrictive myopathy (Fig. 9.6(a) & (b)) follows hypertrophy of the muscles as they become fibrosed and necrotic. The muscles most commonly involved are inferior rectus and medial rectus with limitation of elevation and abduction occurring respectively, along with the resultant diplopia. Initial treatment is with Ⓢ Fresnel prisms on the spectacles. No surgery on the muscles should be contemplated until the condition is stable.

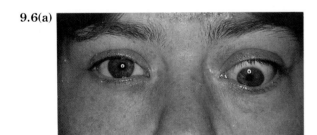

Fig. 9.6(a) Restrictive myopathy – patient looking straight ahead

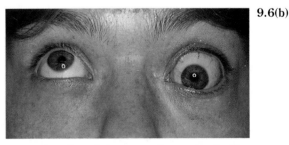

Fig. 9.6(b) Restrictive myopathy – patient looking up

Other orbital disorders include:

Preseptal cellulitis

This presents as an acute swelling and redness of the lids and periorbital tissues and is of similar aetiology to facial cellulitis (*Fig. 9.7*). It may follow an upper respiratory tract infection. The infection is confined to the superficial tissues and does not penetrate the orbital septum to infect the structures of the orbit. The usual organisms are streptococcus, staphylococcus, or *Haemophilus influenzae* in young children. The eye movements are not affected and the eye is not proptosed as in orbital cellulitis (v.i.). Conjunctival and nasopharyngeal swabs are taken. Treatment is with oral antibiotics, e.g. ampicillin or penicillin, as an outpatient, ⓢ with instructions to return promptly if the symptoms do not settle.

9.7

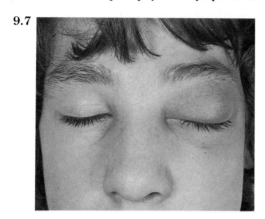

Fig. 9.7 Preseptal cellulitis

Orbital cellulitis

This is a more serious disease than preseptal cellulitis and requires emergency admission to hospital (*Fig. 9.8*). It is an infection of the orbital tissues behind the orbital septum and may arise by infection from the adjacent sinuses.

Symptoms and signs: Acute onset of painful proptosis, restriction of eye movement, chemosis, fever and malaise and sometimes visual impairment.

Management: Admit. Urgent nasal, conjunctival, ⓢ pharyngeal and blood cultures are taken and treatment with broad-spectrum, intravenous antibiotics commenced. Plain radiography may show sinus disease in which case an ENT opinion should be sought. If an orbital abscess develops, it must be drained. Cavernous sinus thrombosis is a potentially life-threatening complication of post-septal orbital cellulitis.

9.8

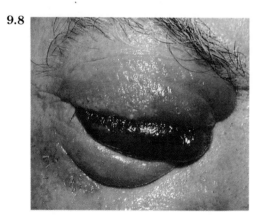

Fig. 9.8 Orbital cellulitis

Tumours of the orbit

These present as pain, proptosis, optic nerve compression and diplopia as mentioned previously. Sometimes there is rapid enlargement due to haemorrhage into the tumour. Orbital tumours are rare in childhood, when the types seen are:

- **Dermoids and epidermoid cysts** (see pp. 72–73, 240)

- **Capillary haemangioma** (see pp. 49, 240)

- **Optic nerve glioma**, which represents a hamartomatous malformation, rarely metastasising, more common in neurofibromatosis.

- **Rhabdomyosarcoma** (*Fig. 9.9*) , which may present as orbital cellulitis.

- **Neurofibroma**

- **Metastatic neuroblastoma**

- **Leukaemic infiltration**

Orbital tumours seen in adulthood include:

- **Cavernous haemangioma**, which is usually well encapsulated and may be removed by lateral orbitotomy.

- **Secondary tumours**, e.g. from bronchus, breast, kidney, prostate and gastrointestinal tract.

- **Lacrimal gland**

- **Meningioma**, e.g. sphenoid wing, which occurs in middle-aged women, is locally invasive and causes hyperostosis on the skull radiograph and optic nerve meningioma which is also slow-growing and locally invasive.

- **Lymphoma**

  The differential diagnosis includes thyroid eye disease and orbital pseudotumour.

9.9

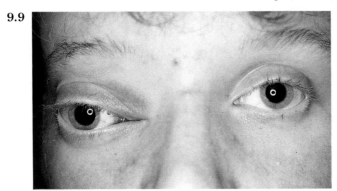

Fig. 9.9 Rhabdomyosarcoma on the right, showing deviation of the globe laterally and inferiorly in primary gaze (Courtesy of Mr. C. Dean Hart)

(S)*Management:* Urgent referral to a specialist eye centre for investigation and treatment. In the presence of proptosis, the cornea is at risk of exposure keratitis. If this is developing, frequent instillations of artificial tear drops, with lubricating ointment and closure of the eyelids by tape at night should be carried out without delay.

Orbital pseudotumour

This is an idiopathic inflammatory condition which can mimic a variety of orbital diseases depending on its site (*Fig. 9.10(a)–(c)*). It is often bilateral in children and unilateral in adults. It presents as a painful proptosis with restriction of ocular movements and an injected, chemosed eye. Other forms may present as lacrimal gland enlargement, myositis, or an orbital apex syndrome. Other inflammatory or neoplastic disorders should be excluded, e.g. sarcoidosis, tuberculosis, polyarteritis nodosa, Wegener's granulomatosis, orbital tumours, thyroid eye disease, lymphoma and other haematological proliferative diseases.

Management: Investigations are carried out to exclude other orbital diseases. A biopsy is performed to confirm the diagnosis before treatment is begun. This will show lymphocytic infiltration. Treatment is with high dose oral steroids. Radiotherapy is used in cases in which this is not effective.

9.10(a)

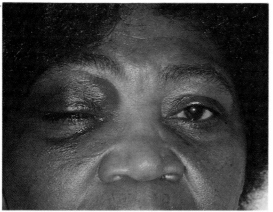

Fig. 9.10(a) Orbital pseudotumour – eventual diagnosis sarcoidosis

9.10(b)

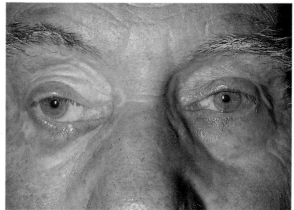

Fig. 9.10(b) Orbital pseudotumour – plus xanthelasma – in Wegener's granulomatosis

9.10(c)

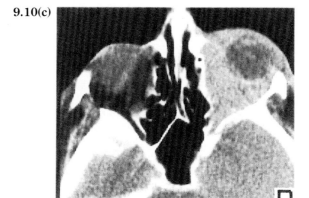

Fig. 9.10(c) CAT scan of another patient with (R) orbital pseudotumour

Orbital lymphoma

Orbital lymphoma can present in an identical fashion. Histology and systemic investigation will generally distinguish the two conditions. Treatment is with radio- and/or chemotherapy.

Ⓢ

Orbital varices

These present as a proptosis which is intermittent and can be induced by a Valsalva manoeuvre or compression of the external jugular vein on the side in question (*Fig. 9.11(a) & (b)*). Sometimes there is an external indicator – a dilated vein periorbitally, which similary fills on increasing venous pressure.

9.11(a)

9.11(b)

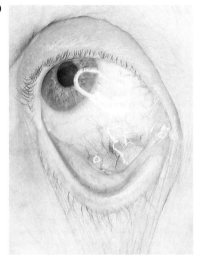

Fig. 9.11(a) Varix

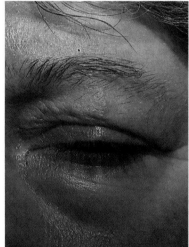

Fig. 9.11(b) Varix appearing as dilated vein on upper lid

Caroticocavernous fistula

This is a communication between the internal carotid artery and the venous blood in the cavernous sinus (*Fig. 9.12*). It is seen following severe head trauma, often after an interval (*see Fig. 12.23*). There is dilatation and tortuosity of the superficial conjunctival vessels due to raised venous pressure and a pulsatile proptosis with bruit.

9.12

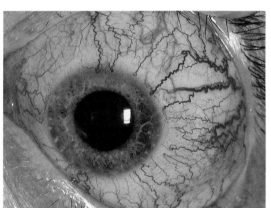

Fig. 9.12 Left caroticocavernous fistula (Courtesy of Institute of Ophthalmology)

Lacrimal gland tumour

This presents as a swelling in the lacrimal fossa (*Fig. 9.13(a) & (b)*). It may be an inflammatory disorder (v.s.), or a benign or malignant tumour. Features suggesting a malignant tumour include pain and localised bony
ⓢ destruction. Treatment consists of excision and/or radiotherapy if complete excision is not possible.

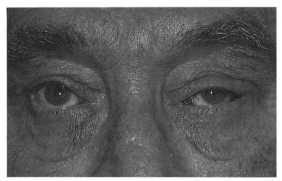

9.13(a)

Fig. 9.13(a) Lacrimal gland tumour (Courtesy of Mr. R. Humphry)

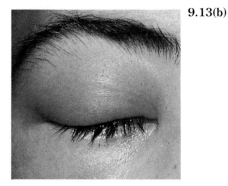

9.13(b)

Fig. 9.13(b) Dacryoadenitis – inflammation of the lacrimal gland

Medial wall lesions

Swellings of the medial orbital wall may be due to mucocoeles or carcinomas of the paranasal sinuses. Mucocoeles appear as smooth, bluish swellings arising from the supero-medial orbital margin. Radiography will demonstrate co-existent sinus disease.

Retrobulbar (orbital) haemorrhage

(see p. 224)

Disorders of the lacrimal system

Dry Eyes

(See pp. 96–98)

Tear drainage

(*See Fig. 5.35*)
Watery eyes may be due to **lacrimation**, a reflex hypersecretion of tears due to, e.g. corneal irritation, or to **epiphora**, in which there is failure of tear drainage. This may either be due to a blockage of the drainage system or malposition of the puncta or even failure of the lacrimal pump, formed by the action of orbicularis.

Epiphora

Symptoms: Painless, watery eye.

Signs: Dry eyes leading to reflex hypersecretion must be excluded. The puncta are examined for malposition and narrowness of opening. The inner canthus is palpated for masses that may lead to obstruction and to exclude a mucocoele, which is a mucus-filled, dilated lacrimal sac caused by nasolacrimal duct blockage, which exudes mucus from the punctum upon pressure.

The site of blockage is determined by inserting a lacrimal cannula into the lower canaliculus after local anaesthetic has been instilled. Punctal stenosis or canalicular blockage will quickly become evident. A 2ml, saline-filled syringe is connected to the cannula and the saline is injected. Regurgitation through the upper punctum signifies common canaliculus obstruction, whereas palpable expansion of the lacrimal sac indicates blockage of the nasolacrimal duct. Further investigations include dacryocystogram, which will demonstrate the site of blockage.

Management: Syringing the tear ducts may be sufficient ⓟ to relieve an obstruction. Further minor lid procedures ⓢ may be performed to enlarge a narrow punctum or repair a medial ectropion. A dacryocystorhinostomy is performed if the patient is very symptomatic and otherwise fit, since a general anaesthetic is preferable. This procedure creates an opening between the lacrimal sac and the lateral wall of the nose, bypassing a blocked nasolacrimal duct. Tubes may be left in to maintain patency of the system until the new passages have epithelialised.

Dacryocystitis

This is an infection of the lacrimal sac, usually associated with a blocked nasolacrimal duct (*9.14*).

Symptoms and Signs: Acute, red, tender, inflamed swelling below the inner canthus. Pus may regurgitate from the lower punctum on gentle pressure over the swelling.

ⓡ *Management:* Broad-spectrum antibiotics by mouth. If the infection does not settle, parenteral antibiotics may be necessary. Incision is not usually carried out because of the risk of later fistula formation. After the acute infection has settled a dacryorhinocystostomy is performed.

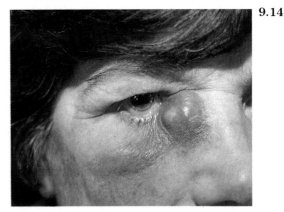

9.14

Fig. 9.14 Right dacryocystitis

PART II
SPECIALISED TOPICS

Key

Ⓟ Family Practitioner and Casualty Officer or Emergency Physician

Ⓡ Eye Casualty Officer or Resident in Ophthalmology

Ⓢ Ophthalmologist or Specialist

10 The eye in systemic disease

Diabetes mellitus

This is a systemic disorder of glucose metabolism whereby insufficient insulin is produced for the metabolic needs of the patient. There are two types, insulin dependent and non-insulin dependent, and ocular complications are seen in both types. These ocular complications are:

- **Intermittent blurring of vision**, which is due to alterations in lens shape and thus refraction owing to fluctuations of glucose levels and osmotic load.

- **Early cataract formation**. This may be an osmotic cataract that forms rapidly in poorly controlled diabetics or early onset, senile-type cataract.

- **Third nerve palsy (pupil-sparing)**, also fourth and sixth nerve palsies.

- **Retinopathy** – three types:

(a) **Background diabetic retinopathy** (*Fig. 10.1*) – dot and blot haemorrhages, microaneurysms, small exudates, cotton wool spots (see pp. 142–43)
(b) **Diabetic maculopathy** – ischaemic changes, oedema and exudate formation at the macula
(c) **Proliferative retinopathy** (*Fig. 10.2(a) & (b)* – disc new vessels, new vessels elsewhere often along the temporal arcades of blood vessels, vitreous haemorrhage, and in advanced stages, tractional retinal detachment

- **Optic neuritis and atrophy** (rare)

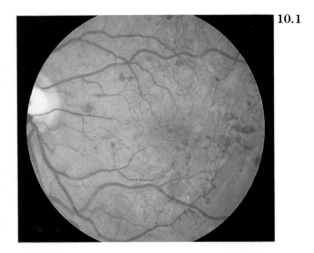

10.1

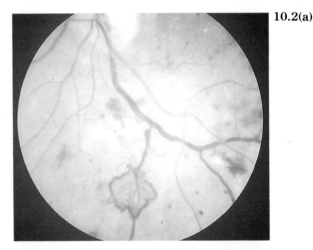

10.2(a)

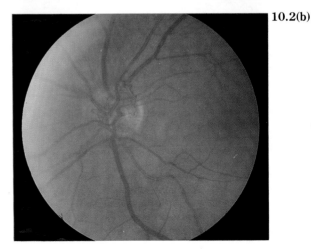

10.2(b)

Fig. 10.1 Background diabetic retinopathy
Fig. 10.2(a) & (b) Proliferative retinopathy – **(a)** new vessels in the periphery, **(b)** disc new vessels

- **Central and branch vein or artery occlusion** (*Fig. 10.3*)

- **Rubeosis iridis** (*Fig. 10.4*) (proliferation of iris blood vessels, often seen initially as a pupillary frill). May lead to rubeotic glaucoma.

10.3

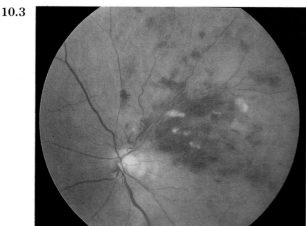

Fig. 10.3 Branch vein occlusion

10.4

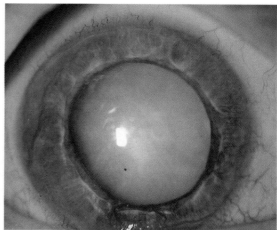

Fig. 10.4 Rubeosis iridis

Diabetic retinopathy

Diabetic retinopathy is the most common cause of blindness between the ages of 20 and 65 years. Diabetics should have regular fundal examination for retinopathy (with dilating drops) by the specialist looking after the diabetes, and referred for treatment to an ophthalmologist when any worrying signs develop. It is beyond the scope of this book to describe features to look for in routine follow-up, however one important situation encountered in eye casualty is:

ⓡ Sudden unilateral loss of vision

- **Vitreous haemorrhage** is one of the most common causes, especially in diabetics with known neovascularisation. This often occurs during the night or after exertion. It causes a rosy haze over the vision and often profound loss of vision. The fundal view is hazy with almost no fundal detail discernible. In patients with known proliferative diabetic retinopathy and previous vitreous haemorrhage, once the diagnosis is made, the patient is advised to rest in bed for a few days, sleeping semi-upright to allow the haemorrhage to settle. Once the haemorrhage has settled, fundoscopy should be performed by an ophthalmologist to determine the site of bleeding and to carry out treatment (laser photocoagulation) at some convenient stage. Sometimes vitreous haemorrhages may take weeks to clear. If there is no history of proliferative retinopathy, the patient should be referred immediately as there is a chance the vitreous haemorrhage has another cause (e.g. retinal tear), unrelated to the diabetes.

- **Central retinal vein thrombosis** (see p. 154) or **branch retinal vein occlusion** affecting the macula region (see p. 156), **central retinal artery occlusion**

- **Unilateral cataract** unrealised previously.

- **Diabetic maculopathy**

- **Other causes not particularly related to diabetes**, e.g. optic neuritis, disciform macular degeneration and so on.

Hypertension

Hypertension may present in an eye casualty as central or branch retinal vein occlusion or retinal artery occlusion, or on routine fundoscopy. The ocular findings are graded according to severity:

I Mild, generalised and focal arteriolar constriction with altered light reflex. Mild to moderate hypertension. Appearances also in arteriosclerosis without hypertension.

II 'AV nipping' whereby the column of venous blood appears to be attenuated at an arterial crossing point by the abnormal arteriole. Increased arteriolar constriction and occasional small haemorrhage and exudate. Moderate hypertension.

III Flame-shaped haemorrhages (haemorrhages in the nerve fibre layer), retinal oedema and cotton wool spots (infarcts in the nerve fibre layer) signify severe, often accelerated hypertension. Life expectancy approximately two years from diagnosis. Similar appearances in severe anaemia, hyperviscosity states, leukaemia, diabetes mellitus and subacute bacterial endocarditis.

IV III plus disc swelling indicates malignant hypertension (*Fig. 10.5(a) & (b)*). If prolonged, there is often hard exudate formation at the macula (macula star). Life expectancy approximately 10 months from diagnosis.

10.5(a)

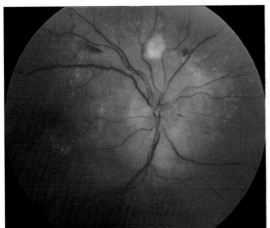

10.5(b)

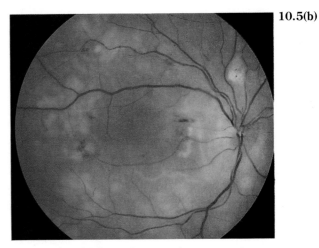

Fig. 10.5(a) Malignant hypertension showing cotton wool spots, haemorrhages, exudates, disc swelling and choroidal infarcts

Fig. 10.5(b) Malignant hypertension – same patient as **Fig. 10.5(a)** – showing choroidal infarcts

Table 1 Ocular disease associated with systemic disease

Systemic disease	Ocular manifestations
Systemic infections	
Cytomegalic inclusion disease	Acquired – retinitis with necrosis, haemorrhages, vascular sheathing, retinal destruction Congenital – cataract, uveitis, microphthalmos, anophthalmos, uveitis, optic nerve hypoplasia, chorioretinitis
Measles	Focal macular chorioretinitis, papilloedema, optic atrophy, nystagmus, cortical blindness
Rubella	Congenital syndrome – cataracts, microphthalmos, 'salt and pepper' retinopathy around macula
Acquired immunodeficiency syndrome	Retina – cotton wool spots, flame-shaped haemorrhages, vascular sheathing, Kaposi's sarcoma of lid or conjunctiva, Cytomegalovirus retinitis
Syphilis	Acquired – iris vascular inflammatory response, papules and gummas. Localised or diffuse chorioretinitis Congenital – interstitial keratitis, 'salt and pepper' retinopathy, uveitis, Argyll–Robertson pupils, optic atrophy
Histoplasmosis	Presumed ocular histoplasmosis syndrome – multifocal choroidal scars, peripapillary chorioretinal atrophy, haemorrhagic disciform maculopathy, linear streaks of chorioretinal atrophy
Candidiasis	Chorioretinitis, focal vitreous exudates
Toxoplasmosis	Acquired – rare Congenital – necrotising focal chorioretinitis, vitritis, optic neuritis, anterior uveitis
Toxocariasis	Chronic, destructive endophthalmitis (children 2–9 years), localised posterior pole or peripheral granuloma
Systemic granulomas	
Sarcoidosis	Acute and chronic anterior uveitis (secondary cataract, glaucoma, band keratopathy), lacrimal gland involvement, conjunctival granulomas, retinopathy (periphlebitis, neovascularisation, 'candle wax' exudates, vitreous haze, choroidal granulomas, optic neuritis)
Tuberculosis	Anterior uveitis, choroiditis
Connective tissue disorders	
Rheumatoid arthritis	Keratoconjunctivitis sicca (KCS), peripheral corneal melting syndrome, nodular, diffuse or necrotising scleritis
Systemic lupus erythematosus	Skin eruption involving lids, KCS, peripheral corneal melting syndrome, necrotising scleritis, hypertensive retinopathy
Polyarteritis nodosa	Necrotising sclerokeratitis, choroiditis, ischaemic optic neuropathy
Wegener's granulomatosis	Nodular or diffuse scleritis, marginal corneal infiltrates, obstruction of nasolacrimal duct, uveitis, retinopathy (cotton wool spots, haemorrhages and oedema)
Seronegative arthritides	
Ankylosing spondylitis	Acute anterior uveitis
Reiter's disease	Conjunctivitis, keratitis, acute anterior uveitis
Psoriatic arthritis	Conjunctivitis, acute anterior uveitis, KCS
Behçet's Disease	Anterior uveitis, conjunctivitis, retinal vasculitis, massive retinal exudation, retinal vessel vasodilation
Juvenile chronic arthritis	Chronic iridocyclitis, secondary cataract, band keratopathy
Metabolic disease	
Galactosaemia	Infantile cataract
Fabry's disease	Cornea verticillata, spoke-like lens opacities
Hypercalcaemia	White, subepithelial deposit of calcium as band in cornea
Wilson's disease (*Fig. 10.6*)	Kayser-Fleischer ring in cornea, sunflower cataract
Cystinosis	Corneal crystalline deposits
Mucopolysaccharidoses	Corneal opacification, retinal pigmentary degeneration, optic atrophy

Table 1 cont.

Systemic disease	Ocular manifestations
Diseases of the skin	
Acne rosacea	Keratitis with vascularisation and corneal thinning, blepharo conjunctivitis
Contact dermatitis	Involvement of lids or cheek, following cosmetics or therapeutic drops
Atopic dermatitis	Blepharitis, keratoconjunctivitis, vernal catarrh, keratoconus, anterior subcapsular cataracts
Cicatricial pemphigoid	Conjunctival shrinkage
Stevens-Johnson syndrome	Bullous conjunctivitis, with occasional secondary infection
Pseudoxanthoma elasticum	Angioid streaks (cracks in Bruch's membrane), macular disease
Blood dyscrasias	
Anaemias	Retinal haemorrhages with white centre (Roth's spots), cotton wool spots
Leukaemias	Posterior polar retinal haemorrhages (Roth's spots), vascular sheathing, neovascularisation, orbital involvement in children, optic nerve infiltration, acute iritis, hyphaema
Haemoglobinopathies (Fig. 10.7)	SC and SThal diseases associated with most severe retinopathy – peripheral arteriolar occlusion and arteriovenous anastamosis, neovascularisation, vitreous haemorrhage, traction, retinal detachment
Hyperviscosity syndrome	Dilation and tortuosity of veins, superficial and deep haemorrhages, cotton wool spots, central vein occlusion
Infectious mononucleosis	Follicular or membranous conjunctivitis, subconjunctival haemorrhage, nummular keratitis, episcleritis, uveitis, retinal oedema, papillitis
Thyroid dysfunction	
Graves' disease	Lid retraction, infiltrative ophthalmopathy producing exophthalmos, optic
Toxic goitre	neuropathy, exposure keratitis
Thyroiditis	

10.6

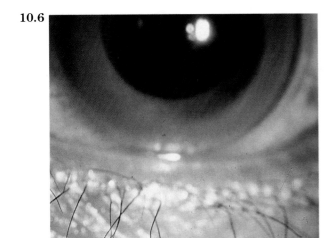

Fig. 10.6 Kayser-Fleischer ring in Wilson's disease

10.7

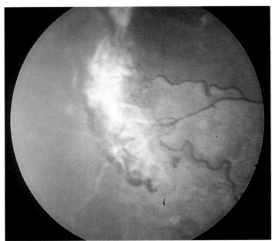

Fig. 10.7 Sickle cell-thalassaemia retinopathy showing proliferative changes in the periphery

Sarcoidosis

This is a granulomatous disorder of unknown aetiology that commonly causes bilateral hilar lymphadenopathy and lung fibrosis. The ocular manifestations include:

• **Uveitis** (see pp. 104–11), often associated with mutton-fat keratic precipitates, retinal vein periphlebitis and chorioretinitis. Also disc and retinal granulomata.

• **Nodules in the lids and episclera**

• **Inflammation of lacrimal gland**

Syphilis

Congenital syphilis gives rise to ophthalmia neonatorum, often associated with a nasal, mucopurulent discharge and interstitial keratitis. This keratitis is associated with vascularisation of the cornea which does not become manifest until the age of 5–25 years, gives rise to a 'salmon patch' on the cornea and subsequently resolves to leave ghost vessels. Other ocular manifestations include chorioretinitis, 'salt and pepper' appearance, or retinitis pigmentosa-like pigment spicules, congenital cataract and iritis.

Acquired syphilis causes iritis, iris nodules and vascular loops, chorioretinitis with appearances similar to retinitis pigmentosa, optic neuritis and pupillary abnormalities, e.g. Argyll Robertson pupil.

Neurofibromatosis

Neurofibromatosis (Von Recklinghausen's disease) is one of a group of disorders called phakomatoses which also includes tuberose sclerosis, Sturge–Weber syndrome and others. It is dominantly inherited. The ocular manifestations include:

• lid neurofibromas (see p.42) – hamartomas, which are localised or diffuse, e.g. a plexiform neurofibroma which resembles a 'bag of worms' on palpation. When they involve the upper lid they may give rise to a mechanical ptosis and a characteristic S-shaped deformity of the upper lid. If they develop in childhood, there is a danger of amblyopia, if the visual axis is impeded.

• iris nodules (melanocytic naevi)

• glaucoma, often in association with plexiform neurofibromas and facial hemiatrophy

• choroidal naevi and, more rarely, retinal astrocytomas (also seen in tuberose sclerosis)

• proptosis, which may be pulsating in the case of bony defects in the greater wing of the sphenoid, orbital tumours, e.g. plexiform neurofibroma, neurilemmoma; optic nerve glioma and meningioma.

The diagnosis is made on associated manifestations elsewhere in the body:

• café au lait spots (*Fig. 10.8*) and axillary freckling (greater than five is supposed to be diagnostic)

• peripheral skin fibromas and neurofibromas – these may later undergo sarcomatous change

• tumours of the central nervous system, e.g. dumbbell neurofibromas, gliomas, meningiomas

• internal tumours, e.g. phaeochromocytomas

• bone defects

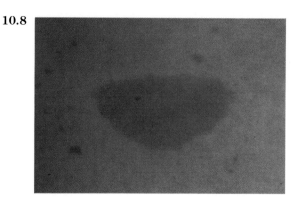

10.8

Fig. 10.8 Café au lait patch in neurofibromatosis

11 Neuro-ophthalmology

Pupils

Normally the pupils are symmetrical and react briskly to light and accommodation.

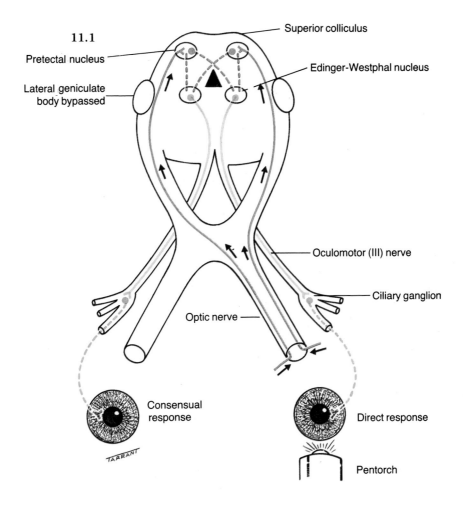

Fig. 11.1 Pathway for light reaction

Pathway for light reaction

See Fig 11.1

● **First neuron** – travels from the retina to the pretectal nucleus in the midbrain via the optic nerve. Nasal retinal fibres cross in the chiasm and reach the contralateral nucleus. Temporal fibres pass to the ipsilateral nucleus.

● **Second neuron** – passes from each pretectal nucleus to both the ipsilateral and contralateral Edinger-Westphal nuclei (parasympathetic nuclei associated with the III cranial nerve).

- **Third neuron** – travels with the oculomotor nerve (III nerve) to the ciliary ganglion. Since pupillomotor fibres are relatively superficial in the nerve between midbrain and cavernous sinus, they are vulnerable to compression, e.g. by aneurysms. Leaving the cavernous sinus, the pupillomotor fibres are deeper and may be spared in compressive lesions.

- **Fourth neuron** – passes from the ciliary ganglion to innervate the sphincter pupillae via the short ciliary nerves.

Near reaction

This involves synchronous convergence, pupil constriction and accommodation. The exact centre for near reaction is not known; the final pathway is identical to the light reaction third and fourth neurons (above). A lesion causing light-near dissociation, which leaves accommodation intact but light reaction defective, probably lies in the dorsal midbrain (at the site of the second neuron). Cases are rare and may occur in neurosyphilis (Argyll Robertson pupil) and pinealoma.

Pupillary abnormalities

Simple (physiological) anisocoria

About 20–25% of normal individuals have asymmetric pupil size with differences of up to 3 mm. Sometimes even the side may alternate. Often it is suddenly noticed, but can be shown to have been there for longer than is imagined if old photographs are consulted. Physiological anisocoria is maintained in all levels of illumination (unlike both Horner's, which is more pronounced in low levels of illumination, and III nerve palsy anisocoria, which is more pronounced in bright light (*see Fig. 11.2(b)*) and the pupil is round, regular and briskly reactive to light and accommodation. The pupil also responds readily to constricting and dilating drops. No further investigation is required.

Adie pupil

This benign cause of anisocoria (*Fig. 11.2(a)*) is common and mainly affects women in their 20s to 40s. It is unilateral at onset in 90% of cases. The affected pupil is a 'tonic' pupil which is virtually unresponsive to light and slowly reactive to accommodation. The lesion is located in the ciliary ganglion, thus affecting the response to both light and near stimulus. Direct trauma (orbital surgery) and viral infection may be responsible in some cases.

11.2(a)

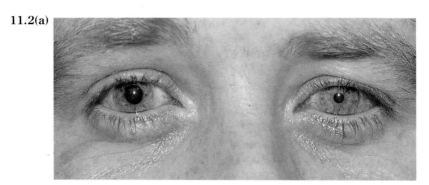

Fig. 11.2(a) Right Adie pupil (Courtesy of Mr. R. Humphry)

Symptoms: The patient or relatives notice one larger pupil. Occasionally the patient experiences difficulty in accommodation.

Signs: In bright illumination the Adie pupil is larger than its fellow; in low illumination it may be smaller as it takes time to dilate. The pupillary border undergoes worm-like or 'vermiform' movements as small segments contract normally (seen well under slit lamp illumination). It is often associated with absent knee and ankle reflexes – the Holmes–Adie syndrome.

Test: Instil a drop of 0.125% pilocarpine (mix one drop of 1% pilocarpine with 7 drops of sterile saline) into both eyes. The Adie pupil will constrict briskly owing to denervation supersensitivity and the normal pupil will show no reaction.

Management: Usually no treatment is required. On ⓢ occasions when good cosmesis is needed, e.g. for photographs, a drop of 0.125% pilocarpine may be used beforehand or, if good accommodation is needed, the drops may be used t.d.s. With time, the anisocoria becomes less marked as the pupil becomes miosed and may need to be differentiated from a Horner's syndrome (see pp. 186–87). In the acute stages it needs to be differentiated from a third nerve palsy (see pp. 192–93).

11.2(b)

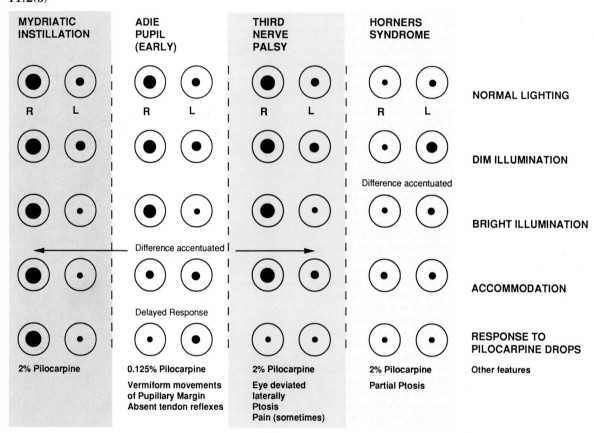

In each case the pupillary abnormality is shown in the Right Eye.

Fig. 11.2(b) Table of four common causes of anisocoria and their differential diagnosis

Other causes of light-near dissociation:

• **Argyll Robertson Pupils** seen in tertiary neuro-syphilis are small, irregular and asymmetrical pupils. They react poorly to light, with an intact near response in the presence of adequate visual acuity. They are usually bilateral. Argyll Robertson pupils are miosed in dark illumination in contrast to other causes of light-near dissociation, e.g. Adie pupils, midbrain pupils and amaurotic pupils, which are not miosed. The possible site of the lesion is at the neurons connecting the pretectal and Edinger–Westphal nuclei. Syphilis serology: VDRL, TPHA, and FTA and cerebrospinal fluid examination may be required to determine if treatment is necessary.

• **Midbrain** lesions, e.g. pinealomas, lead to light-near dissociated pupils which are larger than normal and sometimes eccentric. They may be associated with impaired upgaze and convergence-retraction nystagmus.

• **Amaurotic pupils** are caused by optic nerve lesions where there will obviously be no light reflex, but there is an intact near response.

Horner's syndrome

This syndrome is due to a loss of sympathetic innervation to the eye (*Fig. 11.3*).

Symptoms: The patient or their family usually notice the drooping lid.

Signs: The classical signs are:

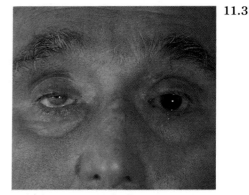

11.3

Fig. 11.3 Horner's syndrome

• **Ptosis**. This is partial rather than total and is due to loss of innervation to the sympathetic part of levator palpebrae superioris (also called Müller's muscle)

• **Miosis**. The affected pupil is smaller than the other, owing to lack of sympathetic innervation to the dilator fibres of the iris sphincter, but it constricts normally. The difference in pupil size may be only 0.5–1.0 mm, but it is more pronounced in dim illumination.

• **Enophthalmos**. This is more apparent than real, owing to narrowing of the palpebral fissure.

• **Skin changes**, e.g. warm, dry, flushed skin of the ipsilateral face. This is usually transient.

• **Heterochromia iridis**. This usually only occurs with Horner's syndrome that is congenital or acquired in the infantile period.

Differential diagnosis: Simple anisocoria, congenital ptosis, myasthenia gravis.

(S) *Investigations:* Once the provisional diagnosis has been made, prompt referral to a neurologist or neuro-ophthalmologist is necessary for urgent investigation.

Confirmation of the diagnosis of Horner's syndrome may be made by instillation of 4% cocaine drops into both eyes, repeated one minute later. The **normal** pupil will dilate, but the Horner's pupil will not. Cocaine acts to block reuptake of noradrenaline at the synaptic cleft. Thus, if there is no noradrenaline production, the pupil will not dilate.

Pre-ganglionic and post-ganglionic lesions may be distinguished by the use of hydroxy-amphetamine 1% drops. A pupil with a **pre-ganglionic** (first or second order neuron) lesion will dilate, whereas a **post-ganglionic** Horner's pupil will not. Hydroxyamphetamine releases packets of noradrenaline from an intact post-ganglionic neuron.

• If the cocaine test has been used, it is necessary to wait 48 hours before the hydroxyamphetamine test can be carried out.

- There is no pharmacological test that distinguishes between a first or second order pre-ganglionic lesion. Clinically, the first order neuron lesion will be associated with brainstem signs and the second order neuron lesion with spinal cord or lung apex signs.

Initial investigations include chest radiograph (to exclude a Pancoast lesion – apical bronchial carcinoma), cervical spine series and head CAT scan.

Anatomy of the sympathetic innervation of the eye

See Fig. 11.4

- **Neuron 1** arises in the posterior hypothalamus and descends the lateral brain stem, adjacent to the lateral lemniscus and medial to the spinothalamic tract in the cervical cord, to synapse in the ciliospinal centre of Budge at the level of C8-T2.

- **Neuron 2** exits the cervical cord via the ventral root and ascends to synapse in the superior cervical ganglion, passing in close relation to the apex of the lung and the subclavian artery.

- **Neuron 3**, the 'post-ganglionic neuron', travels as a plexus on the common, then internal carotid artery. It has a short extracranial course and then enters the skull, passing via the cavernous sinus, where the fibres leave the carotid artery, to join the nasociliary

branch of the ophthalmic division of the trigeminal nerve. The long ciliary nerves convey the final fibres to the iris. The sympathetic innervation to the skin of the face travels up the external carotid artery. Thus, if sweating is affected, the lesion is located as being pre-ganglionic.

The lesion may occur anywhere along the sympathetic pathway from the hypothalamus to the eye. More common causes include: brainstem ischaemia in the elderly, giving rise to a lateral medullary syndrome and involving neuron 1; malignancy involving the cervico-thoracic spine or lung apex, which affects the second 'pre-ganglionic' neuron; and trauma to the neck giving rise to secondary common or internal carotid artery dissection.

11.4

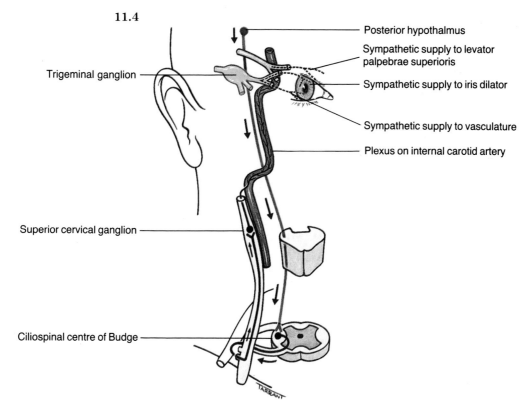

Fig. 11.4 Anatomy of sympathetic innervation to the eye

⑤ Ocular assessment of the unconscious patient

The doctor may be called upon to assess the ocular status of an unconscious patient either with regard to neurological signs or development of ocular pathology, e.g. exposure keratitis.

Caution: Do not use mydriatics to examine the fundus in this instance as the pupil responses will be impossible to assess subsequently.

Care of the eye in the unconscious patient

Corneal exposure can occur in the unconscious patient, resulting in damage to the epithelium with its risk of infection and corneal abscess formation. The management includes regular culture for organisms, antibiotic cover, lid taping and/or goggles.

Neuro-ophthalmological assessment

Pupillary reactions are of vital importance, and size of the pupils may indicate the site of the lesion. Pinpoint pupils are seen in pontine or some cerebellar lesions and mid-dilated pupils are seen in midbrain lesions. In drug overdose or metabolic coma the pupils are usually small, but reactive to light. In the endstages of metabolic coma the pupils may become dilated which is a poor prognostic sign. Unequal pupils are important – the non-reactive pupil is the pathological one. The fixed, dilated pupil implies a third nerve lesion, or drug instillation, for example for fundal examination (see below). Beware a few pitfalls – glaucoma treatment with pilocarpine leads to a miosed pupil; previous cataract surgery may lead to an enlarged, poorly-reactive pupil (with normal consensual response); anterior uveitis may lead to anterior synechiae formation; and local trauma to the eye may cause traumatic mydriasis.

Extraocular movements are also helpful. Oculocephalic (doll's head) and caloric responses indicate the level of the lesion. The doll's head reflex is elicited by rapid, passive movement of the head to one side (or vertically), (not carried out if neck pathology is suspected). The eyes move in the opposite direction if the pontine gaze mechanisms are intact. Caloric testing is performed by tilting the patient's head 30° to the horizontal and syringing cold water into the external auditory canal (not performed if there is otorrhoea). A slow, tonic deviation is seen towards the side of the irrigation and the fast phase of nystagmus away from that side (COWS – Cold Opposite, Warm Same) if the pontine gaze mechanisms are intact.

The fixed, dilated pupil

This is an important physical sign which may present in life-threatening situations to many clinicians. It is due to an interruption in the efferent pupillary response either in the third nerve or through paralysis of the pupil itself (mydriatic agents), leading to **an absence of direct light and near response, but a preservation of consensual response.**

The fixed, dilated pupil in the unconscious patient

Until proved otherwise, the unconscious patient who suddenly develops a fixed, dilated pupil has a third nerve lesion due to temporal lobe herniation and requires urgent neurological assessment and a brain CAT scan. The pilocarpine test described below may be helpful in excluding a pharmacological cause. In optic nerve lesions, e.g. following orbital trauma, even in those severe enough to sever totally the optic nerve on one side, the pupil sizes will be **equal** due to afferent input from the other eye and an intact efferent pathway to both eyes. It is only by carefully testing for an afferent defect that optic nerve damage will be discovered.

The fixed, dilated pupil in the conscious patient

In an otherwise well patient with an isolated, fixed, dilated pupil, but no history of trauma or previous ocular disease, the differential diagnosis is between: third nerve palsy (see pp. 192–93), which requires immediate referral to a neurosurgical unit for brain CAT scan, angiography and so on; Adie pupil (see pp. 184–85); and mydriatic instillation. If none of the associated features of third nerve palsy (limitation of extraocular movement, ptosis) or Adie pupil is present, accidental or deliberate instillation of dilating agents is possible. Common agents include atropine, certain plant products containing bella-donna or similar alkaloids, and some cosmetics or perfumes. This is more common in medical personnel. A useful diagnostic adjunct, the pilocarpine test, is described below. Transient mydriasis, sometimes unilateral, is also seen in the post-ictal phase in epileptics.

Test: Instillation of **1% pilocarpine** to both eyes will cause rapid constriction of the normal pupil and the abnormal pupil, dilated due to a third nerve lesion or an Adie pupil, but **not if mydriatics have been instilled**. This is extremely important in the unconscious patient who may have received a dose of atropine during anaesthesia, which has long since been forgotten.

Disorders of extraocular movement
Principles of identifying extraocular muscle dysfunction

11.5

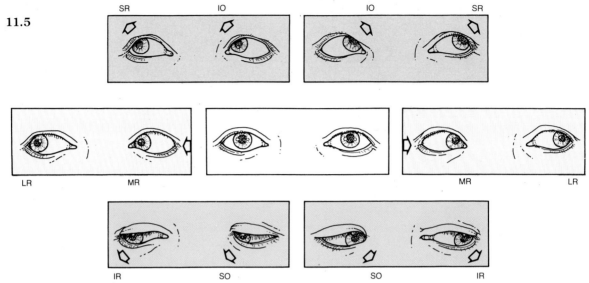

Fig. 11.5 Extraocular movements. SR – superior rectus, IR – inferior rectus, LR – lateral rectus, MR – medial rectus, IO – inferior oblique, SO – superior oblique

● In order to test individual muscle function (*Fig. 11.5*), the maximal line of action of that muscle must be known and any secondary action eliminated.

● The four rectus muscles are inserted in front of the equator and run parallel to the line of the orbit, which is at 23° to the optical axis.

● The **primary position of gaze** refers to the eye looking directly to the front.

● The horizontal recti move the eye medially (medial rectus) and laterally (lateral rectus) from the primary position of gaze around the vertical axis.

● The superior rectus elevates the eye in the abducted position (maximally at 23° to the primary position) and this is its **line of maximal action**. The inferior rectus depresses the eye in the same abducted position.

● The oblique muscles are inserted behind the equator and at 51° to the optical axis in the primary position. Their lines of maximal action are thus with the eye adducted (by 51°), when the superior oblique acts as a pure depressor and the inferior oblique as a pure elevator. The description of the superior oblique as the 'down and out' muscle refers to the actions from the primary position of gaze and is confusing.

● Thus, six positions of gaze are all that are required to test the individual muscles of extraocular movement:
1 Horizontal movement to the right – R. LR and L. MR
2 Horizontal movement to the left – R. MR and L. LR
3 Dextroelevation   – R. SR and L. IO
4 Dextrodepression   – R. IR and L. SO
5 Laevoelevation   – R. IO and L. SR
6 Laevodepression   – R. SO and L. IR

There is no need to test, e.g. elevation in the primary position. It is best to use an 'H'- shaped scheme for testing ocular muscle function, via the six diagnostic positions of gaze shown above.

Diplopia is horizontal when the medial and lateral recti are involved and is vertical when the obliques and superior or inferior recti are affected. It is experienced maximally in the direction of the maximal line of action of the affected muscle. The image which is farther away is that coming from the eye with the defective muscle (determined by covering each eye in turn). Red–green goggles, which have one red lens and one green lens, are of great assistance in determining the eye which is seeing a particular image, making the two images easier to differentiate. If horizontal diplopia is experienced, this suggests a lateral rectus palsy (since an isolated, medial rectus palsy would be extremely unusual). If a head tilt is adopted, it is most commonly due to a superior oblique palsy.

A **Hess** chart or Lees screen (*Fig. 11.6, see also Fig. 11.13*) is extremely useful in demonstrating the underacting muscle, usually with corresponding over-action of the paired yoke muscle of the opposite eye. The two eyes of the patient are dissociated using a mirror with the Lees screen or red–green goggles with the Hess chart. They may also be used to monitor progress of a muscle palsy.

Disorders of extraocular movement may be divided into:

- Supranuclear
- Cranial nerve palsies III, IV and VI
- Myasthenia gravis
- Myopathies

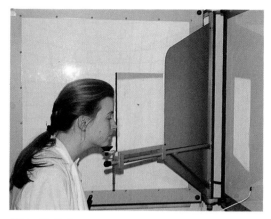

Fig. 11.6 Lees screen

Supranuclear

Horizontal gaze palsy: There are two types of horizontal, conjugate (both eyes moving in the same direction) eye movements, these being smooth pursuit and saccades. Smooth pursuits are slow, steady movements of both eyes, usually to follow a slowly moving target. Pursuit movements to a particular side are controlled by the ipsilateral occipital cortex. Saccades are rapid, fixational eye movements, some-times in response to an object of interest in the peripheral field of view to gain central fixation, or in response to a command, e.g. "look to the left". Fibres from the contralateral frontal cortex control saccadic movements to a given side. Thus, an irritative lesion in the right frontal cortex will give rise to deviation of the eyes to the left.

Both types of horizontal eye movements are mediated through the horizontal gaze centre in the pontine paramedian reticular formation and thence to the ipsilateral sixth nerve nucleus and the contralateral third nerve nucleus. These are connected via the medial longitudinal fasciculus (MLF). A lesion of the MLF will cause defective adduction to the ipsilateral side associated with nystagmus on abduction on the contralateral side – internuclear ophthalmoplegia. Unilateral lesions are usually due to brainstem vascular lesions, while bilateral lesions are usually due to multiple sclerosis.

Vertical gaze palsy (*Fig. 11.7*): This is due to lesion in the pretectal region of midbrain which sends information to the third and fourth nerve nuclei, controlling vertical muscle movements. It leads to defective upgaze, light-near dissociation and convergence-retraction nystagmus.

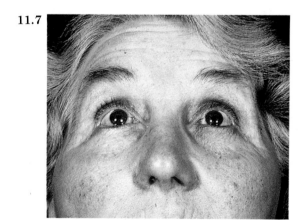

Fig. 11.7 Patient with vertical gaze palsy attempting upgaze (Courtesy of Mr. C. Dean Hart)

Cranial nerve palsies III, IV and VI

Third (oculomotor) nerve palsy

See Figs. 11.8–11.10

Anatomy (Fig. 11.8): The third nerve arises in the midbrain at the level of the superior colliculus as a cluster of nuclei anterior to the aqueduct. There is a single midline nucleus for both levator palpebrae superioris, thus a nuclear third nerve lesion causes bilateral ptosis. Superior rectus is innervated from contralateral nucleus and medial and inferior rectus, together with inferior oblique, from ipsilateral nuclei. Efferent fibres pass anteriorly out from the midbrain, closely related to the posterior cerebral and superior cerebellar artery and posterior communicating artery, and traverse the base of the skull over the tentorial edge to the cavernous sinus. Here the third nerve passes through the lateral part of the cavernous sinus, with the internal carotid artery lying medial to it, and enters the orbit through the superior orbital fissure, when it divides into superior and inferior branches. The superior branch supplies levator palpebrae superi-

oris and superior rectus, whilst the inferior branch supplies medial rectus, inferior rectus and inferior oblique and contains the parasympathetic pupillomotor supply.

The **pupillomotor fibres** lie in a vulnerable, superficial position in the third nerve before it reaches the cavernous sinus. Thus compressive lesions, e.g. posterior communicating artery aneurysms, will cause a complete third nerve palsy without sparing the pupil. The pupillomotor fibres have a different blood supply from the rest of the third nerve via the pial vasculature and may be spared if the main supply is involved in a microangiopathic process, e.g. in diabetes the so-called 'medical' or pupil-sparing third nerve palsy. After the cavernous sinus, surgical compressive lesions may also be pupil-sparing owing to the deeper position of the pupillomotor fibres.

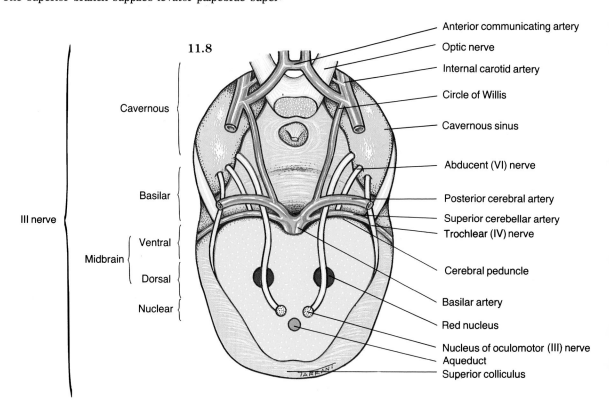

Fig. 11.8 Anatomy of the third cranial nerve

Symptoms: Ptosis, diplopia (when eyelid is lifted), poor accommodation.

Signs: Almost complete ptosis due to paralysis of levator palpebrae superioris (except sympathetic part), the eye is deviated outwards and on attempted down-gaze is seen to intort owing to the intact superior oblique muscle. There is failure of elevation, adduction and depression. The pupil may be dilated with no direct light or accommodation response, but an intact consensual response to light.

11.9

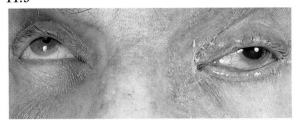

Fig. 11.9 Left third nerve palsy patient looking up (Courtesy of Mr. C. Dean Hart)

11.10

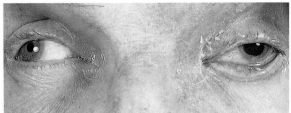

Fig. 11.10 Left third nerve palsy patient looking to the right (Courtesy of Mr. C. Dean Hart)

Fourth (trochlear) nerve palsy

See Figs. 11.11–11.13

Anatomy (Fig. 11.11): The fourth nerve arises in the midbrain nucleus as a caudal continuation of the third nerve nucleus, level with the inferior colliculus. It decussates posteriorly, leaves the brainstem from the dorsal aspect and winds around the brainstem beneath the free edge of the tentorium cerebelli. It has a long intracranial course, making it vulnerable to traumatic damage. It passes through the cavernous sinus and the superior orbital fissure to enter the orbit outside the muscle cone and supply the superior oblique.

11.11

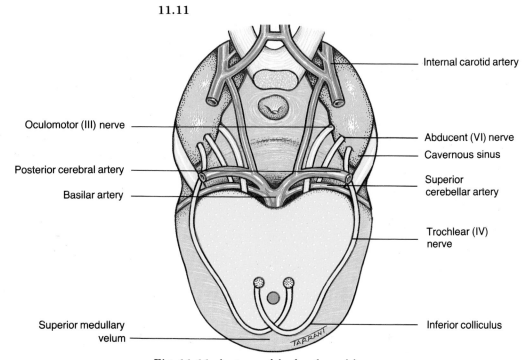

Fig. 11.11 Anatomy of the fourth cranial nerve

Symptoms: Diplopia or difficulty reading and walking downstairs.

Signs: Head tilt away from the side of the lesion to compensate for the torsional effect of the fourth nerve palsy. There is impaired depression of the affected eye in adduction. If the head is tilted **towards** the side of the lesion, marked elevation of the affected eye is seen (positive Bielschowsky test). This is due to attempted intorsion of the affected eye to compensate for the abnormal head posture. Since the superior oblique cannot accomplish this, the secondary intorter, the superior rectus on that side, contracts. Since this muscle is much more effective at elevation than intorsion, the eye is seen to shoot upwards.

11.12

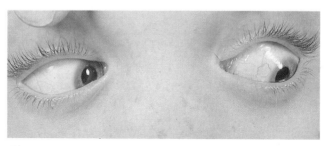

Fig. 11.12 Right fourth nerve palsy, best shown with patient looking down and to the left (Courtesy of Orthoptic Department, Bristol Eye Hospital)

11.13

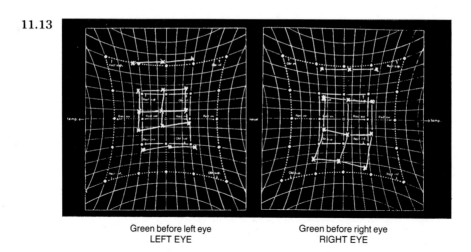

Green before left eye
LEFT EYE

Green before right eye
RIGHT EYE

Fig. 11.13 Left fourth nerve palsy – Hess chart showing underaction of left superior oblique, compensating overaction of right inferior rectus, contracture (overaction) of left inferior oblique, and corresponding underaction of right superior rectus

Sixth (abducent) nerve palsy

See Figs. 11.14–11.16

Anatomy: The sixth nerve arises from a nucleus in the mid-pons, around which the seventh nerve courses. It exits from the pontomedullary junction and courses forwards, ventral to the pons, where it may be involved in a base of skull fracture. It passes to the petrous tip of the temporal bone where it may be damaged in raised intracranial pressure because, as the brainstem descends, the nerve is stretched over the petrous tip. It then passes under the petroclinoid ligament and enters the cavernous sinus. Positioned in the middle of the sinus close to the carotid artery, it is here more vulnerable than the third and fourth nerves to involvement in cavernous sinus thrombosis. It enters the orbit through the superior orbital fissure to supply the lateral rectus.

Symptoms: Diplopia on lateral gaze.

Signs: Defective abduction of the eye.

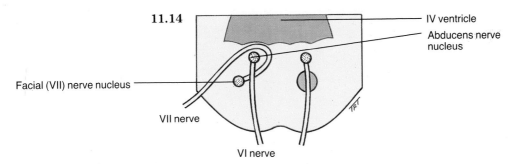

Fig. 11.14 Anatomy of the sixth cranial nerve

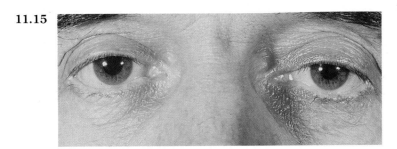

Fig. 11.15 Right sixth nerve palsy – patient looking straight ahead

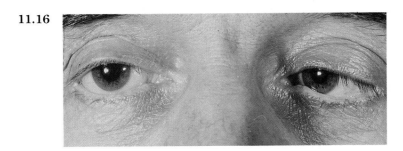

Fig. 11.16 Right sixth nerve palsy – patient looking to the right

Investigation of third, fourth and sixth nerve palsies

The most common causes of third, fourth and sixth nerve palsies are:

● **Trauma** – relatively minor trauma, usually closed head injuries, can lead to fourth nerve palsies. Base-of-skull fractures may lead to sixth nerve palsies and rapid rise in intracranial pressure, giving rise to descent of the temporal lobe which compresses the third nerve and in turn leads to the ominous sign of a unilateral, fixed, dilated pupil and a need for urgent CAT scanning. Orbital trauma is discussed elsewhere (see pp. 222–24).

● **Vascular** – diabetes, hypertension and athero-sclerosis may all lead to an interruption of the micro-vascular supply to the third, fourth or sixth nerves. This type of palsy has a high recovery rate after the cause has been treated. Diabetes may actually present with an isolated third nerve palsy (pupil-sparing). A rare form of migraine, ophthalmoplegic migraine, may cause temporary unilateral ophthalmoplegia.

● **Aneurysms** – e.g. posterior communicating artery aneurysm, leading to a painful, complete third nerve palsy. Immediate neurological referral for investigation by brain CAT scanning and angiography is required. A carotid aneurysm or carotico-cavernous fistula in the cavernous sinus affects the sixth nerve initially.

● **Inflammation** – e.g. basal meningitis, sarcoid, T.B., syphilis, *Herpes zoster*, temporal arteritis, cavernous sinus thrombosis. Multiple sclerosis can rarely cause isolated cranial nerve palsies.

● **Tumour** – e.g. meningioma, chordoma, pontine glioma, acoustic neuroma. An early acoustic neuroma will cause unilateral sensorineural deafness, with tin-nitus and vertigo, sometimes associated with an ipsi-lateral sixth nerve palsy before cerebellar, seventh, or sensory fifth disturbance may be noticed. Loss of corneal reflex is an important early sign.

● **Idiopathic** – after all other causes have been eliminated, this accounts for 25% of cases, of which 50% recover spontaneously.

Summary of basic investigations

● Examination to determine muscle and deduce nerve involvement (Hess chart)

● Examination of other cranial nerves, especially corneal reflex, facial sensation, seventh and eighth nerves

● Examination for proptosis (orbital disease)

● Blood pressure

● Skull radiograph and orbital views

● Full blood count and viscosity

● Urine for glycosuria and fasting blood glucose

Further investigations include exclusion of myopathies, myasthenia gravis and dysthyroid eye disease as relevant.

Myasthenia gravis

This disorder affects any age and both sexes, but classically younger women and older men. It is limited to ocular muscles in 30% of cases. It presents with variable ptosis and diplopia with fatiguability. A positive Tensilon test is seen. Here, 5–10mg of edrophonium bromide is injected intravenously and leads to transient reversal of clinical signs. Definitive diagnosis is esta-blished by serological testing for the presence of antibodies against acetylcholine receptors. Thymoma is present in 15% of cases.

Myopathies

Ocular myopathy (progressive external ophthalmoplegia): This is a collection of myopathies of the extraocular muscles (*Fig. 11.17(a)–(f)*), such as ocular and oculopharyngeal dystrophies, some of which are clearly inherited. Many have mitochondrial metabolic abnormalities. Some have important associated conditions, for example, Kearns-Sayre syndrome is associated with cardiac conduction defects and pigmentary retinopathy. Ptosis, often asymmetric initially, is followed by involvement of medial rectus, then elevators (causing a chin-up posture to be adopted) and finally the depressors, leading to the eyes becoming 'frozen' in their sockets.

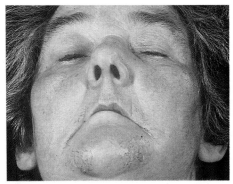

11.17(a)

Fig. 11.17(a) Ocular myopathy – patient in natural position looking straight ahead. Note chin-up posture to compensate for marked ptosis (Courtesy of Mr. F. Larkin)

11.17(b)

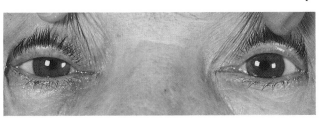

Fig. 11.17(b) Same patient as (**a**) looking straight ahead, eyelids held up (Courtesy of Mr. F. Larkin)

11.17(c)

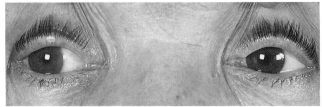

Fig. 11.17(c) Looking to the right (Courtesy of Mr. F. Larkin)

11.17(d)

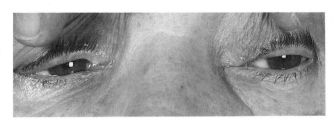

Fig. 11.17(d) Looking to the left (Courtesy of Mr. F. Larkin)

11.17(e)

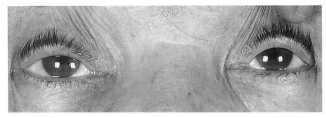

Fig. 11.17(e) Attempting upgaze (Courtesy of Mr. F. Larkin)

11.17(f)

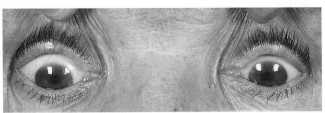

Fig. 11.17(f) Attempting downgaze (Courtesy of Mr. F. Larkin)

Myotonic dystrophy: This is a dominantly inherited condition, characterised by generally increased muscle tone with difficulty in relaxation (handshake), ptosis and poor facial expression, cataracts, frontal baldness, diabetes mellitus, hypogonadism and cardiac abnormalities.

Dysthyroid eye disease (*q.v.*)

Swelling of the optic disc

The three most common mechanisms which induce disc swelling are:

- **Raised intracranial pressure** (*Fig. 11.18(a) & (b)*): This gives rise to bilateral disc swelling – **papilloedema**. The visual acuities are relatively normal (see p. 201).

- **Inflammation of the optic nerve** (*Figs. 11.19 & 11.20*): This causes unilateral, occasionally bilateral disc swelling with a marked drop in visual acuity – **papillitis** (see p. 202).

- **Infarction of the optic nerve head** (*Fig. 11.21*): This is caused by inflammatory or arteriosclerotic changes in the blood supply to the optic nerve head. Unilateral, sometimes progressing to bilateral, pallid swelling of the optic disc with profound loss of vision – **anterior ischaemic optic neuropathy** (see pp. 202–3).

Other important causes of disc swelling include:

- Lesions compressing the optic nerve e.g. optic nerve schwannoma (neurofibromatosis), meningioma of optic nerve sheath (*Fig. 11.22*)

- Malignant hypertension (see p. 179)

- Optic disc vasculitis

- Chronic panuveitis (see p. 109)

- Infiltration of the optic nerve, e.g. tumour – glioma, leukaemia, lymphoma, and metastatic deposits; granulomatous disease – tuberculosis and sarcoidosis

- Ocular hypotony due to trauma or postoperatively

- Leber's optic neuropathy – a rare, X-linked inherited, optic neuropathy occurring in young, adult males.

- Pseudopapilloedema, e.g. hypermetropic disc, optic disc drüsen (see p. 141), distinguished by the presence of normal venous pulsation.

Management of optic disc swelling: All cases of optic ⑤ disc swelling should be referred immediately to a specialist eye centre. In the setting of normal acuity and visual field, when papilloedema is the most likely diagnosis, a neurological referral would be appropriate.

11.18(a)

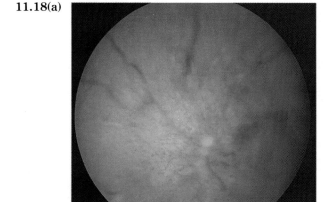

Fig. 11.18(a) Papilloedema – right disc

11.18(b)

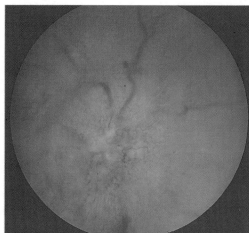

Fig. 11.18(b) Papilloedema – left disc in the same patient as **11.18(a)**

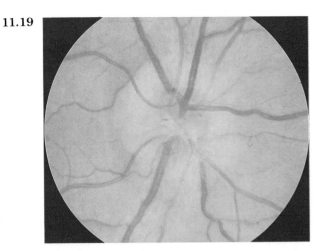

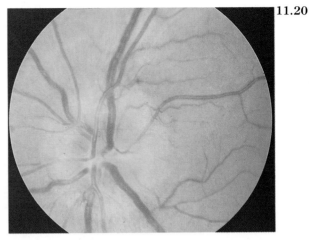

Fig. 11.19 Bilateral papillitis – right disc

Fig. 11.20 Bilateral papillitis – left disc – same patient as in **Fig. 11.19**

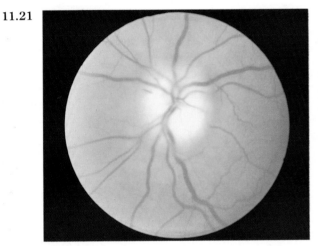

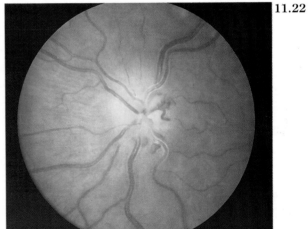

Fig. 11.21 Anterior ischaemic optic neuropathy due to temporal arteritis (Courtesy of Mr. R. Humphry)

Fig. 11.22 Optic nerve sheath meningioma – demonstrating opticociliary shunt vessels

Papilloedema

This is bilateral disc swelling due to raised intracranial pressure.

Symptoms: Headaches, nausea and vomiting (worse in the morning), vague visual symptoms such as "rosiness" or "patchiness" of vision, with **obscurations** of vision – a unilateral or bilateral transient loss of vision, often on change of posture, which recovers after a few seconds.

Signs: **Early papilloedema** (*Fig. 11.23*) – hyperaemia of the disc with blurring of the inferonasal margin. Spontaneous venous pulsation can be seen in a high proportion of normal individuals and its loss is a useful sign to look for in possible early papilloedema. However, if it is present, papilloedema is unlikely. Usually the presence or absence of spontaneous venous pulsation is bilaterally symmetrical and thus, loss of spontaneous venous pulsation on only one side is significant.

Acute papilloedema – pronounced swelling of the disc with congestion of the blood vessels and flame-shaped haemorrhages on the disc margin. Chronic papilloedema (*Figs. 11.26(a) & (b)*) – 'champagne-cork' appearance due to marked swelling of the disc and absence of the central cup. Late changes include optic atrophy (*Fig. 11.24*). Field loss, e.g. bitemporal hemianopia, may indicate the site of the lesion.

Ⓡ Ⓢ *Management:* Routine investigations, e.g. blood pressure, urinalysis, visual field assessment, full blood count and ESR or viscosity and skull and chest radiography, as appropriate. Immediate referral to neurological centre for urgent investigation, including CAT brain scan (*Fig. 11.25*).

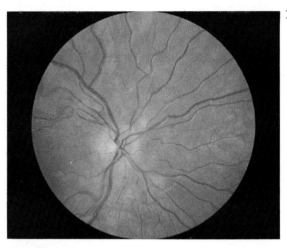

Fig. 11.23 Early papilloedema

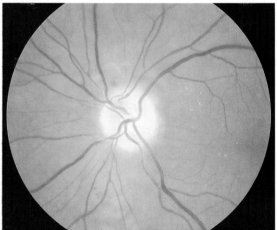

Fig. 11.24 Secondary optic atrophy

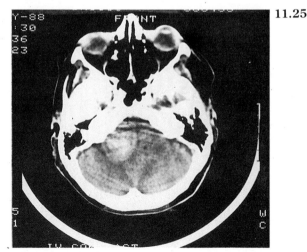

Fig. 11.25 CAT scan showing large acoustic neuroma

Benign intracranial hypertension (pseudotumour cerebri, otitic hydrocephalus)

This is characterised by raised intracranial pressure and chronic papilloedema (*Fig. 11.26(a) & (b)*). In children it may be associated with transverse sinus obstruction, secondary to severe middle ear infections and mastoiditis. More characteristically, it affects women in the third or fourth decade who are overweight and often have menstrual disturbance. It is also associated with cortical venous thrombosis, as in pregnancy, or secondary to oral contraceptive drugs, Addison's disease, hypoparathyroidism, hypercapnia, other drugs including tetracyclines, hypervitaminosis A and steroids.

Symptoms: Mild to severe headaches, dizziness, obscurations of vision. Children may be feverish and unwell.

Signs: Chronic papilloedema. Cranial nerve palsies, e.g. sixth. Field loss, including enlarged blind spot due to optic nerve damage.

Management: Urgent neurological referral for investigation to rule out other causes for raised intracranial pressure. Treatment is carried out to reduce intracranial pressure, e.g. using diuretics or acetazolamide, and steroids. Surgical decompression of the optic nerve sheaths is occasionally required for deteriorating vision and to prevent progressive optic nerve damage. (R) (S)

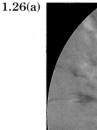

1.26(a)

11.26(b)

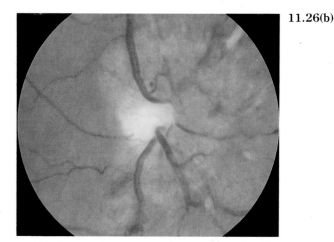

Fig. 11.26(a) Chronic papilloedema – right disc

Fig. 11.26(b) Chronic papilloedema – left disc in same patient as **11.26(a)**

Optic neuritis

This is an inflammation of the optic nerve. In children it is often bilateral and of postviral immunological aetiology. In adults it is usually unilateral during any one attack and is associated with multiple sclerosis in 20–80% of cases (according to different sources), either as a presenting feature or as a manifestation of the previously established disease. The remaining cases include various vasculitides, e.g. syphilis (*Fig. 11.27*) and systemic lupus erythematosus, or occur in otherwise normal individuals. It is often subdivided into papillitis, when disc swelling is observed, and retrobulbar neuritis, when it is not. The latter is more common in adults.

Symptoms: Progressive loss or blurring of vision, associated with an aching around and behind the eye which is worse on eye movements. Subjectively dimmer vision or colour desaturation noticed, i.e. a red colour will look grey and washed out. Vision deteriorates to its lowest level by the end of the first week, usually starts to recover by the end of the following week and is commonly back to normal by the end of the fourth week. Multiple sclerosis may be manifested in other neurological symptoms or as exacerbation of visual loss when body temperature is raised, e.g. in the bath or during exercise (Uhthoff's phenomenon).

Signs: Mild to severe drop in visual acuity, sometimes down to perception of light only. In visual field testing, the red target will look darker and a central scotoma is discernible. A relative afferent pupillary defect is present, elicited using the swinging torchlight test (see p. 20). In papillitis, the optic disc is swollen, sometimes with haemorrhages, but is normal in retrobulbar neuritis.

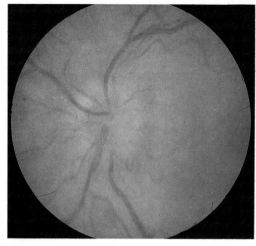

Fig. 11.27 Syphilitic optic neuritis

Management: The patient should be referred initially to an ophthalmologist. A full blood count, ESR or plasma viscosity and VDRL should be done to exclude a vasculitic disease. The patient should be informed that this is an 'inflammation of the optic nerve' and reassured that there is a 75% chance of full recovery of vision with a low risk of significant residual impairment. If this is an isolated attack, any further hint at a possible association with multiple sclerosis may be withheld.

N.B. Steroids are not indicated in optic neuritis except when there is severe, bilateral loss of vision. There is no evidence that they improve eventual visual outcome or lessen the frequency of recurrence. They act only to shorten the attack.

Anterior ischaemic optic neuropathy (AION)

This lesion of the anterior optic nerve is caused by impaired blood supply from the posterior ciliary arteries (*Figs. 11.22, 11.28*). Visual loss is permanent owing to subsequent optic atrophy. The lesion occurs in the elderly and the most common causes are atherosclerosis (often associated with hypertension) and arteritis, usually giant cell arteritis, which must be considered in each case.

Symptoms: Painless loss of vision in one eye (initially). In giant cell arteritis this may be closely followed by involvement of the second eye. May be associated with other symptoms of giant cell arteritis:

- Headache, often temporal or over the scalp, frequently severe

- Jaw claudication – **pathognomonic of giant cell arteritis** – characteristic pain in the jaw area on chewing, relieved by rest, sometimes pain in the tongue

- Polymyalgia rheumatica – aching in the proximal limb muscles

- Malaise and weight loss

Signs: Tender, nonpulsatile temporal arteries. Profoundly decreased visual acuity with altitudinal field defect. Relative afferent pupillary defect. Pale, swollen optic disc +/− disc haemorrhages. A raised ESR > 40mm/h is suspicious of giant cell arteritis, in which it is often elevated to > 100mm/h. *N.B.* occasionally a normal ESR is found in this disease. Hypertension is found in 50% of atherosclerotic AION.

Management: **This is an ocular emergency.** If Ⓢ Ⓡ symptoms and signs suggest giant cell arteritis, immediate treatment is essential with i.v. hydrocortisone 200mg, followed by high dose steroids, e.g. prednisolone 60–80mg daily p.o. as a starting dose. This should be carried out as an inpatient and followed by a temporal artery biopsy. The temporal artery biopsy will still be positive up to five days (sometimes even longer) after starting steroids. Delay in beginning steroids may result in irreversible involvement of the other eye.

As the condition comes under control, as judged by the dramatic improvement of symptoms and lowering of ESR, the steroids may be reduced. Gradually, under close, outpatient supervision, the steroids may be reduced, but they often cannot be stopped for a period of two years. If there is no evidence for giant cell arteritis, the diagnosis is assumed to be atherosclerotic, and, after hypertension has been excluded, there is no further treatment. In 40% of cases of arteriosclerotic anterior ischaemic optic neuropathy the second eye is subsequently found to be affected.

11.28

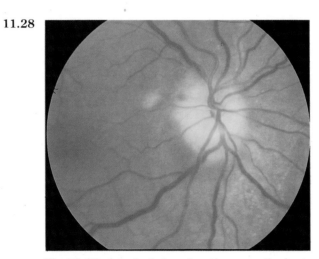

Fig. 11.28 Anterior ischaemic optic neuropathy due to temporal arteritis

Nystagmus

This is defined as involuntary oscillations of the eyes. There are two types of oscillations: jerk nystagmus, where there is a slow (pathological) phase, a fast (corrective) phase and the **direction of the nystagmus is by convention towards the fast phase**; and pendular nystagmus, where the phases are of equal velocity. Nystagmus may be horizontal, vertical or rotatory.

Types of nystagmus

Physiological nystagmus: End-gaze nystagmus is a small-amplitude, horizontal nystagmus seen in normal individuals on extreme lateral gaze. As a rule the examiner testing eye movements should aim to take the edge of the iris of the adducting eye to the caruncle, but no further. If the object is moved too fast, nystagmoid jerks will be elicited.

Optokinetic nystagmus is a jerk nystagmus elicited by presenting moving, repetitive, visual stimuli, where the slow phase is the eyes following the target and the fast phase is the repositioning to centre to pick up the next target. This may be tested using an optokinetic drum (*Fig. 11.29*).

Caloric testing elicits a physiological nystagmus and is a test of intact vestibular function. When warm water is poured into the left ear canal there will be a left jerk nystagmus and when cold water is used there will be a right jerk nystagmus (COWS – Cold-Opposite Warm-Same)

Congenital nystagmus: This presents from birth as a pendular nystagmus, usually with compensatory head nodding in the opposite direction to maintain fixation. It is often familial and is associated with variable visual impairment. It is different from spasmus nutans, which is an acquired, uniocular, pendular nystagmus with onset in the first year of life, also associated with nodding, but which resolves by the age of three years. It is essential to exclude any ocular abnormality since similar eye movements occur in children with grossly impaired vision, e.g. due to congenital cataracts, macular hypoplasia, ocular albinism and Leber's congenital amaurosis. Indeed, pendular nystagmus may develop with sensory deprivation up to the age of six years.

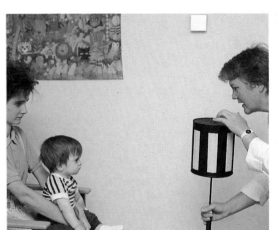

Fig. 11.29 Optokinetic drum

Vestibular nystagmus: In peripheral vestibular disease there is usually a horizontal or rotatory nystagmus with the direction away from the side of the lesion, associated with vertigo, e.g. acute labyrinthitis. In central balance disorders the nystagmus may also be vertical and reflects brainstem and cerebellar involvement, e.g. multiple sclerosis.

Cerebellar nystagmus: Nystagmus is often absent in cerebellar disease, although it may be detectable electrically with the eyes closed. When present it is towards the side of the lesion.

Other types of nystagmus:

- Down-beat nystagmus (vertical nystagmus with the fast phase downwards) is pathognomonic of a lesion of the medulla at the foramen magnum.

- Up-beat nystagmus (vertical nystagmus with the fast phase upwards) occurs in brainstem disease or drug intoxication.

- Rotatory nystagmus may be congenital or acquired and may reflect brainstem or vestibular disease.

- Ocular bobbing is not true nystagmus. It is characterised by rapid downwards jerks of both eyes followed by a slow corrective upwards drift to normal. It occurs in pontine lesions and the patients are often comatose.

- Drugs may induce most forms of nystagmus. Common ones are phenytoin and other anticonvulsants, barbiturates and other sedative drugs, and alcohol – especially in Wernicke's encephalopathy.

Visual fields

Visual field assessment (see pp. 22–23) is of vital importance in neuro-ophthalmology. Advanced field testing is not appropriate in an emergency setting, but accurate fields to confrontation will detect a central scotoma, centrocaecal scotoma and altitudinal and hemianopic field defects and are essential in the following circumstances:

- Blurred vision or loss of vision; perception of blind spot or bumping into objects at the side; dimming of vision or alteration of colour perception.

- Recent onset of neurological symptoms, e.g. headaches, seizures, multiple sclerosis and amaurosis fugax with continued loss of vision.

More accurate perimetry is required for:

- Optic disc abnormalities, e.g. cupping, pale ischaemic swelling of the disc, pallor; proptosis, e.g. in thyroid eye disease, and orbital tumours.

- Abnormalities on skull radiograph or CAT scan, e.g. enlarged sella (*Fig. 11.30(a) & (b)*), enlarged optic foramen, hyperostosis of sphenoid wing and demonstrable intracranial or orbital tumour.

11.30(a)

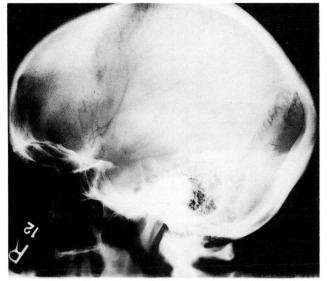

Fig. 11.30(a) Enlarged pituitary fossa shown in lateral skull radiograph (Courtesy of Dr. W.D. Jeans)

11.30(b)

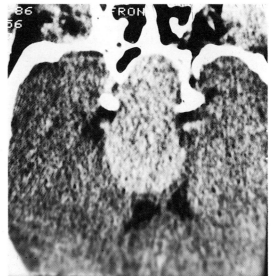

Fig. 11.30(b) Head CT scan of same patient, showing the mass arising from the fossa (Courtesy of Dr. W.D. Jeans)

A diagram of the normal visual field of the right eye is shown (*Fig. 11.31*), demonstrating the isopters of same target threshold. The outer limit of the field is approximately 50° superiorly, 60° nasally, 70° inferiorly and 90° temporally. For many purposes the central 30° of the field is plotted (*Fig. 11.32*) to show details of central field loss and scotomas. The normal blind spot is situated between 15° and 20° temporal and slightly inferior to central fixation.

11.31

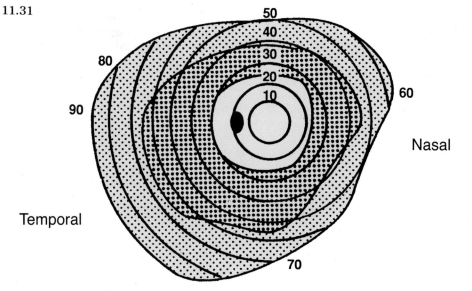

Actual shape of visual field

Fig. 11.31 Normal visual field

11.32

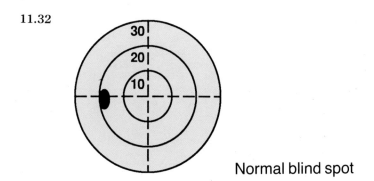

Normal blind spot

Fig. 11.32 Central 30° of normal visual field

Field defects

Here is an outline of the more common field defects seen:

- Monocular field defects with normal other eye
- Binocular field defects.

Monocular field defects with normal other eye

Illustrated for simplicity as the left eye. **T** = Temporal, **N** = Nasal.

T   N

11.33

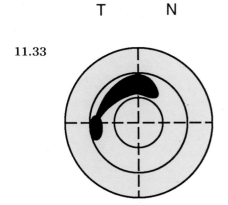

Fig. 11.33 **Superior arcuate scotoma** (inferior nerve fibre bundle defect), e.g. chronic glaucoma (also inferior branch retinal artery or vein occlusion).

11.34

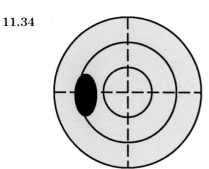

Fig. 11.34 **Enlarged blind spot**. Optic nerve disorders, e.g. optic neuritis.

11.35

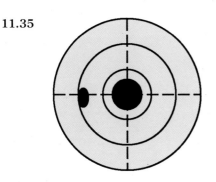

Fig. 11.35 **Central scotoma**. Macula disorders, optic nerve compression, optic neuritis.

T   N

11.36

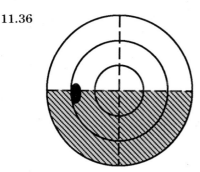

Fig. 11.36 Inferior altitudinal field loss. Anterior ischaemic optic neuropathy, superior hemispheric branch retinal artery or vein occlusion, chronic glaucoma.

11.37

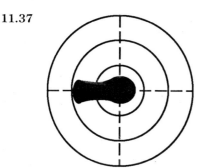

Fig. 11.37 Centrocaecal scotoma. Toxic damage to optic nerve, e.g. tobacco amblyopia, demyelination, infiltrative optic nerve lesions, compressive optic nerve lesions. *N.B.* If associated with contralateral upper temporal field defect, this indicates prechiasmal compression.

11.38

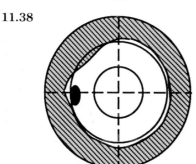

Fig. 11.38 Generalised constriction of visual field. This is more significant if uniocular, e.g. peripheral retinal disorder – retinitis pigmentosa, optic nerve sheath meningioma.

Tubular field. If Bjerrum field remains a constant size, even while the patient is being moved further away from the screen, it is characteristic of a hysterical, constricted field.

Binocular field defects

Congruity implies the edge of the field defect in each eye is identical in shape and is characteristic of the optic radiations. If the edges are steep or vertical, this is more likely to be due to infarction; if the edges are sloping, this implies compression. The macula may be spared because of its dual blood supply by the posterior and middle cerebral arteries and large, bilateral area of representation.

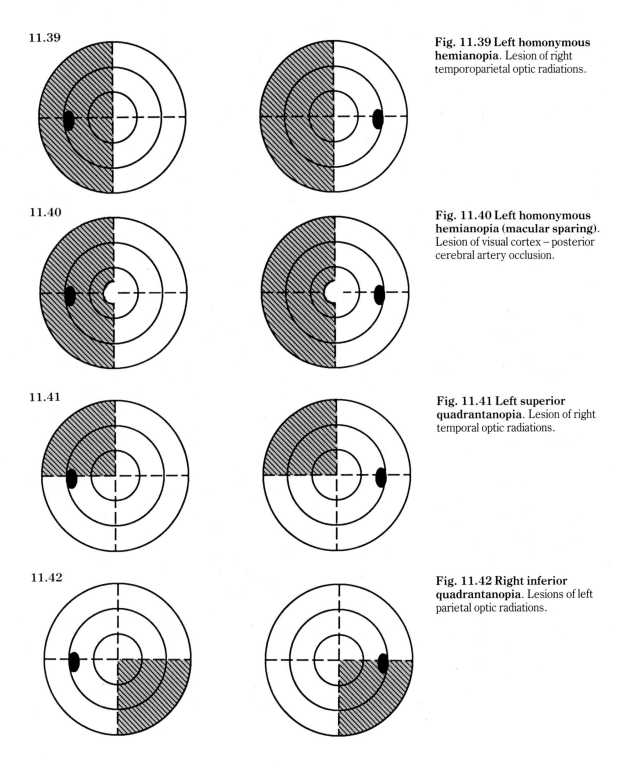

11.39

Fig. 11.39 Left homonymous hemianopia. Lesion of right temporoparietal optic radiations.

11.40

Fig. 11.40 Left homonymous hemianopia (macular sparing). Lesion of visual cortex – posterior cerebral artery occlusion.

11.41

Fig. 11.41 Left superior quadrantanopia. Lesion of right temporal optic radiations.

11.42

Fig. 11.42 Right inferior quadrantanopia. Lesions of left parietal optic radiations.

11.43

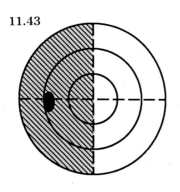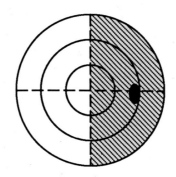

Fig. 11.43 Bitemporal hemianopia. Most common cause – chiasmal compression by pituitary tumour. Other causes – tilted discs, bilateral retinal detachments, drug toxicity, e.g. chloroquine and sectorial retinitis pigmentosa.

Other characteristic pituitary field defects include:

• Bitemporal superior quadrantanopia (*Fig. 11.44*) – compression of chiasm from below, e.g. pituitary tumour.

• Bitemporal inferior quadrantanopia – compression of chiasm from above, e.g. suprasellar cyst or craniopharyngioma.

11.44

11.45

11.46

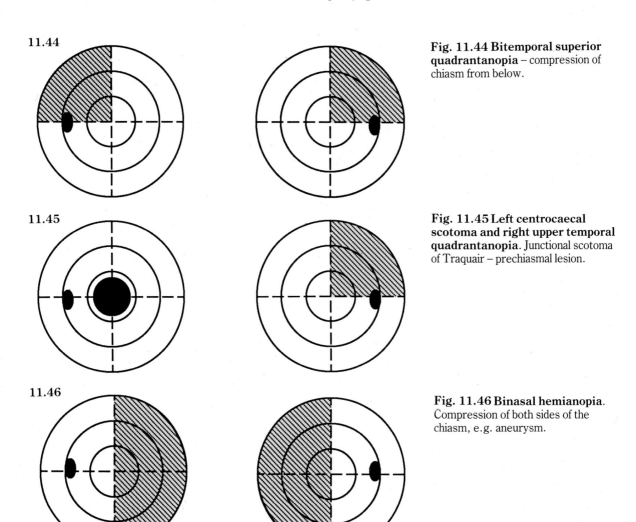

Fig. 11.44 Bitemporal superior quadrantanopia – compression of chiasm from below.

Fig. 11.45 Left centrocaecal scotoma and right upper temporal quadrantanopia. Junctional scotoma of Traquair – prechiasmal lesion.

Fig. 11.46 Binasal hemianopia. Compression of both sides of the chiasm, e.g. aneurysm.

12 Trauma to the eye

In the assessment of trauma to the eye the following factors are important:

- Exact mode of injury
- Extent of injury to the eye – a penetrating injury requires emergency referral to a specialist eye centre
- Extent of other injuries
- Tetanus prophylaxis
- Previous ocular, medical and drug history including hepatitis/HIV status

- Visual acuity at presentation – even in the case of severe trauma it is vitally important to know, for example, if the visual ability to count fingers is present.

Subconjunctival haemorrhage

This flat, bright-red haemorrhage (*Fig. 12.1*) under the conjunctiva may occur spontaneously, with raised venous pressure as in coughing, straining or playing a trumpet, or with minor or major trauma. Occasionally, a severe haemorrhage may form a boggy, dark-red mass that spills over the lower lid margin. Subconjunctival haemorrhage is asymptomatic, unless associated with a haemorrhagic conjunctivitis.

(P) *Management:* With no other ocular signs the spontaneous subconjunctival haemorrhage, or that associated with minor trauma, requires no treatment. It will resolve in 2–3 weeks. In the case of recurrent, spontaneous, subconjunctival haemorrhages, haematological investigations should be performed. If trauma with a sharp object is suspected, local exploration under the conjunctiva is necessary to look for signs of scleral perforation. This may be carried out at the slit lamp after instilling local anaesthetic drops or, if perforation is strongly suspected, in the theatre. Fundal examination through a dilated pupil is carried out to look for signs of contusion or perforation.

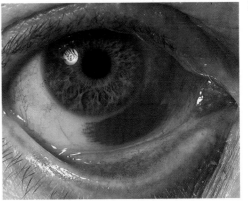

12.1

Fig. 12.1 Right subconjunctival haemorrhage (Courtesy of Mr. R. Humphry)

Tetanus status needs to be checked. In a case of major trauma, where there are subconjunctival haemorrhages which are bilateral or with no posterior margin, a basal skull fracture must be suspected.

Conjunctival laceration

A sharp injury, for example with a rose thorn, may produce a superficial, conjunctival laceration with a subconjunctival haemorrhage. The edges of the laceration will stain brilliantly with fluorescein. After the instillation of local anaesthetic drops, the conjunctiva should be gently explored to see if the laceration is of full or partial thickness. A search for a possible perforation must be made by opening up the conjunctiva to allow adequate exposure of the sclera. A partial thickness conjunctival laceration requires no suturing, but, if Tenon's capsule has been torn, this requires suturing with 8/0 dexon. Tetanus status (R) needs to be checked.

Corneal abrasion

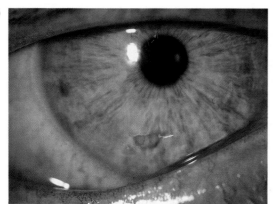

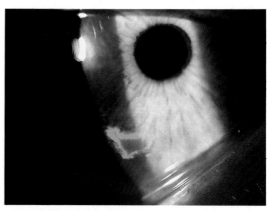

Fig. 12.2(a) Corneal abrasion – before staining

Fig. 12.2(b) Corneal abrasion – staining with fluorescein

Corneal abrasion is one of the most common injuries to the eye (*Fig. 12.2(a) & (b)*). It is often caused by a finger nail or a twig catching the eye. There is immediate intense pain, lacrimation, foreign body sensation, photophobia and blepharospasm. Instillation of local anaesthetic, e.g. benoxinate 0.4% drops, may be required to examine the eye. There is ciliary injection and an area of epithelial loss that stains bright green with fluorescein (seen especially well with a cobalt blue filter).

ℙℝ *Management:* Any loose epithelium, seen as white tags, or any foreign matter is removed using a 21-gauge needle along the side of the bevel after instillation of benoxinate 0.4% drops. A **moist**, sterile cotton-tip may be used for the purpose, but care is needed not to strip off further large areas of epithelium.

Chloramphenicol 0.5% and homatropine 2% drops are instilled and the eye firmly padded (see p. 35) for 24 hours and reviewed the next day. The epithelial cells will spread over the surface of the cornea and by the next day the area of epithelial loss should be considerably smaller. If any epithelial defect is still present, further antibiotic and homatropine drops are instilled and the eye padded for a further 24 hours. When the epithelium is almost healed, seen as a linear, sometimes branched defect, chloramphenicol drops q.d.s. are instilled for 4 days and the pad kept off.

Sometimes a secondary iritis develops with large abrasions. Initial treatment with topical antibiotics, homatropine and padding is used, but cycloplegics, e.g. cyclopentolate drops 0.5% t.d.s. with chloramphenicol, are used whilst there is an iritis present. A fundal check is necessary. Steroids should not be used until the epithelium has healed because of the danger of infection.

Recurrent corneal abrasions

This may occur weeks or months after the original corneal abrasion and presents as a recurrence of the original symptoms of pain, lacrimation, photophobia and foreign body sensation. It occurs as a result of inadequate cell-junction formation between the new epithelial layer and the tissues underneath, such that minimal trauma will cause loss of the top surface again.

The majority of corneal abrasions are noticed upon waking. Overnight the tears have failed to keep the surface between the cornea and the eyelid well lubricated and, either during rapid eye movement sleep or upon opening the lids first thing in the morning, friction occurs and thence a recurrent abrasion.

Signs: An area of abnormal epithelium with a part of it staining brightly with fluorescein. Treatment consists of a single application of chloramphenicol ointment and firm padding for 24 hours, followed by twice daily chloramphenicol ointment for a week and nightly chloramphenicol or lubricating ointment for one month.

Some people recommend debriding the abnormal (S)(R) area to restart the healing process from scratch. Recurrent abrasions may continue for up to two years. Sometimes they are associated with a corneal dystrophy. Recalcitrant abrasions may need to be treated with soft contact lens wear.

Corneal foreign body

The most common foreign body found on the cornea is a metallic, often rusty particle associated with a history of grinding 1–3 days previously. Alternatively, a sudden event such as an explosion, may scatter small fragments on to the cornea.

Symptoms: Photophobia, lacrimation, foreign body sensation.

Signs: Small metallic foreign body seen, often surrounded by rusty infiltrate, especially if left there 2–3 days. There may be associated anterior chamber activity.

Investigations: If there is a history of chiselling metal on metal or other high velocity situation, a fundal examination and X-ray of orbit are obligatory to exclude an intraocular foreign body. The presence of anterior chamber +/− posterior chamber activity increases the likelihood of such a possibility.

(R) *Management:*

- Metallic foreign bodies should always be removed, even if deeply embedded. In the case of deeply embedded fragments of inert materials, for example glass, it is often safer to leave them *in situ*.

- A cotton tip should not be used to remove a corneal foreign body as it may cause an abrasion.

Procedure for removing a metallic foreign body: (R)

1. Instil 2–3 drops benoxinate 0.4% as local anaesthetic.
2. With an orange needle, using the magnification of a loupe or slit lamp, gently prise off the foreign body. Once removed, the rust ring should be scraped away. If the tissues are too resistant, the eye may be padded overnight with chloramphenicol ointment and the rust ring tackled the following day.
3. Instil homatropine 2% drops, chloramphenicol ointment and pad for 24–48 hours.
4. When comfortable after this period, use chloramphenicol 0.5% drops q.d.s., or more frequently if the infiltrate is large. If there is anterior chamber activity, keep the pupil dilated with cyclopentolate 1% drops t.d.s. until quiet.

Blunt trauma to the eye

Blunt trauma, including squash ball injury, assault, injury from elasticated luggage straps, airgun pellets and, in the elderly, a fall against a piece of furniture, may lead to anything from mild anterior uveitis to a ruptured globe.

Traumatic anterior uveitis

This may occur from a minor blow even 2–3 days previously and may accompany a corneal abrasion (v.s.).

Symptoms: Aching, photophobia and mild blurring of vision.

Signs: Ciliary injection, flare and cells in the anterior chamber and a poorly reactive, semi-dilated pupil (traumatic mydriasis). A fundal check with a dilated pupil is mandatory to exclude lens dislocation, vitreous haemorrhage or retinal damage (v.i.).

- In the long term, **traumatic iridoplegia** may occur, when the poorly reactive semi-dilated pupil continues. This may cause problems with blurring of vision and glare from light sources. Occasionally, miotics may be of benefit.

Management: Steroid drops q.d.s. (prednisolone Ⓡ 0.5% for mild uveitis or betamethasone for more severe uveitis) and mydriatics, e.g. cyclopentolate 1% t.d.s., until the inflammation has settled, after which the treatment may be tailed off.

Hyphaema

In this the trauma causes bleeding from the iris root into the anterior chamber and a fluid level of blood is formed (*Fig. 12.3*).

Symptoms: Dull ache and reduced visual acuity initially, improving as the blood settles.

Signs: Ciliary injection and a hyphaema with traumatic mydriasis are seen. There may be associated anterior segment damage, e.g. iris dialysis where the iris is torn away from its insertion. In less severe injuries, even though a **macroscopic** hyphaema is not seen, the anterior chamber will show activity with red cells +/– white cells, the red cells appearing as rusty particles moving with the currents in the anterior chamber. This is referred to as a **microscopic** hyphaema. The intraocular pressure should be measured using applanation tonometry (not digital), as it may rise with a hyphaema. If it is very low, a ruptured globe should be suspected. A prolonged, severe hyphaema may lead to staining of the cornea with blood.

Ⓡ *Management:* If a macroscopic hyphaema is present, the patient is admitted for bed rest, the eye is kept padded and betnesol drops q.d.s. are used to prevent anterior uveitis. Controversy rages about whether the pupil should be dilated. Some ophthalmologists do not dilate the pupil until the hyphaema has settled for fear of inducing a secondary hyphaema which may be harder to treat. Others dilate the pupil using atropine 1% drops t.d.s. to allow a fuller fundal view initially and comfort to the eye.

Abrasions are treated in the usual way. Raised intraocular pressure is treated with g Timolol drops 0.5% b.d. (if there are no contra-indications) and acetazolamide 250 mg q.d.s. p.o., with an i.v. dose of acetazolamide 500 mg initially if the pressure is greater than 35 mmHg. Gonioscopy looking for angle recession and fundal examination should be carried out after the hyphaema has settled and before discharge. Annual follow-up for pressure measurement is necessary if there has been significant (greater than 180°) angle damage. Patients with microscopic hyphaemas can rest at home in bed for 4–5 days, provided that they return if the pain increases (possible secondary hyphaema). They should use g betnesol q.d.s. At re-examination on day five, if their hyphaema has settled, gonioscopy and fundal examination are performed.

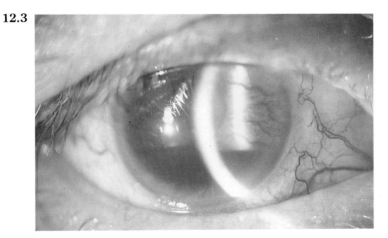

Fig. 12.3 Hyphaema

An **iris dialysis** (*Figs. 12.4, 12.5*) requires no immediate treatment but suggests that the injury has been severe and secondary hyphaemas will be more common. There may be associated retinal dialysis. If patients remain symptomatic, for example with dazzle and monocular diplopia, they may be repaired after a year.

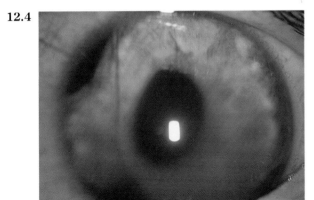

Fig. 12.4 Iridodialysis with continued bleeding producing hyphaema

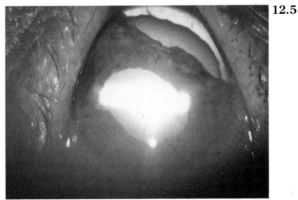

Fig. 12.5 Iridodialysis (Courtesy of Mr. C. Dean Hart)

Damage to the lens

Blunt trauma or a penetrating injury (*Figs. 12.6, 12.7*) may result in a **traumatic cataract**. At the time of minor injury, small anterior lens opacities develop which may not progress. More severe trauma leads either to central posterior opacities, which develop within hours of injury and usually progress, or peripheral lens opacities, which often stay static. In either case, the best policy is to wait six months before contemplating surgery to allow the cataract to show its progression and any retinal pathology to settle.

More severe trauma may lead to dislocation of the lens, either anteriorly into the anterior chamber, or posteriorly. This may be complicated by an acute pressure rise in anterior dislocation and requires immediate i.v. acetazolamide 500 mg, dilation of the ⑤ pupil with atropine drops 1% t.d.s., steroid drops to control the uveitis and positioning the patient supine to allow the lens to fall back into its correct position. If this fails, immediate surgery is required to reposition the lens or remove it, preceded by i.v. mannitol 1.5 g/kg to bring the pressure down.

Posterior dislocation of the lens into the vitreous may be asymptomatic, in which case the management is conservative. However, secondary glaucoma, uveitis, vitreous inflammation or visual loss due to cataract formation, with intermittent obstruction of the visual axis, may occur, in which case removal of the lens will be necessary.

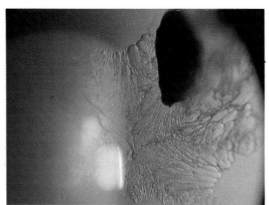

Fig. 12.6 Red reflex outlining 'sunflower' cataract and an embedded metallic foreign body (Courtesy of Institute of Ophthalmology)

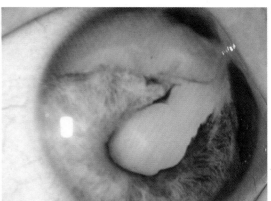

Fig. 12.7 Traumatic cataract and avulsion of iris root

Retinal injury

Purtscher's retinopathy

This occurs after crush injuries to the chest. It appears as widespread areas of white exudate and haemorrhages around the disc. It seems to be ischaemic in origin and resolves leaving some loss of vision.

Retinal detachment

This occurs secondary to a tear or dialysis forming at the time of injury, and may be immediate or delayed ⑤ by 1–2 weeks (in the case of a dialysis). It is managed by supporting the tear with indentation and cryotherapy.

Retinal dialysis

This is a disinsertion of the retina peripherally and is most common in the superonasal or inferotemporal quadrants. It may either settle spontaneously or progress to bullous retinal detachment. If it settles, the treatment is cryotherapy to the affected areas. If ⑤ it starts to progress to retinal detachment, indentation with a plomb or encirclement is carried out in the usual way.

Commotio retinae

Direct, blunt trauma to the eye often leads to an area of diffuse oedema of the retina which appears as a greyish sheen and is referred to as commotio retinae (*Fig. 12.8*). Depending on the site of the trauma, it may be a localised area in the periphery or may extend to involve the macula, giving rise to macular oedema and profound central visual loss. There may be a corresponding area of field loss in commotio retinae. (R) A careful search using the indirect ophthalmoscope is important to exclude any holes or a coexisting retinal dialysis or detachment. The patient is instructed to rest at home and the oedema usually settles, although macular oedema may be complicated by lamellar hole formation. A repeat fundal examination, with application of a three-mirror contact lens, is carried out 10–14 days later to check that the commotio has settled and to ensure that no new holes or tears have formed.

Choroidal rupture

These are localised, crescent-shaped tears in the choroid (*Fig. 12.9*) and may occur in the posterior pole (concentric configuration) or peripherally (radial configuration). Often there is associated macular oedema. There is no treatment for an isolated, small, (S) choroidal rupture, but it may be complicated by choroidal haematomas which, in turn, may give rise to vitreous haemorrhages. Patients with choroidal haematomas should be managed on bed rest for a few days. Choroidal effusions, macular disciforms and choroiditis are further complications.

N.B. If there is a **vitreous haemorrhage** following (S) trauma, patients should always be admitted for bed rest and observation as there may be an underlying retinal detachment.

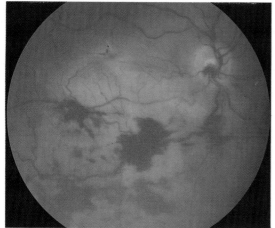

Fig. 12.8 Commotio retinae

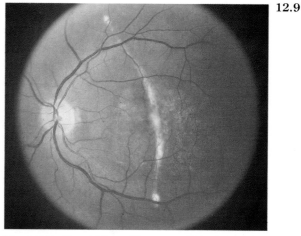

Fig. 12.9 Choroidal tear (Courtesy of Mr. S. Cook)

Evulsion of the optic nerve

Severe trauma to the eye can lead to evulsion of the optic nerve behind the optic nerve head. There is usually either no perception of light or perception of light only. There is also a total afferent pupillary defect, as shown by no direct or consensual response when light is shone at the affected eye, but an intact, consensual response when light is directed at the other eye. The retina shows infarction with large blot haemorrhages. Sometimes a cleft is seen adjacent to the disc, but more often this is obscured by preretinal haemorrhage. It is important to diagnose as the (S)(R) patient may then be given a definite statement regarding the poor visual prognosis.

Penetrating ocular injury

Any injury which perforates the outer layer of the eye, cornea or sclera is referred to as a penetrating eye injury. It may be due to sharp trauma, e.g. compass or pencil points in children, and knives or high velocity metallic or glass fragments in adults, leading to a retained, intraocular foreign body. Blunt trauma can lead to a posterior rupture of the globe.

N.B. All cases of **suspected** penetrating injury or intraocular foreign body require emergency referral to a specialist eye centre. On no account should an attempt be made to remove a protruding object from the eye before referral as further damage may be caused.

®Ⓢ *Initial assessment*

This should be carried out after any life-threatening complications have been managed.

- The patient is assessed initially lying on a couch, when the visual acuity should be measured. If there is perception of light, the ability to detect direction should be noted. Snellen charts, suitable for use at the bedside, are used.

- A pen-torch or examination light by the bedside is used to assess obvious external injury to the eye, e.g. corneal or scleral laceration with iris prolapse, protruding foreign body or collapsed globe. In this instance the eyelids should be **gently** opened and no undue pressure applied to the eye as this may lead to prolapse of the intraocular contents through an open wound. A red reflex is looked for and may outline a traumatic cataract. If the wound is large or a ruptured globe is suspected, **no further examination in the casualty area is carried out**. The eye is lightly padded and protected with a shield and the patient prepared for examination and repair under anaesthesia.

- Sometimes perforation has occurred in the absence of obvious signs, e.g. in penetration by small metallic fragments at high velocity.

- In less severe cases, where no obvious injury is seen, the eye may be assessed at the slit lamp. Here other **signs of perforation** may become apparent:

(a) small, corneal entry site that may leak aqueous from the anterior chamber. Here, a drop of fluorescein placed on the cornea over the possible entry site will become diluted by the issuing aqueous and turn green and brightly fluorescent (positive Seidel's test). A small, corneal perforation may show a knuckle of iris tissue incarcerated in the wound and a scleral perforation may show vitreous leakage. *N.B.* a subconjunctival haemorrhage may be covering a site of entry.

(b) hypotony as measured by applanation tonometry (never digitally). This may also be present in severe contusion injuries without perforation.

(c) shallowed anterior chamber

(d) pupil abnormalities, especially deviation of pupil from central location

(e) lens capsule rupture and early cataract formation

Corneal and scleral lacerations

After the initial assessment has revealed the presence of a corneal or scleral laceration (*Figs. 12.10 & 12.11*), the patient should be kept nil by mouth, started on systemic, broad-spectrum antibiotics, given analgesics and antiemetics as necessary and tetanus status should be checked. If there is even the remotest possibility of an intraocular foreign body, a skull and orbital radiography is mandatory. In theatre, using the operating microscope, gentle cultures are taken from the eye and the wound is cleaned using vitreous sponges and a syringe with a fine cannula containing Hartmann's solution. The scleral wound must be explored to its posterior limit. Prolapsed uveal tissue is replaced into the wound if viable, or excised if non-viable. The scleral/corneal laceration is carefully realigned (at the limbus if appropriate) and repaired using 9/0 nylon for the sclera and 10/0 nylon for the cornea. The viscoelastic substance, sodium hyaluronate, is used to keep the iris from prolapsing through the wound. Increasingly nowadays, more radical procedures are undertaken at a primary stage, e.g. removal of lens. After surgery the pupil is dilated with atropine 1% and a subconjunctival injection of methicillin given. In the postoperative period, detailed fundoscopy is carried out. At a later date further procedures may be necessary, e.g. lens removal, if there is extensive cataract formation. Primary repair is attempted on all but the most severe injuries, repair of which would not lead to any acceptable vision or cosmetic appearance. In this case, enucleation is necessary for quick rehabilitation and should be carried out within two weeks of injury to try to prevent sympathetic ophthalmitis developing.

12.10

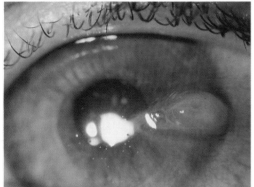

Fig. 12.10 Corneal perforation

12.11

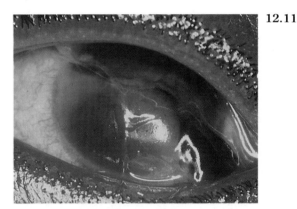

Fig. 12.11 Perforated cornea with uveal prolapse (Courtesy of Mr. F. Larkin)

Ⓢ Ruptured globe

The initial management is similar to that of corneal and scleral lacerations, but the prognosis is worse as the lens, vitreous and sometimes the retina have prolapsed through the wound and there is extensive haemorrhage within the eye (*Fig. 12.12*). Primary repair and reformation of the posterior segment is carried out. Secondary haemorrhage is common, but occasionally some useful visual function remains. Enucleation is the only course if the eye continues to deteriorate.

12.12

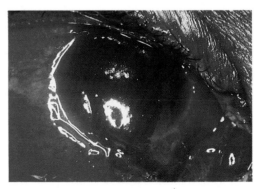

Fig. 12.12 Ruptured globe (Courtesy of Mr. F. Larkin)

Intraocular foreign body

The most common cause of intraocular foreign body (*Figs. 12.13, 12.14, 12.15, 12.16*) is from hammering or chiselling (usually steel on steel, but also on concrete or stone) when a fragment of metal flies up and enters the eye. Other causes include explosions or airgun pellets (*Fig. 12.17(a) & (b)*).

12.13 **12.14** **12.15**

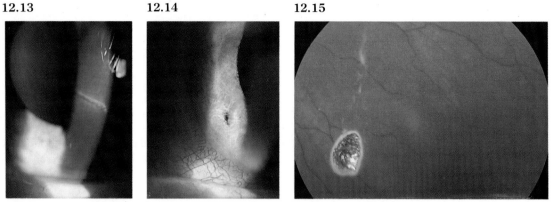

Fig. 12.13 Entry of foreign body through cornea
Fig. 12.14 Entry of foreign body through iris

Fig. 12.15 Foreign body on retina

12.16

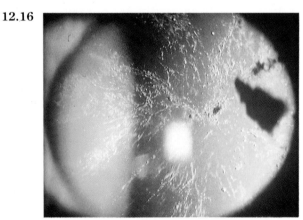

Fig. 12.16 Foreign body in lens with early cataract (Courtesy of Mr. S. Cook)

12.17(a) **12.17(b)**

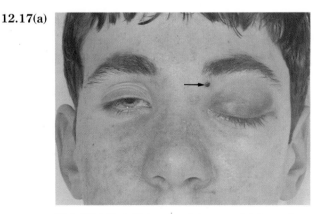

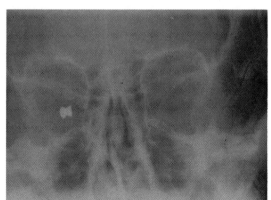

Fig. 12.17(a) Entry site of air gun pellet (arrow)

Fig. 12.17(b) Skull radiograph demonstrating air gun pellet (Courtesy of Mr. C. Dean Hart)

S) Management: The initial management is similar to that of any perforating injury, except that accurate location of the foreign body is carried out using plain radiology and CAT scanning (using a contact lens localizing ring). Ultrasound may be helpful. It is often difficult to determine whether an object at the posterior pole is lodged within the retina or just outside the eye. MRI scanning may become a more accurate method for localising **non-magnetic**, metallic, intraocular foreign bodies, with elimination of the scatter from metallic objects seen with CAT scanning. A piece of identical material should be tested inside the magnet first.

Signs: With large objects, there is obvious disruption of the anterior segment with a site of penetration, possible hyphaema and/or stellate cataract formation. The object may be seen lodged deep in the cornea or in the lens, vitreous or retina. With smaller objects, there may be few symptoms or signs.

N.B. Any history of hammering or chiselling accompanying even trivial eye injury should be investigated with a plain radiograph of the orbit (two views should be taken to eliminate artefact) and a fundal examination with the pupil fully dilated.

The entry site is sutured primarily and then a planned removal of the foreign body is carried out if feasible. Metallic foreign bodies should be removed within 24 hours unless vitrectomy procedures are being planned, in which case removal is delayed to allow time for posterior vitreous detachment to occur. Corneal and anterior chamber foreign bodies can be removed by corneal section whilst a lensectomy is carried out for those lodged in the lens. Posterior foreign bodies may be removed with the aid of a magnet, but vitrectomy procedures and use of foreign body forceps to extract the object have greatly improved the prognosis. Some foreign bodies are inert and do not need to be removed, e.g. eyelashes in the anterior chamber (*Fig. 12.18*), glass, stone, some plastics and certain metals such as gold, silver, platinum. Others are toxic, e.g. vegetable matter and metals such as copper, iron, aluminium and zinc. Retained, iron foreign bodies may lead to deposition of iron salts in the eye and to consequent retinal toxicity. This condition is called siderosis bulbi and an alteration in iris colour may be seen (*Fig. 12.19(a) & (b)*).

12.18

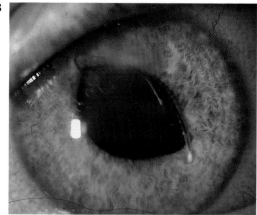

Fig. 12.18 Eyelashes in anterior chamber (Courtesy of Mr. C. Dean Hart)
Fig. 12.19(a) Siderosis bulbi – affected eye
Fig. 12.19(b) Siderosis bulbi – normal eye

12.19(a)

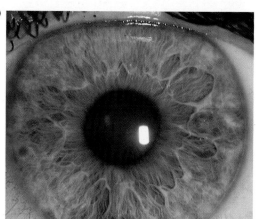

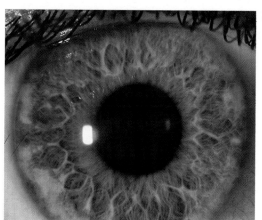

12.19(b)

Orbital fractures

Fracture of the inferior orbital margin

This common orbital fracture is caused by a direct blow to the orbit leading to the classical 'black eye'. The bone fractures at its weakest point – the canal for the infraorbital nerve.

Signs: Periorbital haematoma and infraorbital anaesthesia. There is no disturbance of ocular movements unless there is an associated fracture of the orbital floor. The eye should be examined for anterior segment or retinal damage. The diagnosis is confirmed by orbital radiography (occipito-mental view).

Management: No treatment is required for this type of fracture.

'Blow-out fractures'

This type of fracture (*Figs. 12.20, 12.21(a)–(c)*) is caused by direct impact of an object just larger than the orbital rim, transmitting force within the orbit to the walls, which fracture at their weakest point, namely the orbital floor, or less commonly, the medial wall.

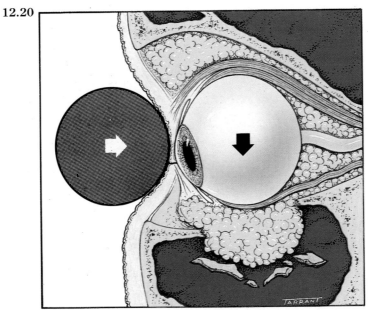

Fig. 12.20 An artist's impression of a blow-out fracture caused by the impact of a ball

Signs: There is usually **periorbital and lid bruising**, together with **surgical emphysema**, which often occurs alarmingly when the patient sneezes or blows his nose. The latter sign suggests a fracture involving a sinus, usually ethmoid or maxillary. There is **enophthalmos** (measurable with an exophthalmometer after the periorbital swelling has diminished), **infraorbital anaesthesia, restricted elevation** and sometimes **depression** leading to **diplopia**, due to entrapment of the orbital fat, the inferior rectus and inferior oblique muscles. The diplopia may be assessed using a Hess chart and a binocular field of single vision. An occipito-mental skull radiograph shows the classical 'tear-drop' sign of prolapsed orbital soft tissue in the maxillary sinus, bony disruption of the orbital floor or fluid in the maxillary sinus. Further views, including tomography or orbital CAT scanning, may be helpful if surgical correction is contemplated (*Fig. 12.22*).

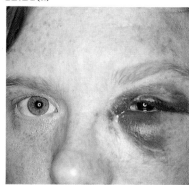

Fig. 12.21(a) Periorbital haematoma

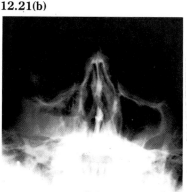

Fig. 12.21(b) Blow-out fracture –
skull radiograph showing a fluid level in
the right maxillary sinus

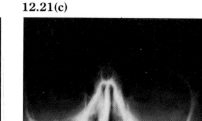

Fig. 12.21(c) Blow-out fracture –
skull radiograph showing prolapse of
orbital contents inferiorly – tear drop
sign

(S) *Management:* This depends on the extent of the injury
and the treatment preferred by the centre. The
symptoms often settle rapidly in the first few days. In
general the more serious blow-out fracture, with
significant entrapment of soft tissue, enophthalmos
(greater than 2 mm) and severe diplopia five days after
injury, is corrected surgically at 5–10 days post-injury,
with freeing of the trapped tissue and silastic implant
to restore the orbital floor. Less severe cases are
treated conservatively in the first instance, with later
surgical intervention considered if symptoms remain
disturbing.

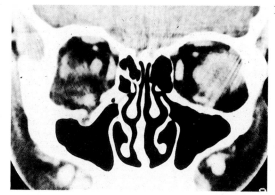

Fig. 12.22 A CT scan of a blow-out fracture of the
orbit showing a fragment of bone angled down into
right antrum (Courtesy of Dr. W.D. Jeans)

Other fractures

Medial wall fractures seldom require surgical intervention unless the medial rectus muscle is caught in
the fracture.

Orbital roof fractures result from a severe direct
blow and may be accompanied by a cerebro-spinal
fluid leak. There is a risk of meningitis and antibiotic
cover (e.g. sulphadimidine) should be given. The
superior rectus and levator muscles may also be
involved.

Lateral wall fractures occur after severe trauma
and are often accompanied by ocular damage and
orbital haemorrhage (v.i.).

Severe head injuries may be accompanied by the
development of a caroticocavernous fistula (*Fig.
12.23*).

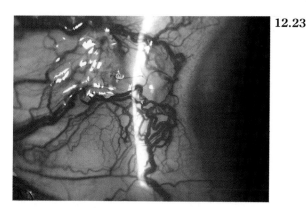

Fig. 12.23 Left caroticocavernous fistula (detail)

Optic nerve compression secondary to orbital haemorrhage

In severe orbital trauma there may be intraorbital bleeding. Since the orbit is a closed space, this will lead to **proptosis** and **optic nerve compression**. Progressive loss of visual acuity occurs in the absence of obvious ocular injury. A relative afferent pupillary defect is seen, signifying optic nerve involvement (the pupils will be of equal size, but there will be a deficient direct response to light on the affected side compared with the normal (see p. 20)). Retinal examination shows congestion of the retinal veins and diminished retinal arterial circulation. The treatment is orbital decompression which is only successful in the first few hours of optic nerve compromisation.

Skin lacerations around the eye

Simple skin lacerations in the periorbital area (*Figs.12.24(a)–(c)*) may be stitched with interrupted sutures under direct vision, using a fine non-absorbable suture material, for example 6/0 black silk or nylon. Tetanus prophylaxis should be given if necessary. The sutures are removed at four days. Extensive wounds around the eye or those involving the lid margin should be referred to an eye centre. Upper lid lacerations with resulting ptosis need exploration to exclude damage to the levator palpebrae superioris and/or retained foreign material, e.g. pieces of twig.

12.24(a)

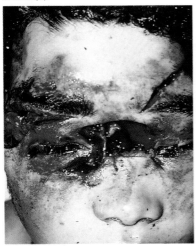

12.24(b)

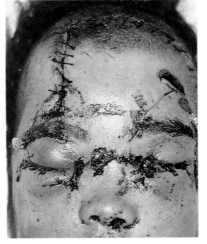

12.24(c)

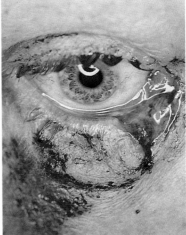

Fig. 12.24(a) Extensive facial lacerations in road traffic accident victim – patient not wearing a seat belt (Courtesy of Mr. C. Dean Hart)

Fig. 12.24(b) Same patient as in Fig. 12.24(a) after suturing (Courtesy of Mr. C. Dean Hart)

Fig. 12.24(c) Avulsion of right lower lid (Courtesy of Mr. C. Dean Hart)

Repair of a full-thickness lid margin wound

12.25

Lid margin
sutures

Skin
sutures

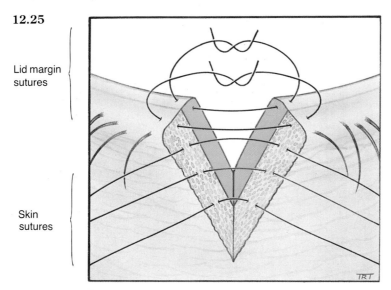

Fig. 12.25 Method of suturing a lower lid laceration.
N.B. Sutures to tarsal plate deep to skin have been omitted
for clarity.

Repair of such a wound (*Fig. 12.25*) should be carried out under sterile conditions preferably using an operating microscope, or at least a pair of operating loupes. It is essential to create perfect lid margin alignment otherwise lid notching and deformity will occur. With extensive lacerations, general anaesthesia is preferable. Tetanus status should be checked.

● The skin is infiltrated with local anaesthetic, e.g. 2% lignocaine with adrenaline (unless the patient is under general anaesthetic). The area is prepared with antiseptic and sterile drapes are applied.

● The wound edges are cleaned with physiological solutions and apposed to plan the suture positioning.

● The lid margin is aligned using an absorbable suture, e.g. 6/0 vicryl, which is passed subcutaneously through the orbicularis muscle and tarsal plate (but not out through the conjunctival side) on one side and then through the tarsal plate and finally the orbicularis muscle on the other side. This suture is placed as close to the lid margin as possible. A single throw is placed to test correct alignment. The correct positioning is vital for the rest of the procedure and the suture is replaced if the position is unsatisfactory.

● Two further subcutaneous, absorbable sutures, e.g. 6/0 vicryl, are placed similarly in the tarsal plate, further away from the lid margin and spaced at regular intervals. These are then tied. The uppermost, absorbable suture may now be tied if the appearances are satisfactory.

● The lid margin suture is now placed. A 6/0 black silk suture is passed through the grey line on either side of the wound, either as a mattress suture or as a simple interrupted suture. If the position is satisfactory, the suture is tied and the ends left long (about 2 cm). Ideally, the lid margins should pout up on either side of the repaired wound as this avoids later lid notching.

● The skin is sutured from the lid margin downwards using 6/0 black silk interrupted sutures. Catching the long ends of the lid margin suture in the second throw of the first skin suture, a final throw is placed and both may then be trimmed.

● A single dose of antibiotic ointment is given and a course of oral, prophylactic antibiotics if necessary.

● The skin sutures are removed at five days, but the lid margin sutures should remain 10–14 days.

Lid lacerations involving the upper canaliculi are sutured as a primary procedure with no consequent problems from epiphora since the lower canaliculus is still functioning. However, lacerations through the lower canaliculus may lead to persistent epiphora. Care is needed for precise alignment of the two cut edges. Some surgeons use stents to support the canaliculus during repair and healing, whilst others are of the opinion that this leads to more scarring and favour a simple, primary repair and subsequent drainage surgery if required. Avulsion of the medial canthal tendon requires a deep suture attaching the medial lower lid to periosteum to prevent subsequent sagging of the tissues.

13 Paediatric eye conditions

General points

Paediatric ophthalmology presents certain problems not present in adult ophthalmology. There is often delayed presentation since children may not notice a gradual visual loss. Examination and treatment of children requires great patience and patient cooperation (not always readily achieved except under general anaesthetic). It is usually best to take a history from the parent before attempting to examine the child as this relaxes both parent and child. Babies are often best examined when wrapped up in a blanket, which cuts down on the number of moving parts. Paediatric eyelid retractors are an extremely useful and atraumatic way of looking at the eye, e.g. to assess injury. Eye movements are often successfully elicited with the child positioned over the parent's shoulder. Fundoscopy in babies is best achieved using an indirect ophthalmoscope, with the baby positioned lying down on the parent's knee, head outwards, feet in towards the parent and head held still by positioning between the knees. In general, ointment is easier for parents to use than drops as one can be sure a dose has reached the right place. Chloramphenicol drops should not be used in babies owing to significant absorption by this route and the risk of haematological abnormalities. Atropine drops or ointment should not be used in young babies because of systemic side-effects. Atropine ointment is preferable to drops in all children as there is less risk of overdose and dangerous toxicity. Tropicamide 1% is an adequate dilating drop for all children and cyclopentolate 0.5% or 1% is an adequate cycloplegic (and dilating drop) for refraction in young babies. In older children, atropine may be used for cycloplegic refraction, but some specialists also use cyclopentolate for such cases.

Common problems

Trauma

Corneal abrasion

This is a common injury (*see Fig. 12.2(a) & (b)*) in babies and toddlers, often caused by a finger-nail or toy. The eye becomes red and the child will start rubbing it. The abrasion will stain brilliantly with a drop of fluorescein. Unless the history is clear, the eyelid should be everted to exclude a subtarsal foreign body. This is best achieved by wrapping the child in a blanket, pulling the top lid downwards and using a glass rod in the tarsal crease to push down whilst the lid margin is flipped back. A cotton tip bud should be handy for swift removal of the subtarsal foreign body. The corneal abrasion is treated with antibiotic ointment q.d.s. for 3–4 days and the patient should be seen daily until healed (usually 1–2 days). A pad will not be tolerated and should not be attempted with young children.

Corneal foreign body

Ⓡ Sometimes a piece of grit etc. becomes embedded in the cornea and if it is only loosely attached, a quick dab with a moist, cotton wool bud may remove it after some benoxinate 1% drops have been applied. Care should be taken not to touch the cornea as an abrasion may be induced. Clearly, needles are too dangerous to be used in young children who cannot be relied upon to keep still. The best approach for embedded objects is a trial of chloramphenicol ointment applied q.d.s. This often softens the cornea and the foreign body will fall off after a few days. If the foreign body is still firmly embedded, a short general anaesthetic may be required to remove it.

Corneal ulcer

Ⓡ Ⓢ This presents as a sticky, red eye, often with a white speck (infiltrate) on the cornea. This may stain with fluorescein. The lids must be everted to exclude a subtarsal foreign body. This is best managed in an eye centre. Conjunctival swabs and, if possible, a corneal scrape should be taken. Depending on the results, frequent application of antibiotic drops, e.g. two-hourly, together with antibiotic ointment at night, is started.

Non-accidental injury

A careful history is necessary with all paediatric injuries and if there is any suspicion of child abuse, the child is admitted and a general paediatric opinion is sought. The "At Risk Register", a register compiled of families at risk, is consulted. Injuries include cigarette burns or bruising around the face and eyes and retinal and vitreous haemorrhages following repeated head shaking.

Developmental anomalies

Hypertelorism

This is an increased distance between the lateral orbital margins, usually measured clinically as the interpupillary distance. If the distance between the medial canthi is increased, this is referred to as telecanthus or sometimes hypertelorism. It is associated with craniofacial abnormalities and sometimes congenital abnormalities elsewhere.

Epicanthic folds

This (*Fig. 13.1*) is a common finding in normal, young children, especially those of oriental origin. There is a broad fold of skin arising from the medial aspect of the upper lid that partially obscures the nasal aspect of the globe. It may give the false impression of convergent squint and the symmetry of the corneal reflexes is a useful guide here.

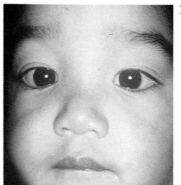

13.1

Fig. 13.1 Epicanthic folds (Courtesy of the Orthoptic Department, Bristol Eye Hospital)

Aniridia

This literally means an absent iris (*Fig. 13.2*), although remnants can be seen on gonioscopy. There is usually associated macular hypoplasia with poor vision, and glaucoma may develop.

The condition may be dominantly inherited or a spontaneous mutation, often associated with a chromosome abnormality. It has an important association with Wilm's tumour (nephroblastoma) and all children with aniridia should be screened at regular intervals with intravenous urography to exclude this.

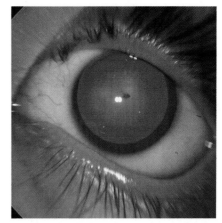
13.2

Fig. 13.2 Aniridia (Courtesy of Institute of Child Health)

Coloboma

Colobomas are developmental defects of various parts of the eye. **Lid colobomas** are usually full-thickness defects and may be associated with other facial abnormalities, e.g. dermoids and cleft palate. They are repaired early if there is a risk of exposure keratitis. Otherwise repair is delayed until the child is a few years old.

Iris colobomas (*Fig. 13.3*) are often associated with more posterior colobomas of the chorioretina (*Fig. 13.4*) as they are due to failure of the optic fissure to close correctly during development. Iris colobomas do not cause any visual problems, but the more posterior defects may. They may also be associated with other systemic disorders. Cosmetic appearances may be improved with a tinted contact lens.

Persistence of the foetal hyaloid system include a persistent hyaloid artery, Bergmeister's papilla, which is a remnant at the optic disc, and Mittendorf dot, a remnant at the posterior lens surface. Persistent primary hyperplastic vitreous (see p. 235) is the most extreme example.

13.3
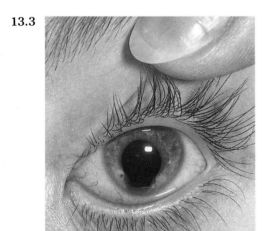

Fig. 13.3 Iris coloboma (Courtesy of Mr. R. Humphry)

13.4
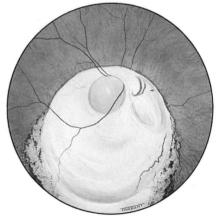

Fig. 13.4 Artist's impression of coloboma of the chorioretina

Blocked nasolacrimal duct

This presents in the first few months of life, sometimes in the newborn period. It is due to blockage of the distal end of the nasolacrimal duct.

Symptoms: Lacrimation, recurrent sticky eyes and occasionally dacryocystitis, seen as a red, inflamed swelling, medial to the inner canthus.

Signs: The eye has a mucoid discharge which tends to crust on the lashes. It is not usually associated with an inflamed conjunctiva. Pressure over the lacrimal sac may produce regurgitation of mucoid material from the puncta. Occasionally a dacryocoele is present from birth. This appears as a bluish swelling filled with mucoid material which is medial to the inner canthus.

Management: Most cases will eventually resolve (s) spontaneously as the nasolacrimal duct canalises, usually by the age of one year. Interim treatment consists of massage of the lacrimal sac to expel the mucoid contents and antibiotic drops or ointment. Dacryocystitis is treated with systemic antibiotics in addition. True congenital dacryocoeles may be probed in the neonatal period, but the majority are probed if they have failed to resolve after one year.

Systemic disease affecting the eye
Juvenile chronic arthritis (JCA)

This seronegative arthritis, which by definition affects children under the age of 16 years, is associated with chronic uveitis. The uveitis is often asymptomatic until the later complications have arisen and thus it is important to **screen** the children at risk. Occasionally the uveitis precedes the arthritis.

There are three types of JCA which refer to the type of presentation:

● **Systemic JCA**, which presents as a systemic illness with fever, rash, lymphadenopathy, hepatosplenomegaly and minimal, if any, joint involvement initially. Uveitis is very rarely associated.

● **Pauciarticular JCA**, which presents as arthritis affecting fewer than five joints. Uveitis affects about 20% of patients in this group. High risk factors include positive antinuclear antibody and female sex. There is a high prevalence of HLA-B5 in those with uveitis.

● **Polyarticular JCA**, which presents as arthritis affecting five or more joints. Uveitis is rare in this group.

Symptoms: Initially asymptomatic. When complications develop, e.g. cataract formation, there is loss of visual acuity.

Signs: The eye is invariably white and there is often bilateral involvement. The complications seen are:

● Band keratopathy – a band-shaped deposition of calcium in Bowman's membrane, commencing at three and nine o'clock and spreading inwards to the centre

● Chronic uveitis with keratic precipitates, cells and flare in the anterior chamber, posterior synechiae formation and vitreous activity

● Complicated posterior subcapsular cataract

● Glaucoma

● Cystoid macular oedema, which should be looked for in any patient with reduced visual acuity

Investigations: If there is any doubt about the aetiology of the uveitis, the child should have routine screening tests for uveitis (see p. 108) including a full blood count and viscosity, chest radiograph, and tests for syphilis and tuberculosis if applicable. A test for antinuclear antibody is helpful.

Ⓢ *Management:* The uveitis is initially controlled with topical steroid, e.g. betamethasone drops q.d.s. or in mild cases prednisolone drops 0.5% q.d.s. until the inflammation is under control. The dosage is then reduced slowly. Mydriatics, e.g. cyclopentolate drops 0.5% or 1% t.d.s., are used. In severe cases oral steroids are used, preferably in alternate day therapy to prevent adrenal suppression and growth retardation. This is carried out in conjunction with a paediatrician. Subconjunctival injections can only be carried out under general anaesthesia in children. Band keratopathy may be treated for visual or cosmetic reasons. Under general anaesthetic the corneal epithelium is gently scraped off over the band and sodium versonate drops applied to leach out the calcium deposits. Antibiotic ointment, cycloplegic drops and a pad are then applied. The cataracts are removed by extracapsular cataract extraction when visual symptoms require this.

Leukocoria

Leukocoria or a white pupillary reflex (*Fig. 13.5*) is one of the most important presentations of eye disease in children. It requires immediate referral for accurate diagnosis. The differential diagnoses are:

- **Congenital cataract**
- **Retinoblastoma**
- **Retinopathy of prematurity**
- **Persistent primary hyperplastic vitreous**
- **Toxocara** and **Toxoplasma** or any cause of severe posterior uveitis
- **Retinal detachment**
- **Retinal dysplasia**
- **Coat's disease**
- **Large chorioretinal coloboma**

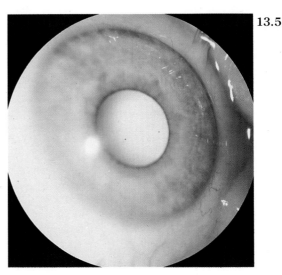

13.5

Fig. 13.5 Leukocoria

Congenital cataract

Congenital (or infantile) cataracts (*Fig. 13.6*) are lens opacities that present at birth or within infancy. They usually present as a white pupillary reflex, but less dense opacities appear as white opacities in the lens. They may be unilateral or bilateral. Many congenital cataracts are hereditary, but they are also commonly associated with the following conditions:

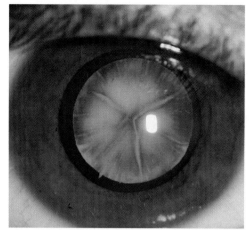

Fig. 13.6 Congenital cataract

Intrauterine infections

Rubella infection in the first nine weeks of gestation can lead to congenital cataracts and is often associated with other congenital abnormalities, e.g. sensorineural deafness, mental retardation, microcephaly, congenital heart defects, hepatosplenomegaly, thrombocytopenia and pneumonitis. Other ocular manifestations include rubella retinopathy (*Fig. 13.7*), microphthalmos and uveitis. Any of the congenital infections screened for in the "TORCH'S" (Toxoplasmosis, Other, Rubella, Cytomegalovirus, *Herpes simplex*, Syphilis) test may also give rise to cataracts.

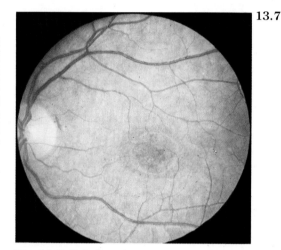

Fig. 13.7 Rubella retinopathy

Inherited metabolic disease

Galactosaemia is due to two types of recessively inherited enzyme deficiencies – classical galactosaemia and galactokinase deficiency. They are both associated with a high level of galactose in the blood and the presence of this reducing sugar in the urine. Classical galactosaemia is due to a deficiency of galactose-1-phosphate uridyl transferase (GPUT). Other manifestations in infancy include failure to thrive, hepatosplenomegaly, jaundice, cirrhosis, renal disease, anaemia, mental retardation, deafness and ultimately death if untreated. The treatment consists of a lactose-free diet, i.e., the exclusion of all dairy products. A deficiency of galactokinase (the first enzyme in the pathway of galactose metabolism) leads to cataract formation alone without any systemic manifestations. Both types lead to cataract formation within the first two months of life and may be reversible if treatment is instigated sufficiently early.

One of the other metabolic disorders causing congenital cataract (and congenital glaucoma) is Lowe's syndrome (oculocerebrorenal syndrome). This is an X-linked disorder of amino acid metabolism. It is important to screen for this by looking for amino acids in the urine since the systemic features in infancy may be non-specific failure to thrive, progressing to renal failure and mental retardation.

Metabolic disturbances

These include hypoglycaemia in the neonatal period and hypocalcaemia, e.g. in idiopathic hypoparathyroidism.

Maternal drug ingestion

Steroids taken by the mother during pregnancy may lead to congenital cataracts in the baby.

(S) *Management of congenital cataracts:* All patients with congenital cataracts should have immediate referral to a specialist eye centre as any delay in treatment may lead to the development of amblyopia. A combined assessment with a paediatrician is important. History should include details of maternal health during pregnancy, birth and neonatal problems and family history as well as ocular history. The visual acuities are assessed using the Catford Drum (*see Figs. 1.6(a) & (b)*) or, if available, preferential looking (*see Fig. 1.7*). The eye is examined for signs of inflammation and fundoscopy is carried out with direct and indirect ophthalmoscopes. As well as indicating any fundal abnormality, e.g. rubella retinopathy, or persistent primary hyperplastic vitreous, this gives an indication of the density of the lens opacities. If very dense, no view will be obtained with either type of ophthalmoscopy. If less dense, the indirect ophthalmoscope will give fundal detail, and if insignificant, both types will give fundal detail.

If the cataract is present at birth and unilateral, unless it is operated upon within the first few days of life, there is a very poor prognosis for visual development. Bilateral cataracts have a better prognosis. Screening tests carried out include:

- Serum rubella IgM titres and virus cultures from nasopharynx and urine. A TORCH'S test would screen for all common congenital infections.

- Urine – for reducing substances and amino acids. If reducing substances are present, red cell GPUT and GK levels are taken.

- Blood glucose, serum calcium and phosphate.

For dense cataracts an examination under anaesthetic, followed by cataract extraction by lens aspiration or lensectomy, is carried out. The baby is then fitted with extended-wear contact lenses. This requires highly motivated parents since the lenses are often lost, infections may develop and frequent visits to the eye centre are required, often several times a week. If treatment is persevered with, the eventual visual outcome is much better than before the advent of these lenses. Sometimes, following lens aspiration, the capsule becomes opacified and a capsulotomy is then required.

Later onset cataracts in childhood can be associated with a number of conditions including atopic eczema, treatment with steroids, e.g. for severe asthma or eczema, Down's syndrome and rarer inherited disorders, e.g. Fabry's disease and mucopolysaccharidoses.

Retinoblastoma

This rare tumour (*Fig. 13.8*) has an incidence of about 1 in 20,000 births, but is the most common ocular tumour of childhood. About 94% of all cases of retinoblastoma are spontaneous with no previous family history, although a third of these will then be seen to be of the inherited type, as further siblings and offspring are affected. The long arm of chromosome 13 is thought to be the site of genetic abnormality. Retinoblastoma may be unilateral or bilateral. Bilateral cases are invariably of the inherited type and present earlier, usually by the age of 15 months. Unilateral cases are more common and tend to present later. Almost all present by the age of three years and are 80–90% sporadic with the remainder inherited.

Symptoms and Signs: The most common mode of presentation is an abnormal pupil appearance which has been noticed by the parent, family practitioner or paediatrician. The second most common presentation is the development of a squint. It is therefore mandatory to carry out fundoscopy with full pupillary dilatation with all squints. Other modes are intraocular inflammation, glaucoma, orbital spread with proptosis and metastasis to bone marrow or CNS. Fundal appearances may either show a single, well-defined, solid, white–pink tumour, sometimes with strands radiating into the vitreous, or a total retinal detachment with vitreous haemorrhage or activity.

(R)(S) *Management:* Patients with retinoblastoma are best managed in specialist centres where, as well as surgical or radiotherapy expertise, there is good genetic counselling. Other causes of leukocoria should be excluded. An ELISA (Enzyme Linked Immunosorbent Assay) test for toxocara antibodies is carried out. Plain radiographs and CT scanning of the orbit are performed

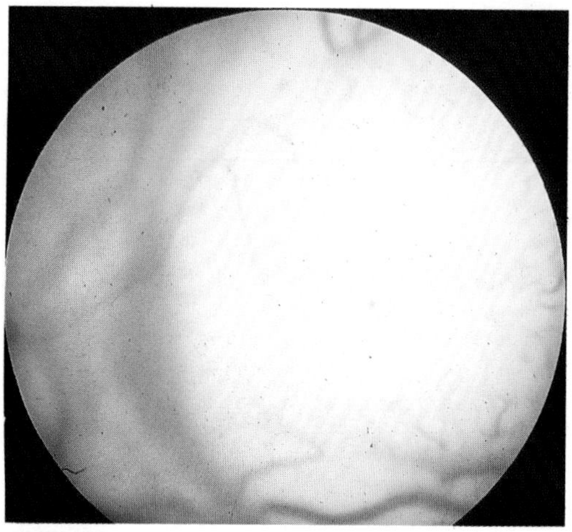

Fig. 13.8 Retinoblastoma (Courtesy of Mr. C. Dean Hart)

to determine the extent of the tumour and any calcification which is suggestive of retinoblastoma. Bone marrow biopsy or CSF examination to look for metastases is performed in some centres. An examination under anaesthesia is performed for diagnosis often prior to enucleation. Enucleation is usually performed in eyes with no useful vision especially if first eyes. Radiotherapy is performed if it is thought that the eye can be saved with some vision. Treatments vary with particular centres, however. The rest of the family should be checked at regular intervals for asymptomatic tumours.

Prognosis: The overall mortality is 15–20%. If there is any extension the prognosis is much worse. Small posterior tumours have up to a 70% survival rate.

Useful figures for genetic counselling

• The risk of an individual with bilateral retinoblastoma or unilateral retinoblastoma with a positive family history passing the condition on to an offspring is 50%. If the retinoblastoma was unilateral and spontaneous, the risk is under 10%.

• The risk of developing a retinoblastoma is 50% for the sibling of an affected child with bilateral retinoblastoma or unilateral retinoblastoma with a positive family history. With unilateral, spontaneous retinoblastoma the risk is about 1%.

- The risk of the unaffected sibling or offspring of a retinoblastoma patient producing an offspring with retinoblastoma is about 6%. If this does occur, the person is then a known carrier and the risk to any subsequent offspring is 50%.

Much of the uncertainty of carrier status will be removed with further advances in genetic mapping.

Retinopathy of prematurity (retrolental fibroplasia)

This is a disease of premature (<36 weeks gestation) and low birth weight babies (usually <1.5kg at birth) who have received treatment with oxygen for respiratory problems (*Fig. 13.9*). It consists of a proliferative retinopathy which can progress to vitreous haemorrhage, tractional retinal detachment and finally a retrolental mass with leukocoria (white pupil). It may, however, stop at any stage or regress if the changes are fairly mild. Milder cases may show the typical appearances of the dragged disc where there is traction of the temporal retinal vessels. In later life there is a higher incidence of rhegmatogenous retinal detachment.

(S) *Management:* The best management is prevention by continuous oxygen monitoring to keep blood oxygen at safe levels in the high risk groups. There is some evidence that Vitamin E may be partly protective. In early stages the condition may regress. If progressive, it may be treated with cyclocryotherapy. Retinal detachment and vitrectomy surgery are sometimes helpful. Careful follow-up is required, even in those individuals with mild ROP, to detect and treat any lesions predisposing to retinal detachment.

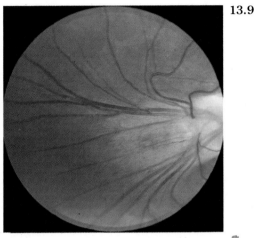

13.9

Fig. 13.9 Retinopathy of prematurity

Persistent primary hyperplastic vitreous

This is a developmental abnormality in which the foetal primary vitreous persists and appears as leukocoria in the young infant. Other causes of leukocoria must be excluded before the diagnosis can be made.

Toxocara

This (*Fig. 13.10,* see pp. 112–13) is extremely rare under the age of two years as the child does not usually come into close contact with dog faeces or puppies until he is independently mobile. In young children, the most common ocular manifestation is a chronic uveitis that may be associated with exudative detachment. In older children (> six years), posterior pole granulomas are seen. Peripheral granulomas may also occur after this age. ELISA test for toxocara antibodies, if positive at 1 in 8, is highly significant. FBC for eosinophil count is helpful.

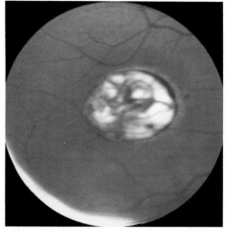

13.10

Fig. 13.10 Toxocara – chorioretinal tear
(Courtesy of Mr. R. Humphry)

Toxoplasmosis

Most childhood cases of toxoplasmosis (see p. 112) are asymptomatic and may appear as a posterior pole chorioretinal scars. They rarely reactivate before the teens. Toxoplasma dye test and indirect fluorescent antibody test are significant if positive on undiluted serum.

Coat's disease

This occurs most commonly in healthy boys and consists of telangiectasia of the retinal blood vessels and widespread exudation (*Fig. 13.11*). It only affects one eye. If untreated with laser or cryotherapy in the early stages, it may progress to total retinal detachment which is a cause of leukocoria.

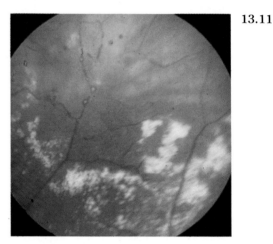

13.11

Fig. 13.11 Coat's disease

Congenital opaque cornea

This may be caused by a number of different conditions and requires immediate specialist referral (*Figs. 13.12, 13.13*). It is due to corneal decompensation and may be caused by:

- **Direct injury with forceps during delivery**

- **Congenital ocular infection including rubella, ophthalmia neonatorum**

- **Mucopolysaccharidoses**, e.g. Hurler's syndrome.

- **Corneal endothelial dystrophy**

- **Congenital glaucoma** (Buphthalmos) (*Figs. 13.14(a) & (b)*). This is associated with diffuse oedema of the cornea and breaks in the corneal endothelium (Haab's striae). The cornea enlarges and the infant will be intensely photophobic with lacrimation. The intraocular pressure can sometimes be measured using a Perkin's hand-held applanation tonometer while the infant is feeding. Gonioscopy, examination of the optic nerve, measurement of corneal diameter and intraocular pressure are carried out under anaesthetic. Treatment is with acetazolamide initially, followed by goniotomy (with or without drops) to lower the intraocular pressure.

13.12

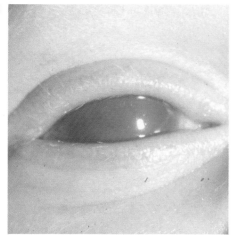

Fig. 13.12 Congenital opaque cornea (Courtesy of Institute of Child Health)

13.13

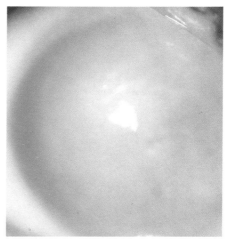

Fig. 13.13 Congenital opaque cornea

13.14(a)

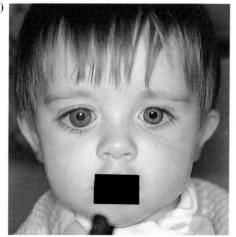

Fig. 13.14(a) Congenital glaucoma (Buphthalmos) showing enlargement of the right (affected) eye

13.14(b)

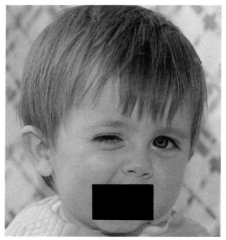

Fig. 13.14(b) Congenital glaucoma (demonstrating closure of the affected eye in response to light)

Ophthalmia neonatorum

This is conjunctivitis occurring within the first month of life (*Fig. 13.15(a)–(c)*). It may be caused by various agents and timing may offer some guide as to the type of infection. Conjunctivitis within hours of birth may be due to **chemical** contamination, e.g. silver nitrate, and this will settle spontaneously. If it occurs within 2–4 days, **gonococcal** infection should be suspected. This is an ophthalmic emergency since penetration of the cornea may occur within 24–48 hours. Congenital syphilis may present with sticky eyes associated with 'snuffles' and systemic disease within the first few days of birth. Other bacterial infections, e.g. Streptococcus, Staphylococcus and *E. coli*, present at 5–7 days. TRIC (chlamydial) conjunctivitis presents at 5–14 days and is the most common cause in the UK Viral infections, e.g. *Herpes simplex* type 2, usually present from one week. Cases with ophthalmia neonatorum should be admitted to hospital and in the UK the disease is notifiable.

13.15(a)

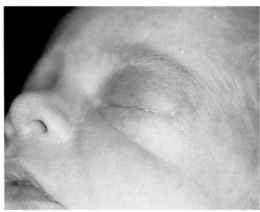

Fig. 13.15(a) Ophthalmia neonatorum
Fig. 13.15(b) Lid oedema in ophthalmia neonatorum (Courtesy of Professor S. Darougar)
Fig. 13.15(c) Chlamydial inclusion bodies in a conjunctival smear stained with giemsa (Courtesy of Professor S. Darougar)

13.15(b)

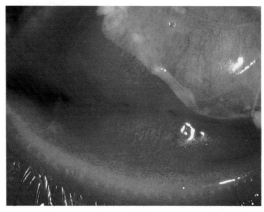

13.15(c

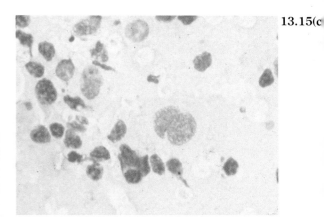

Clinical features

Bacterial conjunctivitis

The most common cause is the gonococcus, with an incubation period, as mentioned, of 2–4 days. The next most prevalent is *Staphylococcus aureus*.

Signs:

• In gonococcal infection there is severe lid oedema and chemosis, with a serosanguinous discharge becoming mucopurulent after six days. Corneal ulceration can occur, leading to endophthalmitis and blindness.

• In conjunctivitis due to *Staph. aureus* there is a moderate lid swelling and conjunctival oedema. Corneal ulceration is rare.

(R) *Investigation:*

• Scrapings (*Fig. 13.15(c)*) show Gram negative cocci in gonococcal conjunctivitis , and Gram positive cocci in infection due to *Staph. aureus*.

• Cultures should be taken sequentially to aid diagnosis and response to treatment.

Management: The following is recommended: (S)

• Gonococcal conjunctivitis.

a. Prophylaxis is by the introduction of a single dose ampoule of silver nitrate 1%, or a single use tube of tetracycline 1% or erythromycin 0.5% ointment. Irrigation with silver nitrate is not employed because of the risk of chemical irritation.
b. Cases must be hospitalised in isolation.
c. IV aqueous benzyl penicillin g 50,000 units/kg/day in two doses daily for seven days.
d. Topical benzyl penicillin in buffered citrate (10,000–20,000 units/ml) intensively until the condition resolves and is culture negative.
e. Saline irrigation.

• Staphylococcal conjunctivitis. This will respond to topical chloramphenicol, erythromycin, tobramycin or neomycin ointment.

Chlamydial ophthalmia neonatorum

Chlamydia trachomatis is the most common cause of ophthalmia neonatorum. The incubation period is 5–14 days.

Signs: Moderate lid and conjunctival oedema, with occasional purulent discharge. Conjunctival scars have been noted.

(R) *Investigations:* Giemsa staining of conjunctival scrapings shows basophilic paranuclear cytoplasmic inclusion bodies. There is now an ELISA for fast diagnosis.

Management: (S)

• Oral erythromycin (30–50 mg/kg/day) four times daily for two weeks (to prevent pneumonia).

• Topical tetracycline ointment (1%) every two hours for the first day, then four times daily.

Herpetic ophthalmia neonatorum

Herpes simplex virus type 2 infrequently causes viral conjunctivitis and may be combined with lesions of the mouth, skin or central nervous system. The ocular signs may appear 2–14 days post partum. Late sequelae may occur, with stromal keratitis, cataract, chorioretinitis and optic neuritis.

(R) *Investigations:*

• Culture of all involved sites for *Herpes simplex* virus

• Serial antibody assays

Management: (S)

• Topical acyclovir 3% ointment two hourly

• Slow IV infusion of acyclovir 5 mg/kg eight hourly for five days. The infant has a red, inflamed eye with mucopurulent discharge. Examination of the cornea for ulceration is important. A subtarsal foreign body must be excluded.

Other tumours of childhood

Dermoid

This is a congenital inclusion of abnormal epithelial elements and is most frequently situated at the limbus or on the orbital rim in children (see Chapter 3).

(S) **Limbal dermoids** (*Fig. 13.16*) are treated with local excision, and keratoplasty if necessary. They are present in Goldenhar's syndrome which also includes orbital dermoids, pre-auricular skin tags, coloboma of the upper lid and vertebral, cardiovascular, renal, genitourinary and gastrointestinal abnormalities.

Orbital dermoids are most commonly situated at the superotemporal margin of the orbit. Even if well-defined on palpation, they may extend a long way posteriorly, making it advisable to carry out an orbital (S) CT scan before exploration and excision.

Conjunctival lipodermoid (*Fig. 13.17*) is a congenital tumour of adipose tissue that often causes great alarm to the parents when first discovered.

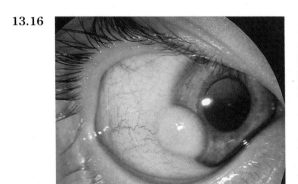

Fig. 13.16 Limbal dermoid

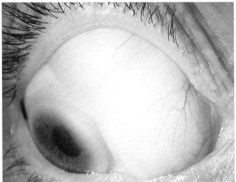

Fig. 13.17 Conjunctival lipodermoid

Juvenile xanthogranuloma of iris

This yellowish, benign, vascular tumour (*Fig. 13.18*) may lead to spontaneous hyphaema and glaucoma in children, commonly in the first year of life. It may be associated with similar yellowish tumours in the (S) skin. It is excised or treated with steroids or irradiation.

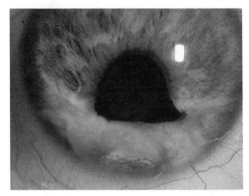

Fig. 13.18 Juvenile xanthogranuloma of iris (Courtesy of Institute of Ophthalmology)

Haemangiomas

Naevus flammeus and strawberry naevus

For a full discussion see p. 49. Haemangiomas of the retina are seen in Von Hippel-Lindau syndrome, associated with cerebellar haemangiomas, renal and epididymal tumours and cysts, pancreatic cysts and phaeochromocytoma.

Strabismus

The evaluation of strabismus (squint) is best performed in an ophthalmic clinic and will only be discussed at a basic level in this text.

Definition of terms

A **-tropia** is a manifest squint and a **-phoria** is a latent squint. The direction of squint is indicated by the prefix, i.e. **exo-** is a horizontal deviation outwards (divergent) (*Fig. 13.19*), **eso-** is a horizontal deviation inwards (convergent), **hypo-** is a vertical deviation downwards and **hyper-** is a vertical deviation upwards. Thus an **esotropia** is a manifest, convergent squint and an **exophoria** is a latent, divergent squint.

13.19

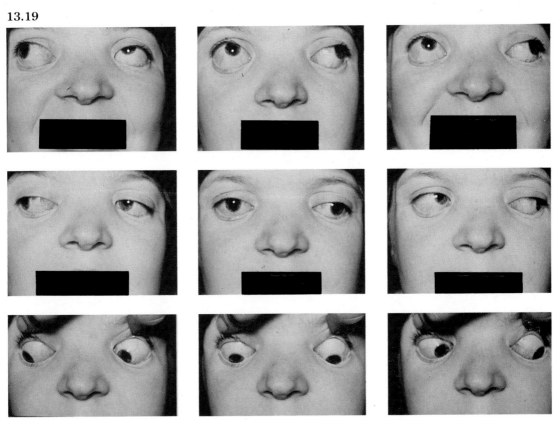

Fig. 13.19 Nine positions of gaze in child with Crouzon's syndrome (craniofacial dysostosis), demonstrating 'V' pattern exotropia (i.e. exotropia which is more marked in upgaze) (Courtesy of Mr. D. Taylor)

A **concomitant** squint is one in which the angle of deviation between the two eyes is equal in all directions, a situation most often seen in childhood squints. An **incomitant** squint is one in which the angle of squint varies depending on the direction of gaze, e.g. in paralysis of the extraocular muscles or restriction of the muscles. *Fig. 13.20* shows the origin of insertion of the extraocular muscles.

Amblyopia is decreased visual acuity in the absence of organic disease and is usually due to lack of foveal stimulation at an early age. The most common causes are strabismus, when the non-fixating eye may develop amblyopia; anisometropia (difference in refractive error between the two eyes) when the patient may suppress the blurred image; and visual deprivation, e.g. in congenital cataract or retinoblastoma. Clues to amblyopia include a worse visual acuity when tested with a group of letters rather than individual letters – called the 'crowding' phenomenon. This is important since the standard visual acuity test for children age 2½ years plus is the Sheridan-Gardiner which only tests individual letters. Also, a marked drop in visual acuity is seen when a neutral density filter is held up in front of the eye, compared with the normal.

13.20

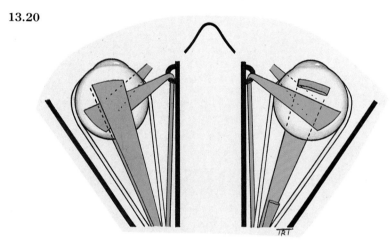

Fig. 13.20 Origin and insertion of the extraocular muscles (pink = superior rectus, green = inferior rectus, blue = superior and inferior obliques, yellow = lateral and medial recti)

Assessment of a child with strabismus

13.21(a)   **13.21(b)**

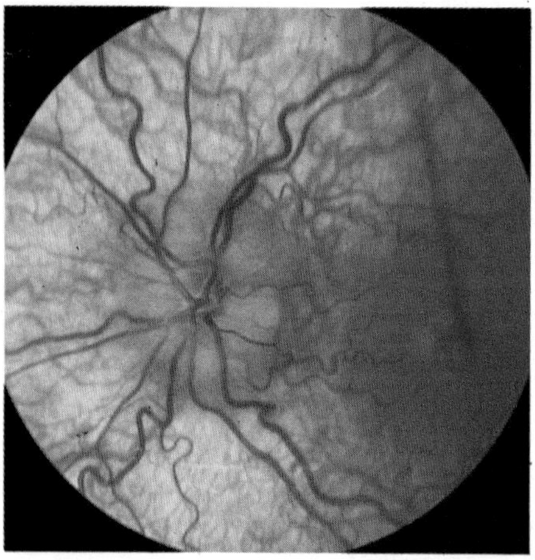

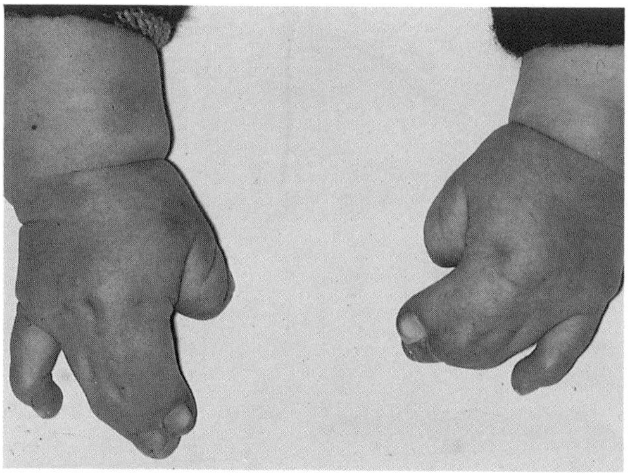

Fig. 13.21(a) Same child as **13.19**. Crouzon's syndrome showing papilloedema as a result of failure of premature fusion of cranial sutures (Courtesy of Mr. D. Taylor)
Fig. 13.21(b) Hand appearance – syndactyly in Apert's syndrome (craniofacial dysostosis) (Courtesy of Mr. D. Taylor)

History includes age of onset, progression and nature of squint, details of pregnancy, birth, congenital abnormalities (*Fig. 13.21(a) & (b)*), postnatal and paediatric illnesses, including neurological abnormalities, trauma, family history and drugs. Previous photographs are often helpful for comparison.

Examination includes looking for a compensatory head posture, e.g. the child will turn the head to the right in a right, lateral rectus palsy as the eyes are then deviated to the left away from the direction of action of the weak muscle. One eye may be closed intermittently to suppress one image of diplopia.

Visual acuity is assessed using the Catford Drum, preferential looking in the <2 year age group, picture tests, e.g. Kay, in the 2–3 year age group and Sheridan-Gardiner in the 2½–5 year age-group until able to use a Snellen chart. This is tested with and without glasses to assess possible amblyopia.

Corneal reflexes are a good indication of true rather than pseudostrabismus such as is found with broad epicanthic folds and facial asymmetry. They will be symmetrical if no manifest squint is present, deviated towards the nose in exotropia and away from the nose in esotropia. A small amount of deviation towards the nose is physiological due to the slight temporal displacement of the fovea from the posterior pole (called a positive angle kappa). They also give a rough indication of angle of squint: each millimetre of displacement corresponds to 7° of squint.

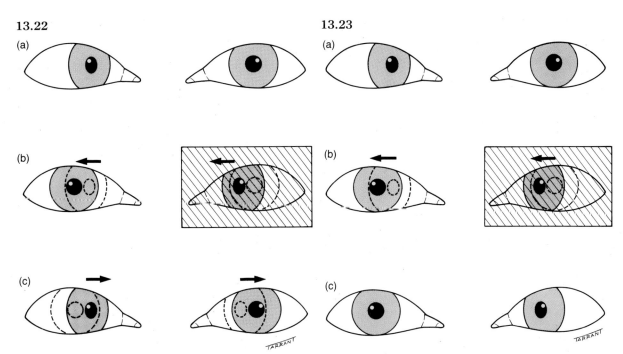

13.22

13.23

Fig. 13.22(a)–(c) Cover test demonstrating a manifest squint. (**a**) Looking straight ahead – right convergent squint (esotropia), (**b**) Cover over left eye – right eye moves to take up fixation, (**c**) Cover removed – left eye takes up fixation again and movement of both eyes to the left is seen

Fig. 13.23(a)–(c) Cover test demonstrating on alternating squint. (**a**) Looking straight ahead – right convergent squint (esotropia), (**b**) Cover over left eye – right eye moves to take up fixation, (**c**) Cover removed – right eye keeps fixation; both eyes have equal or near equal visual acuity

Cover tests – Initially a cover–uncover test is performed to detect a manifest squint (*Fig. 13.22(a)–(c)*). The patient is asked to fix on an interesting target at 1m. The eye that is used for fixation (usually the one with the best visual acuity) will take up fixation. That eye is then covered and the other eye observed to see if it moves to take up fixation. A movement inwards to take up fixation implies an exotropia and a movement outwards an esotropia. The cover is then removed and a movement is seen as the other eye takes up fixation again. The test is repeated on the other side. If both eyes are able to hold fixation this is called an alternating squint (*Fig. 13.23(a)–(c)*).

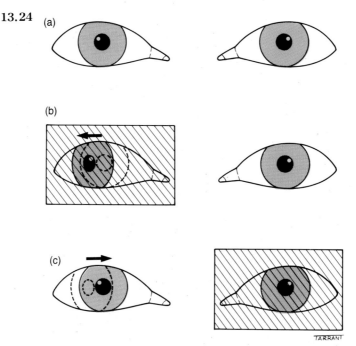

13.24

(a)

(b)

(c)

TARRANT

Fig. 13.24(a)–(c) An alternate cover test demonstrating a latent squint. (**a**) Looking straight ahead – no manifest squint, (**b**) Cover over right eye – right eye drifts out (latent divergent squint or exophoria), (**c**) Cover transferred to left eye – movement of right eye inwards to take up fixation again

If no movement is seen it is possible that a latent squint is present. To detect this the previous test may be used, this time observing the eye that has just been uncovered. Whilst the eye is covered it may drift away from fixation, so that when the cover is removed it is seen to take up fixation once more. An alternate cover test, (*Fig. 13.24(a)–(c)*) in which a card is swiftly placed over each eye in turn several times and the eyes then observed, is a better way to demonstrate latent squints.

If various prisms are used at the same time as the cover test, the angle of squint may be measured as the prism required to prevent any compensatory movement to take up fixation.

Extraocular movements are tested to exclude a paralytic squint. Nystagmus is looked for.

Convergence and **accommodation** are tested. Some convergent squints are due to excessive accommodation effort in hypermetropes.

Tests of binocular visual function are performed, including stereopsis and fusion ability.

Slit-lamp and **fundal examination** with full dilation are carried out to exclude ocular pathology, e.g. retinoblastoma.

Refraction under cycloplegia is carried out for refractive errors.

Ⓢ *Management:* It is essential that children with strabismus are referred swiftly to eye centres since any delay may increase the risk of amblyopia, especially in very young children. Refractive errors are corrected and followed by treatment of amblyopia by occlusion (patching) or penalisation (atropine ointment) of the good eye. Careful follow-up is required to encourage compliance and to ensure amblyopia does not develop in the occluded eye. The timing of surgery is controversial, but in children under two years it tends to be done as early as possible so that the chance of binocular vision developing increases. Surgical techniques vary and depend on a number of factors. In esotropia, the operation involves either bimedial rectus recession (slackening) or medial rectus recession plus lateral rectus resection in the same eye. Exotropia surgery involves either lateral rectus recession with medial rectus resection or bilateral lateral rectus recession. The children must be carefully followed up for development of further squint or refractive errors.

14 Occupational eye disease

The most common injuries to the eye sustained at work are caused by chemical splashes and corneal and intraocular, metallic foreign bodies. Most of these injuries are preventable. In the UK, the Factories Act and the Health and Safety at Work etc. Act 1974, along with the Protection of Eyes Regulations 1974 Statutory Instrument (SI) 1974 1681 as amended by SI 1975 303, set out the areas of risk and the requirements for protection. From 1st October 1989, employers were legally responsible for assessing the risk to health arising from any work process and the precautions needed to prevent or control the risk as outlined in the COSHH (Control of Substances Hazardous to Health) regulations 1988. This includes education of employees of risks and precautions to be taken.

Eye protection

Use of eye protection prevents the following hazards:

- Impact of low or high velocity particles

- Splashes from hot or corrosive liquid

- Contact from irritant or toxic vapours

- Various types of radiation including UV, infrared, and laser beams

Each type of eye protection is designed to guard against specific hazards and must conform both legally and to the British Standards. A choice for each type of job should be made available so that the worker can select the most comfortable to wear. People may not maintain their protection if they are discouraged, for example, by discomfort, restricted view, interference with existing spectacles or hearing aids, inadequate cleaning and maintenance and incorrect guidance on the correct type for use with a given hazard.

Types of eye protection available include:

- **Safety spectacles** provide protection against low hazard particles and physical splashes. They are usually fitted with side pieces and may be tinted, clear or clip-on, or have the worker's prescription included.

- **Goggles** provide both side and top protection to the eye for general purposes or from specific hazards such as chemicals, gas welding, molten metal or laser. They may be sealed to prevent any chemical entry or vented. Again the prescription may be incorporated.

- **Face shields** protect the eye or the whole face. They are most suitable for grinding, welding, furnace work and working with hazardous chemical and biological products.

N.B. Contact lenses, far from protecting the eye against direct splashes, may increase the hazard by absorbing the dangerous chemical onto the surface of the lens, producing a prolonged contact with the cornea and globe. Soft contact lenses take up vapours from the atmosphere and all types should be avoided in the industrial situation.

Injury to the eye at work

This may be divided into:

- Physical
- Chemical
- Biological

Physical

Metallic foreign bodies

Metal foreign bodies (*Fig. 14.1(a) & (b)*) may fly up and hit the eye during nearly every forming process (turning, drilling, milling, welding, grinding, chiselling, hammering and so on) when no protective goggles are worn or when the visor has temporarily been displaced to allow better vision. In general, when a fine dust of particles hits the eye, or when goggles are in place and a metallic particle has blown around the goggles, the metal particle will lodge on the outside of the eye, for example on the cornea or subtarsally. High velocity metallic fragments, e.g. from hammering metal on metal, are extremely dangerous and may penetrate the cornea or sclera to become an intraocular foreign body.

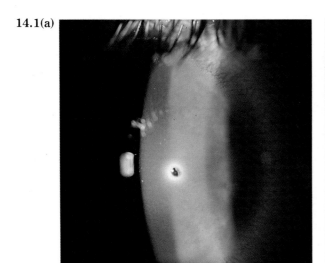

14.1(a)

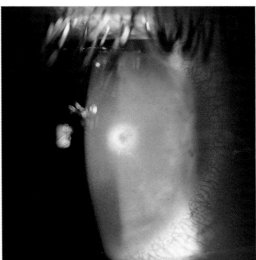

14.1(b)

Fig. 14.1(a) & (b) Corneal foreign body with surrounding infiltrate – **(a)** before removal and **(b)** same patient after removal of the foreign body

(P)(R) *Management:* If a cloud of tiny particles has blown into the eye, the eye should be irrigated to wash out the particles. The eye should then be examined for remaining particles, e.g. subtarsally (see p. 17) and on the cornea. If there is a corneal foreign body present, the patient should be seen at an eye centre where the foreign body can best be removed. The temptation to remove it using a cotton-tip or a handkerchief should be resisted as this may cause an abrasion. If left *in situ*, the particle will rust and a ring of infiltrate will form around it.

The foreign body and surrounding infiltrate may be removed using a 21G needle attached to the end of a cotton tip. Gentle scraping is required under slit-lamp magnification until all the rust is removed. Antibiotic drops and cycloplegic drops (for example homatropine 2%) are instilled and the eye is padded for 24 hours (see p. 35). The patient is then reviewed and treatment with antibiotic drops (for example chloramphenicol 0.5% four times daily) and topical cycloplegics continued until the cornea is completely healed (usually after one week).

Any metal forming injury may lead to an intraocular foreign body. Even if no obvious entry site is seen or a corneal foreign body is found, this does not exclude the possibility and orbital radiography (two views) and fundus examination are mandatory. If there is a large metal foreign body, e.g. a nail, embedded in the cornea, the patient should be sent immediately to a specialist eye centre where removal and repair will be carried out under general anaesthetic. If possible, the nail should not be removed under uncontrolled conditions as this may cause more harm. Instead, a pad or shield should be placed lightly over the eye. The patient must be kept nil by mouth. At the eye hospital, initial assessment and management will be as for a penetrating injury (see pp. 218–19).

Explosions may scatter a myriad of tiny particles onto the surface of the conjunctiva and cornea (*Fig. 14.2(a)*) and intraocular foreign bodies must again be excluded. The skin may also become tattooed (*Fig. 14.2(b)*). With multiple, corneal, epithelial foreign bodies, it is preferable to denude the involved epith-elium, leaving a 1–2mm zone of intact epithelium at the limbus to allow regeneration to take place, rather than picking out individual foreign bodies which will leave multiple scars in Bowman's membrane. This is done with a cotton-tip soaked with alcohol. Antibiotic ointment and mydriatics are instilled initially, then twice daily, and the eye is kept firmly padded for a few days until re-epithelialisation has occurred.

Inert, small, deeply embedded, corneal foreign bodies, e.g. glass, may safely be left as the epithelium regrows over them and only minimal, if any, disturbance of vision results. If there is any leakage from the corneal wound, the foreign body should be removed and the wound repaired.

Blunt trauma to the eye may cause a hyphaema, traumatic anterior uveitis, traumatic mydriasis, irido-dialysis, lens dislocation, contusion cataract, commotio retinae, choroidal haemorrhage and tears, and a rup-tured globe. All cases should be assessed by an ophthal-mologist.

14.2(a)

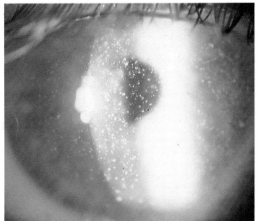

14.2(b)

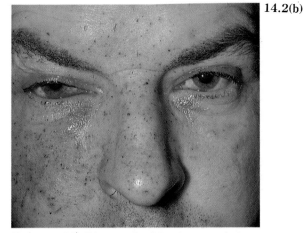

Fig. 14.2(a) Multiple corneal foreign bodies

Fig. 14.2(b) Skin tattooing following an explosion

Thermal injuries

Burns from hot metal objects or liquids usually affect the lids owing to the protective blink reflex. Occasionally in industry hot molten metal may enter the eye and a cast is formed in the palpebral fissure. Immediate damage to corneal and conjunctival tissues occurs. The cornea may be completely opaque from the injury and the rest of the globe may be severely damaged.

(R) *Management of eyelid burns:*

• **Superficial or partial thickness burns** (*Fig. 14.3*) are painful and lead to lid swelling, erythema, blistering and exudation. For minor burns, the treatment of choice is to gently cleanse the affected area with antiseptic solution and leave it dry. For more severe burns, a sterile dressing, changed daily, is used. Antibiotic preparations to the skin are not generally recommended as they may favour super-infection with more virulent organisms. A careful assessment of the eye is required, using topical anaesthetic drops and eyelid retractors to overcome the blepharospasm.

• **Full thickness burns** are less painful, owing to the destruction of the nerve endings, and are associated with coagulative necrosis of the skin. After assessment of the globe, the eyelid wounds are cleansed with antiseptic and a moist sterile dressing is applied which is changed daily. Since it is vitally important to avoid exposure of the globe, the eye must be protected using lubricating ointment and a pad. If large sections of the eyelids are missing, a moist chamber, formed by using a plastic wrap which adheres to the periorbital skin, is used. Skin grafting may be required in the early stages.

14.3

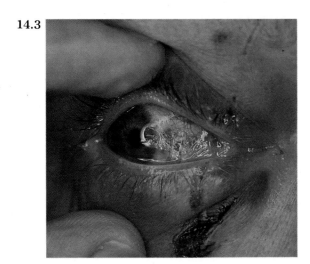

Fig. 14.3 Partial thickness lid burn

(R) *Management of burns to the globe:* Topical anaesthetic is instilled and the eye examined, including subtarsally, to assess the extent of the damage. In minor cases, there may be mild ischaemic necrosis of the conjunctiva and small areas of superficial epithelial loss. Antibiotic ointment and mydriatics are instilled and the eye is padded. If the corneal epithelium is intact, steroid preparations are used to try to reduce conjunctival inflammation and subsequent symblepharon formation. Daily examinations are required to assess healing and subsequent complications, e.g. intraocular pressure rise. In the more severe case of the molten metal, any cast which has formed must be removed with a pair of forceps, usually revealing an area of necrosis of the globe. Antibiotic ointment, mydriatics and steroid as appropriate are applied and the patient is padded and admitted for close observation. Late complications include scarring and symblepharon formation. In the case of molten metal, the cornea may never clear.

Radiation injury

Ionizing radiation

The most common cause of radiation injury to the eye is radiotherapy for malignancies of the eye or orbit. A less common cause is accidental exposure to an industrial radiation leak.

Radiation injuries may cause initial conjunctival hyperaemia, watering, corneal anaesthesia, radiation keratitis leading to areas of persistent epithelial loss and possible corneal necrosis, cataract formation after a latent period of six months to 12 years, papilloedema and retinal damage.

Ⓡ Radiation keratitis is the main concern of the eye casualty officer and is treated with antibiotic ointment and padding until the epithelium is healed. If healing is severely delayed, a lateral tarsorrhaphy is performed.

Ultraviolet radiation

In industry this is most commonly caused by electric arc-welding or gas-welding without protective goggles which leads to "arc eye". Occasionally it may be caused by sun lamps (*Fig. 14.4*).

There may be an initial glare from the intense light, but this is followed 6–10 hours later by ocular irritation, lid swelling, watering and extreme photophobia. Examination reveals lid oedema, conjunctival injection and superficial punctate disturbance of both corneas.

Ⓡ *Management:* This consists of antibiotic ointment, mydriatics, e.g. homatropine 2%, and firm padding for 12–24 hours, coupled with strong reassurance that complete recovery is likely within 24–48 hours.

Infrared radiation

Short exposure to infrared radiation may lead to temporary ocular discomfort due to lid swelling and conjunctival inflammation. Treatment consists of topical antibiotics for a few days until the symptoms have improved. Long-term, unprotected exposure may induce cataracts, as can be seen in glass-blowers or furnace workers. Characteristic splits are seen in the anterior lens capsule which may peel back to form scrolls. If this appearance is seen, it helps to distinguish this type of cataract from a senile cataract.

Microwave radiation

Domestic use is most unlikely to cause cataract formation.

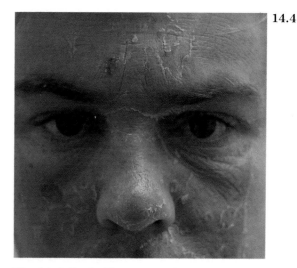

14.4

Fig. 14.4 Sun bed burn

Laser

Laser (**L**ight **A**mplification by **S**timulated **E**mission of **R**adiation) beams are an intense form of electromagnetic energy at selected wavelengths. They are often used therapeutically in medical practice, for example in the treatment of diabetic retinopathy. Stringent safety precautions are necessary to prevent the laser being switched on accidentally and all workers must wear the appropriate protective goggles. The skin and the eye are the areas of the body most commonly affected.

Lasers are divided into four classes according to the type of energy and the hazard they evoke. This combination determines the maximum permissible exposure limits.

- **Class 1:** Lowest powered lasers; incapable of damaging the eye or burning the skin.

- **Class 2:** Lasers that emit visible light; only hazardous if the normal aversion response to bright light is overcome and people deliberately stare at the light for a minute or more. They must be warned against this.

- **Class 3:** Able to cause retinal damage within the natural aversion time (<0.25 s). Considerable safety precautions are necessary.

- **Class 4:** Highest power laser. High risk both to the skin and the eye by direct exposure and by reflection. Also a fire hazard.

Electric shock

Ⓡ This may lead to transient visual loss with macular oedema which usually recovers, or permanent retinal or optic nerve damage which may not. After a latent period of months to years, bilateral cataracts may form.

Chemical

The most serious chemical burns are produced by strong alkalis, e.g. sodium hydroxide, potassium hydroxide, ammonia and lime (calcium hydroxide). Strong acids, with the exception of hydrofluoric acid, tend to produce less serious damage. Many strong alkalis and hydrofluoric acid are lipophilic and can penetrate intact cellular barriers within seconds. The hydroxide ions cause saponification of the fatty acids in the cell membrane which leads to cell death. Acids, e.g. battery acid or acetic acid, tend to precipitate cellular proteins and produce a barrier to deep penetration. Thus, the damage is self-limiting within the first few minutes to hours.

Management: N.B. Chemical (especially alkali) burns Ⓡ are true emergencies. The immediate management in the first seconds and minutes determines the outcome. Therefore treatment must begin at the scene of the accident.

Alkali burns

- **Immediate, copious irrigation** with the nearest available source of water, e.g. hose, shower. There must be no delay whilst physiological solutions are sought. There will be intense blepharospasm, but the eyelids must be held apart whilst water is poured onto the affected eye(s) – a dry cloth is helpful for gripping the lids. This irrigation should be continued for at least 10 minutes and if possible during emergency transport to hospital. Large particles of lime should be removed if possible.

- Emergency transfer to eye casualty department, which should be alerted by telephone in advance so that preparations are made for immediate treatment upon arrival of the patient.

- At the eye casualty, topical anaesthetic drops are instilled and eyelid retractors inserted. Irrigation is continued with physiological solutions, e.g. Hartmann's solution via a blood giving set. Sodium EDTA is often suggested as an irrigant for calcium hydroxide as it acts as a chelating agent, but it may increase the pH because it forms sodium hydroxide. The eyelids must be everted to remove any particles of lime or plaster that continue to cause damage.

- Irrigation is continued for at least 40 minutes. Litmus paper is used to test the pH of the tears after irrigation and should be neutral, i.e. pH 7.3–7.7, on two consecutive tests 20 minutes apart, before irrigation is ceased altogether. Alternatively, 5 ml of 0.1% bromthymol blue can be added to 500 ml of irrigant to act as an indicator for neutralisation: acids are yellow, alkalis blue, neutral is green. Alkali can continue to leach out of the anterior chamber for several hours and it is beneficial to continue irrigation until this ceases.

- Assessment of the extent of ocular injury is performed by an ophthalmologist.

Minor burns

Signs: Conjunctival injection and corneal epithelial loss. If there is no ischaemia and less than half the corneal epithelium is involved, the patient may be managed as an outpatient, but should be reviewed daily.

Treatment: Topical antibiotics b.d. – q.d.s. to act as a prophylactic against infection, topical cycloplegics, e.g. homatropine drops 2% t.d.s., and firm padding.

Moderate to severe burns

Signs: Marked corneal loss or opacification, conjunctival ischaemia, often seen subtarsally or limbally as blanching of the conjunctival blood vessels, intraocular pressure may be elevated owing to damage to the trabecular meshwork or reduced owing to damage to the ciliary body, the lens may start to opacify and lids may have tissue loss due to burns (*Figs. 14.5, 14.6, 14.7*).

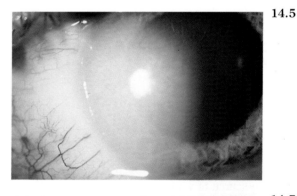

14.5

Fig. 14.5 Alkali burn – limbal ischaemia with blanching of the conjunctival vessels and partial corneal opacification
Fig. 14.6 Alkali burn – total corneal opacification
Fig. 14.7 Alkali burn – corneal vascularisation and scarring as late sequelae (same patient as **Fig. 14.6**)

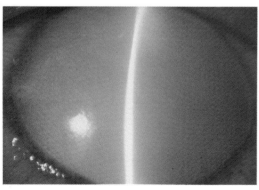

14.6

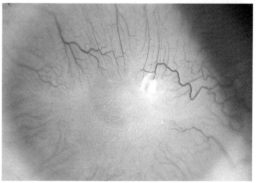

14.7

Ⓟ *Treatment:* The patient is admitted. Topical antibiotics b.d. – q.d.s., atropine drops 1% t.d.s., topical steroid, e.g. betamethasone drops q.d.s., to reduce uveitis and conjunctival inflammation with subsequent cicatrisation. Ascorbic acid, 10% drops in artificial tears 12–14 times a day, is thought to decrease the incidence of corneal ulceration and perforation if used in the acute stages. Ascorbic acid is a natural scavenger of harmful radicals, as well as being important in collagen synthesis, and its level in the anterior chamber is reduced in alkali burns. Systemic ascorbic acid 1–2 g per day may be used in addition. Intraocular pressure is reduced, if necessary, with timolol 0.5% drops b.d. +/− acetazolamide 250 mg q.d.s.. The eye is kept firmly padded.

Late complications include persistent corneal ulceration and perforation, corneal scarring and vascularisation (*Fig. 14.7*), uveitis, dry eye, symblepharon formation, lid scarring with entropion or ectropion formation, glaucoma and cataract. Long-term treatment includes artificial tears, cycloplegics, glaucoma therapy, corticosteroids and corneal grafting (which has a poor prognosis owing in particular to defects in the tear film).

The Roper-Hall classification is useful in grading findings to prognosis:

Grade	Clinical findings	Prognosis
I	corneal epithelial damage; no ischaemia	good
II	cornea hazy; iris details visible; ischaemia <⅓ at limbus	good
III	total loss of corneal epithelium; stromal haze obscures iris details; limbal ischaemia of ⅓–½	guarded
IV	cornea opaque; iris and pupil obscured; ischaemia affects >½ at limbus	poor

Lid or lacrimal involvement worsens prognosis.

Acid burns

Acid burns (*Fig. 14.8*) tend to be less severe and are managed in the initial stages as for an alkali burn. Hydrofluoric acid may penetrate into the anterior chamber and cause problems similar to alkali burns.

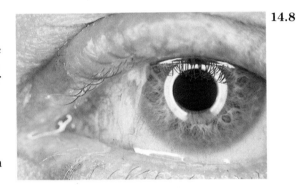

14.8

Fig. 14.8 Minor acid burn showing superficial damage to conjunctiva and a small area of cornea and lids

Biological

There are several micro-organisms thought to be capable of penetrating the conjunctiva, thus providing a route of infection. These include:

- **Leptospirosis** – a hazard to farm workers, sewage workers and those falling into polluted water.

- **Brucellosis** – mainly affecting workers in slaughter houses, those handling meat, and veterinary surgeons.

- **Hepatitis B** – when infected blood products are splashed into the eye. Hospital workers are at risk.

15 Tropical eye disease

This section includes those diseases which may require immediate care, but which have not been referred to previously. Although advanced cataract, glaucoma and severe trauma are often seen, these conditions have been described, together with the emergency treatment where indicated.

The main diseases are nutritional blindness, onchocerciasis, trachoma and leprosy.

Nutritional disease

There are 100,000–200,000 new cases of nutritional blindness per year within the developing world, the most common manifestation being nutritional corneal ulceration. Malnutrition results from vitamin A and protein deficiency, sometimes exacerbated by an attack of measles.

Vitamin A deficiency

The function of vitamin A is the maintenance of healthy epithelial tissues. The effects of deficiency are:

- Loss of conjunctival goblet cells
- Keratinisation of the corneal and conjunctival surface
- Perifollicular hyperkeratosis of the skin

- Night blindness with reduction of adaptation to darkness and loss of ability to see in the dark

The effects of vitamin A deficiency are more pronounced in children because of a greater requirement per unit of body weight than in adults. In addition, children cannot store vitamin A in the liver.

Clinical disease

- Loss of lustre of the corneal and conjunctival surface, with poor wetting by the tear film. The conjunctival surface becomes opaque with loss of definition of the blood vessels. Wrinkles and folds appear.

- There is increased pigmentation of the bulbar conjunctiva.

- Creamy white debris may appear in the tear film.

- Bitot's spots – plaques of material within the lid fissure on the bulbar conjunctiva. They have a foamy, waxy appearance and can be slightly pigmented (*Fig. 15.1*).

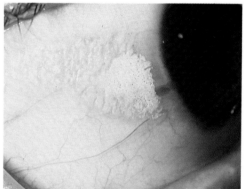

15.1

Fig. 15.1 Bitot's spots in a patient with Vitamin A deficiency

• The surface of the cornea can be rough, dull and irregular, the appearance being known as corneal xerosis. The tear break-up time is less than 10 seconds.

• Corneal ulceration occurs with xerosis in the central part. In keratomalacia, which is the most severe form of xerophthalmia, the cornea melts with minimal inflammatory reaction. A staphyloma involving the anterior uvea can form (*Figs. 15.2 & 15.3*).

• Night blindness is induced by vitamin A deficiency, with poor dark adaptation and night vision.

15.2

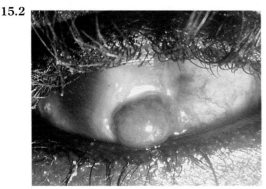

Fig. 15.2 Corneal ulceration with prolapse of iris in a patient with Vitamin A deficiency

15.3

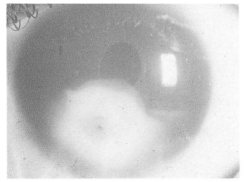

Fig. 15.3 Corneal scarring following ulceration in Vitamin A deficiency (Courtesy of Mr. J. Sandford-Smith)

Protein malnutrition

This retards growth and weakens resistance to infection. In children with vitamin A deficiency as well as protein malnutrition, the eye lesions are more severe. Where measles occurs, the incidence of corneal ulceration becomes higher. It is known that recurrent herpes simplex keratitis is seemingly induced during an attack of measles, thereby adding to the severity and adverse prognosis in these malnourished children (*Fig. 15.4*).

15.4

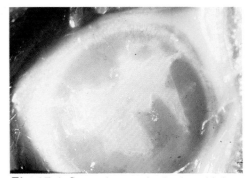

Fig. 15.4 Severe herpes simplex keratitis in association with measles (Courtesy of Mr. J. Sandford-Smith)

Ⓢ *Management:*

• General treatment is required for the nutritional deficiency and local treatment for the eyes. High doses of vitamin A are required, namely 200,000iu on days 1 and 2, followed by 200,000iu at 2 weeks. Prevention within the community requires 100,000iu at 6-monthly intervals up to the age of 12 months and thereafter dosages of 200,000, 4–6 monthly are required.

• Local treatment should be with antibiotics and mydriatics. Where laboratory facilities are available, topical and systemic antibiotics must be given according to the organism and its sensitivity. Padding or lid taping may be necessary, particularly where there is poor lid closure.

Onchocerciasis

This is a disease caused by a filarial worm – *Onchocerca volvulus*. It is transmitted from man to man by a vector, the black fly or *Simulium damnosum*. The eye and skin are mainly affected.

• The black fly lives on fast-flowing rivers and streams, particularly in the savannah zone of west Africa.

• The adult worms occur in skin nodules. The male is less than 5 cm long and 0.4 mm in diameter, while the female can be up to 50 cm long and 0.5 mm in diameter.

• The female releases millions of microfilariae, which are 300 microns long and 8 microns in diameter. These organisms congregate in the skin and the eye.

• The microfilariae are ingested when the black fly bites an infected person. These then go through a number of stages to form a third-stage larva.

• The larva is then injected at the next blood meal and it takes about 12 months to develop into the adult worm, the female of which can live for 10–15 years.

• The adult worms form a nodule and produce millions of microfilariae which disseminate throughout the skin and infect the eye.

The skin is affected in a number of ways.

• Pruritis is common.

• Pigmentation may be decreased or increased. In the pre-tibial areas, the appearance is known as leopard skin, owing to skin atrophy.

• Thickened and roughened skin occurs where inflammation has been induced, following the death of the organisms.

• Nodules containing adult worms, usually over bony prominences.

Eye signs are seen particularly in the anterior chamber and the cornea.

• Keratitis occurs on death of the organisms, producing fine, fluffy, punctate opacities. Following severe infections, a diffuse opacity within the interpalpebral area is produced, known as sclerosing keratitis (*Fig. 15.5*).

• Iritis is seen with a small, inverted, pear-shaped pupil, posterior synechiae and iris atrophy. Peripheral anterior synechiae may induce secondary glaucoma.

• Chorioretinitis, with atrophy of the pigment epithelium temporal to the macula, is seen. There are areas of pigment clumping (*Fig. 15.6*).

• Acute optic neuritis, leading to optic atrophy, is seen.

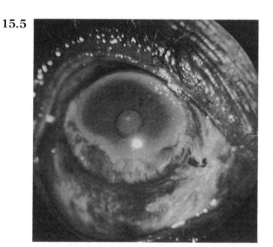

Fig. 15.5 Severe keratitis in a patient with onchocerciasis (Courtesy of Teaching Aids at Low Cost (TALC))

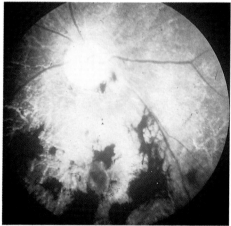

Fig. 15.6 Optic nerve atrophy and inactive chorioretinitis in a patient with onchocerciasis (Courtesy of Mr. J. Sandford-Smith)

Diagnosis:

- Skin snips, taken from the buttocks or shoulder, are placed in a drop of saline and examined 20 minutes later. Microfilariae are seen leaving the biopsy and can be counted, providing some measure of the intensity of the infection.

- The presence of nodules aids diagnosis. Nodules close to the orbit are more often associated with severe ocular infection.

- Microfilariae can sometimes be seen within the anterior chamber or the cornea with a slit lamp.

(P)(S) Control:

- Control of the fly vector is carried out by specific programmes, employing larvicidal compounds on rivers to kill larvae of the black fly.

- The adult worms can be treated with drugs such as suramin, which is macro- and micro-filaricidal, as six-weekly injections. Nodulectomy has been practised, although the effect of this has not been proven.

- Microfilaricidal drugs include diethylcarbamazine, which causes an exacerbation of inflammation and occasional further loss of vision (the Mazotti reaction), or ivermectin (Mectizan), as a single oral dose. The latter has few adverse reactions.

- Iritis is treated according to routine principles, using topical corticosteroid and mydriatics. Optic neuritis is treated with a course of systemic steroid.

Trachoma

Trachoma is a highly infectious disease of the eye, leading to blindness on a vast scale in endemic regions. It is spread between people by flies (*Fig. 15.7*) and is caused by *Chlamydia trachomatis*, which is an obligate intracellular organism, intermediate between bacteria and viruses. The incubation period ranges between 5–14 days but on average is seven days.

Trachoma is a chronic inflammatory condition leading to spontaneous resolution, but often leaving cicatrisation of the conjunctival and subconjunctival tissue. It leads to inwards deviation of the lid margins and aberrant growth of the lashes. This so-called trichiasis results in corneal damage in the form of microerosions on the surface, which themselves can be the portal for entry of other organisms such as pathogenic bacteria.

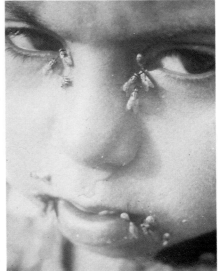

15.7

Fig. 15.7 Transmission of *chlamydia trachomatis* in eye and nasal secretions by fly vector (Courtesy of World Health Organisation)

Symptoms: Photophobia, redness, mucopurulent discharge and watering

Signs:

- Follicles situated on the upper tarsal and upper and lower fornices (*Fig. 15.8(a)*)

- Papillae on the upper tarsal plate (*Fig. 15.8(b)*)

- Limbal follicles which leave scalloped areas at the limbus on resolution, known as Herbert's pits (*Fig. 15.9*)

- Pannus, which is peripheral, superficial vascularisation at the limbus, present in all quadrants, but typically most marked at the upper limbus (*Fig. 15.10*)

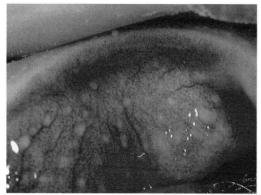

Fig. 15.8(a) Follicles on the upper tarsal plate in a patient with trachoma (Courtesy of Professor S. Darougar)

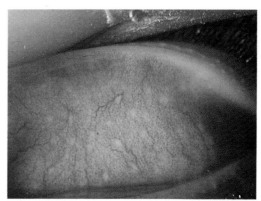

Fig. 15.8(b) Papillae on the upper tarsal plate in a patient with trachoma (Courtesy of Professor S. Darougar)

15.9

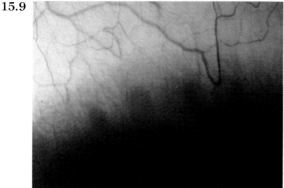

Fig. 15.9 Herbert's pits at upper limbus in trachoma

15.10

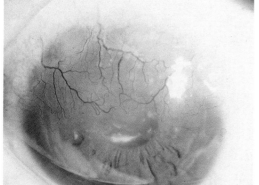

Fig. 15.10 Vascular pannus in trachoma (Courtesy of Mr. J. Sandford-Smith)

15.11

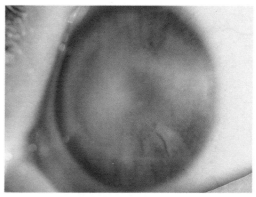

Fig. 15.11 Corneal scarring due to trachoma

● Scarring of the upper tarsal plate – typically stellate and linear. The classical change is a line of scarring about 3mm above the mucocutaneous junction, known as Arlt's line

● Corneal manifestations include superficial punctate keratitis, mostly in the upper part of the cornea (*Fig. 15.11*)

Complications: The complications of trachoma have a greater adverse effect than the original disease.

• Entropion, due to distortion of the tarsal plates, leads to secondary traumatic injury to the corneal surface, with consequent inflammation and loss of corneal transparency due to secondary infection

• Tear deficits are caused by obstruction of the ductules of the lacrimal gland, producing keratoconjunctivitis sicca

• Obstruction of the Meibomian glands and thickening of the tarsal plate

• Cicatricial obstruction of the lacrimal drainage system may compensate for the poor tear secretion, but on the other hand, may cause epiphora

• Conjunctival shrinkage, squamous metaplasia of the epithelium and loss of goblet cells

• Secondary infection by *Haemophilus influenzae*, *Streptococcus pneumoniae*, Moraxella species and *Staphylococcus aureus*

Classification: MacCallan first identified the value of a simple classification of trachoma for descriptive and therapeutic purposes.

Stage 1 Lymphoid follicles and subepithelial lymphoid infiltration. The follicles are hard, small and immature.

Stage 2a In addition to a papillary response, mature follicles appear in the upper palpebral conjunctiva.

Stage 2b The papillary response becomes predominant, so that deep conjunctival vessels in the tarsal plate become obscured.

Stage 3 Follicles are present with early cicatrisation.

Stage 4 Follicles have disappeared, but cicatrisation is noted. The disease is inactive.

The WHO classification records the presence or papillae (P) or follicles (F) and grades activity as mild, moderate or severe.

P0 Normal conjunctiva.

P1 (mild) Papillae are present, but the deep conjunctival vessels are not obscured.

P2 (moderate) In addition to the presence of papillae, the conjunctiva of the upper tarsal plate is infiltrated, so that the deep vessels are not visible.

P3 (severe) Papillary response is marked and there is diffuse conjunctival infiltration and thickening. The conjunctiva is opaque, disguising the deep vessels completely.

The presence of follicles is described according to a series of zones, zone 1 being near the upper margin of the tarsal plate, zone 2 being intermediate and zone 3 being the lowest and adjacent to the middle third of the lid margin.

F0 Normal conjunctiva without any follicles.

F1 Follicles are present, but no more than five in zones 1 and 2.

F2 More than five follicles in zones 1 and 2, but less than five in zone 3.

F3 Five or more follicles in each of the three zones.

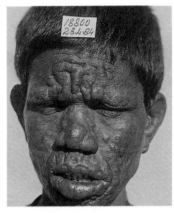

15.12(a)

Management: Chlamydia trachomatis is sensitive to a number of antibiotics.

- The active disease responds promptly to tetracycline hydrochloride 1.5–2.00 g orally per day for three weeks.

- In pregnancy it must be treated with topical tetracycline ointment 1% or erythromycin ointment, twice daily for at least two months.

- In children it must be treated with tetracycline or erythromycin ointment twice daily for 6–8 weeks. Children may also be treated systemically with oral erythromycin (40 mg per kg body weight) for three weeks.

Where there is abnormality of the lids producing entropion or trichiasis, surgical measures should be taken.

Leprosy

Leprosy is a chronic, disfiguring, crippling and blinding disease caused by *Mycobacterium leprae*, an acid-fast, obligate, intracellular parasite (*Fig. 15.12(a)–(c)*). The organism has an affinity for tissue macrophages and involves the skin, nerves and the lymphoreticular system. It tends to be attracted towards the cooler parts of the body.

It is a disease of the developing world, but a high prevalence is found in temperate zones, such as North and South Korea and Argentina. The total number of cases in the world today is estimated to be in excess of 12 million.

15.12(b)

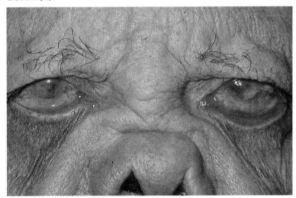

15.12(c)

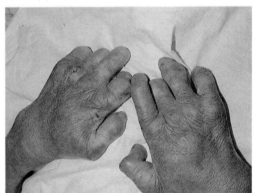

Fig. 15.12(a) Typical facial changes in lepromatous leprosy (Courtesy of Mr. T. ffytche)

Fig. 15.12(b) Severe ectropion of lower lids, corneal scarring and loss of the bridge of the nose in leprosy (Courtesy of Mr. T. ffytche)

Fig. 15.12(c) Loss of phalanges in a patient with leprosy (Courtesy of Mr. T. ffytche)

Pathogenesis

This depends upon the presence or absence of cell-mediated immunity.

There are two types of disease:

● Tuberculoid – where cell-mediated immunity is intense and the reaction is granulomatous, with giant cells, epithelioid cells and lymphocytes. There is early neural involvement and skin lesions are limited with discrete and well-demarcated edges.

● Lepromatous – a more severe type of disease with defective, cell-mediated immunity. There are diffuse and multiple dermal lesions, with plaques, nodules and papules. Neural involvement and sensory loss occurs later in this form of disease.

Eye disease

● Skin: there is loss of eyebrows and thickening of the supraciliary ridges. The lids are thickened and there is tylosis, leontiasis and madarosis. Lacrimal gland involvement leads to keratoconjunctivitis sicca.

Seventh nerve involvement is common in tuberculoid leprosy, inducing decreased blinking, ectropion of the lower lid, lagophthalmos and exposure keratitis. When this is combined with corneal anaesthesia and entropion of the upper lid, the outlook for vision is extremely poor.

● Cornea and conjunctiva (*Fig. 15.13*): punctate superficial keratitis occurs in the upper and outer quadrant of the cornea, with discrete, milky, subepithelial opacities. These may coalesce to form a general haze. Avascular keratitis occurs in the same area. Characteristically, there may be thickening of the corneal nerves, with a beaded appearance, particularly in the lepromatous form. Interstitial keratitis begins at the upper part of the cornea and occasionally deep keratitis occurs. Ghost vessels can occur. The keratitis may eventually involve the visual axis.

● Sclera and episclera: yellowish, gelatinous nodules are seen at the 3 o'clock and the 9 o'clock positions within the interpalpebral zone. Scleritis is induced by the presence of the organisms themselves.

● Uvea: creamy-white aggregations of *M. leprae*, with monocytes, are pathognomonic of leprosy and have been designated iris pearls. Uveitis may be acute or chronic.

a. Acute anterior uveitis is associated with hypopyon, posterior synechiae, seclusio pupillae and cataracts.
b. Chronic uveitis is seen in lepromatous leprosy and leads to blindness. It is asymptomatic initially and associated with iris atrophy.

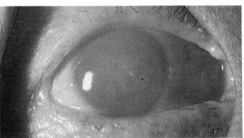

15.13

Fig. 15.13 Diffuse corneal scarring with constricted pupil due to leprosy (Courtesy of Mr. T. ffytche)

Management: It is not usually the ophthalmologist ⓢ ⓟ who makes the diagnosis, but the appearance of avascular keratitis in the superior temporal quadrant, together with beading and thickening of corneal nerves, or iris pearls, will do much to support it. Treatment is as follows:

● Systemic disease is treated with Dapsone, 100mg per day, Rifampicin, 600mg per month and Clofazimine 50mg per day, in courses which last for between six months and life.

● In the tuberculoid form, keratoconjunctivitis sicca is treated with tear replacement and ointments such as Lacri Lube. Topical antibiotics are used as necessary. Uveitis is treated with intensive topical corticosteroid and cycloplegics.

● In the lepromatous form, uveitis is treated with topical corticosteroid and phenylephrine for miotic pupils. Glaucoma is treated with acetazolamide orally and epinephrine drops 1% twice daily.

● Surgical procedures are necessary and include ectropion and entropion procedures, lid-sling surgery for lagophthalmos, sector iridectomy, cataract extraction and tarsorrhaphy. Iridectomy may be required for angle-closure glaucoma induced by seclusio pupillae.

16 Drug induced ophthalmic conditions

Topical eye medication – local and systemic side-effects

Topical steroids

• **Raised intraocular pressure** is seen with the use of steroids in so-called 'steroid responders'. A change to a lower strength or frequency, or use of fluorometholone 0.1%, may stop this. Otherwise, if steroids must be continued, concomitant use of pressure-lowering drugs is indicated, e.g. timolol.

• **Early posterior subcapsular cataract formation** may occur.

• **Reactivation of latent herpes simplex infection** may occur. The steroids must be stopped and topical antiviral, e.g. acyclovir ointment 3% five times a day, used until the ulcer has healed. If further steroid therapy is necessary, it must be used with acyclovir cover.

Antibiotics

• **Drug allergy** is a common complication (*see Fig. 3.27*). The patient may be allergic to either the antibiotic itself or the preservative. One of the most common reactions is to neomycin, often combined with a steroid, e.g. Betnesol N. The clinical features include itching, redness and scaling around the eye, especially inferiorly, and a follicular reaction more marked in the lower lid. The drug should be stopped and another antibiotic used, if treatment needs to be continued. No drug is known to speed up spontaneous resolution of the allergic reaction and it is best left alone.

• **Toxicity** is seen with many antibiotics, especially antiviral agents, e.g. idoxuridine (*Fig. 16.1*) and trifluorothymidine. Punctate corneal epitheliopathy, conjunctival scarring, delayed healing of corneal wounds, follicular conjunctivitis and conjunctival scarring may occur.

• **Bone marrow suppression** has been described rarely with the topical use of chloramphenicol.

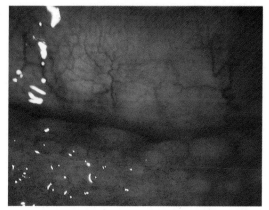

Fig. 16.1 Follicular reaction in idoxyuridine toxicity

Drugs used in glaucoma therapy

● **Pilocarpine** often causes local ocular discomfort and headaches when first instilled. These symptoms usually settle within the first 1–2 weeks of therapy. As there is pupil constriction, the visual acuity may be reduced, especially if there are axial lens opacities. In addition, there may be decreased visual field and difficulty with night driving. If nuclear sclerosis is present, visual acuity may actually improve as the glare is reduced. Nevertheless, some patients find it difficult to tolerate this drug. Occasionally systemic effects of sweating, bradycardia and gastrointestinal upset occur.

● **Adrenaline**-containing drops, e.g. Eppy, may lead to deposition of brown–black adrenochrome pigment subconjunctivally (*Fig. 16.2*). This is harmless, but it is important that it is recognised since it may be mis-diagnosed as a subtarsal foreign body. It may also lead to canalicular stenosis and may cause cystoid macular oedema, especially in aphakic patients. Systemic effects, e.g. tachycardia, may occur.

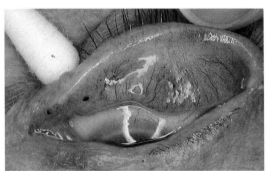

Fig. 16.2 Subconjunctival adrenochrome pigment deposit

● **Timolol** causes very few side-effects in the eye, but may cause corneal anaesthesia. Systemic side-effects occur due to its action as a beta-blocker, e.g. exacerbation of asthma, hypotension, and bradycardia, especially if there are pre-existing conduction defects. Systemic absorption may be minimised by punctal occlusion during drop instillation.

Mydriatics

Any dilating drop may induce angle-closure glaucoma in susceptible individuals. Tropicamide 1% is the shortest acting and thus the safest drop to use. However, even this should be avoided in those with a suggestive history or examination.

Dilating drops cause marked blurring of vision, especially those with cycloplegic (impaired accommodation) as well as mydriatic action (tropicamide is also the drop with least cycloplegic action).

Contact lens solutions

Thiomersal is a commonly used preservative in contact lens solutions and tends to impregnate soft contact lenses. Over a period of months it can lead to contact lens intolerance and keratitis.

Systemic drugs – ocular complications

● **Transient blurring** is commonly seen with anti-cholinergic agents, antihistamines and other systemic drugs, e.g. tricyclic antidepressants and amphetamines (because of mydriasis and cycloplegia). Sedative drugs, thiazide diuretics, carbonic anhydrase inhibitors and many other drugs may also cause transient blurring of vision.

• **Posterior subcapsular cataract** formation (*Fig. 16.3*) is seen with systemic corticosteroids and ACTH treatment either over a long period or in high doses. Busulphan, a drug used in the treatment of chronic myeloid leukaemia, may cause cataracts. Long-term use of chlorpromazine may lead to a fine, stellate deposition of brownish granules on the anterior lens capsule (*Fig. 16.4*). Amiodarone, gold, allopurinol and haloperidol may all lead to usually insignificant lens opacities.

• **Optic neuritis** is seen with ethambutol, isoniazid, streptomycin, chloramphenicol, sulphonamides, chlorpropamide, monoaminoxidase inhibitors, salicylates and others. Prior to commencing treatment with any of the drugs known to cause optic neuritis, especially antituberculous drugs, a full ocular examination including visual acuity, fundoscopy, field tests and colour vision, should be performed. Ethambutol toxicity is more common if there is co-existing diabetes or alcoholism, but is not usually seen if a dose of 15mg/kg/day is used. When visual loss occurs for this reason, it is sudden and severe. If any adverse ocular effects occur, the drugs should be discontinued. In some centres eye examinations, as outlined above for the initial examination, are repeated at 6–12 month intervals.

• **Glaucoma** (open angle) is occasionally seen with systemic corticosteroids. Acute angle closure is sometimes seen in susceptible individuals with drugs which may cause mydriasis, for example, anticholinergics, antihistamines, amphetamines and tricyclic antidepressants.

• **Maculopathy** is seen with quinine, chloroquine, hydroxychloroquine and nicotinic acid. A more generalised retinopathy is occasionally seen with tamoxifen, thioridazine and chlorpromazine. Full ocular assessment, including visual acuity, colour vision, field tests and macula examination, should be performed prior to starting treatment on any quinine derivative, and regular monitoring of these should be carried out.

Early maculopathy, which is often asymptomatic, is reversible if the drug is stopped. A small, paracentral scotoma may be demonstrated on Goldmann Field testing or with an Amsler Grid (see p. 23) and colour vision disturbances may be seen, especially in the more sophisticated 100-hue test. Established maculopathy is often signified by visual loss, scotomas on field testing and pigmentary changes at the maculae (typically 'bull's eye' maculopathy in chloroquine toxicity). The drug should be discontinued if any visual loss starts to occur. Safe doses of chloroquine are a cumulative dose of under 300g (daily dose of 250mg for three years).

16.3 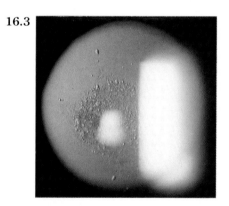 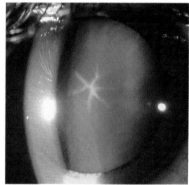 16.4

Fig. 16.3 Steroid induced posterior subcapsular cataract
Fig. 16.4 Stellate cataract in chlorpromazine treatment

• **Corneal deposition of crystals** is seen in treatment with gold, chlorpromazine, chloroquine, indomethacin, and amiodarone. A vortex distribution 'cornea verticillata' (*Fig. 16.5*) is seen with the latter two.

• **Disturbance of colour vision** may occur in digitalis toxicity, cannabis, chlorthiazides, frusemide and ibuprofen.

• **Nystagmus** is caused by anticonvulsants, neostigmine, diazepam (overdosage) or salicylates. Oculogyric crises (when there are sudden, involuntary eye movements) are seen with prochlorperazine, perphenazine, chlorpromazine or barbiturates.

• **Dry eye**, conjunctival and corneal scarring was seen with practolol, but this is rarely used now owing to the severe complications (*Fig. 16.6*).

16.5

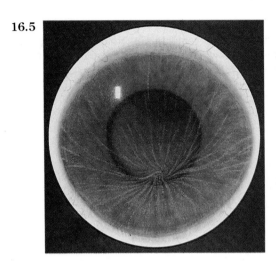

Fig. 16.5 Cornea verticillata in amiodarone treatment

16.6

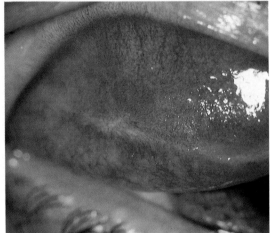

Fig. 16.6 Practolol toxicity

17 Postoperative complications

Patients will occasionally report to their general practitioner or hospital for a variety of complications following ocular surgery. The physician will need to decide whether expert advice is necessary and the following is designed to help make the appropriate decisions and carrying out immediate treatment where it is indicated.

The major operations are performed for cataract, glaucoma, corneal opacification, retinal detachment and lacrimal duct obstruction.

Cataract extraction

Cataracts are removed by two different methods:

• *In toto* (intracapsular extraction), when only the face of the vitreous remains between the anterior chamber and the posterior segment

• The nucleus, cortex and anterior capsule are removed, with the posterior capsule remaining as a barrier between the anterior chamber and posterior segment (extracapsular extraction)

Because the latter is associated with less severe postoperative complications, it is now commonly employed.

Intraocular implants of plastic are introduced to reduce visual complications that result from lens aberrations which occur with high powered spectacle lens corrections.

Postoperative complications are divided into:

• Those occurring during the surgery (operative)
• Those occurring immediately after surgery (early)
• Those occurring sometime after the surgery (late)

Operative complications are not described because they are handled under the direction of special eye units.

Early postoperative complications

Pain

Causes of postoperative pain include:

• Suture ends causing irritation to the upper tarsal plate. The patient complains of a 'foreign body' or 'gritty' sensation' (*Fig. 17.1*)
• Elevation of the intraocular pressure
• Intraocular inflammation

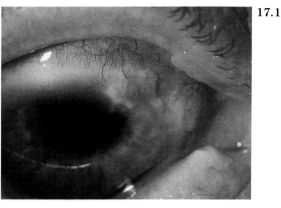

17.1

Fig. 17.1 Stitch abscess in a patient who has undergone a cataract extraction

Blurring of vision

The vision is usually blurred after surgery, particularly if no intraocular lens implant has been introduced. However, sudden loss of vision must be investigated, as it may be due to:

- Dislocation of an implant
- Intraocular haemorrhage

- Severe glaucoma
- Early cystoid macular oedema
- Retinal detachment

Management: The patient must be referred to a ⓈⒻ hospital eye unit immediately.

Wound leakage

- Leaking of aqueous humour through the operative wound can inadvertently lead to a bleb beneath the conjunctival flap formed during the operative procedure. The anterior chamber can be shallow or flat. This complication requires further surgical management.

- Iris prolapse through a poorly sutured wound is a serious complication and requires immediate resuture. The prolapse is seen with the eye depressed and the upper lid gently elevated (*Fig. 17.2*).

ⓇⓈ *Management:* The patient should be referred to a hospital eye unit for repair of the wound.

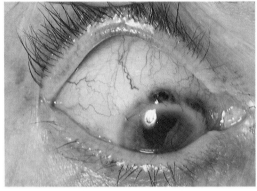

Fig. 17.2 Iris prolapse following a cataract extraction (Courtesy of Mr. R. Humphry)

Flat anterior chamber

This occurs in association with:

- Wound leakage following inadequate suturing (*Fig. 17.3*)

- Choroidal effusion, which is seen with the ophthalmoscope as a peripheral, dark shadow outlined against the red reflex as a smoothly curved contour

- Pupil block glaucoma and rupture of the corneoscleral section; the pupil is obstructed by vitreous following intracapsular extraction, preventing aqueous humour circulation to the anterior chamber, so that the intraocular pressure rises, dehiscence of the section occurs and the anterior chamber is lost

ⓇⓈ *Management:* Referral to hospital eye unit for observation or surgical intervention.

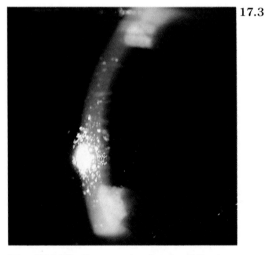

Fig. 17.3 Shallow anterior chamber following a cataract extraction

Endophthalmitis

This serious complication should be recognised and treated promptly.

Symptoms:

- Pain, photophobia and watering
- Visual deterioration

The clinical manifestations are:

- Conjunctival hyperaemia and chemosis
- Lid swelling
- Corneal oedema

- Hypopyon (white blood cells in the anterior chamber forming a fluid level)
- Opacification of the optic media, with loss of the red reflex

Management: Ⓢ Ⓡ

- Refer to eye department
- Samples must be taken by means of an anterior chamber or vitreous tap for Gram stain, culture and sensitivity
- Antibiotic therapy initiated (p. 118)

Raised intraocular pressure

This complication arises by a number of mechanisms. The patient occasionally complains of pain, but often it is asymptomatic. It is difficult to test intraocular pressure using the digital method but, if the pressure is considered high on comparison with the opposite eye, ophthalmological assistance will be required.

Ⓢ *Management:* Medical therapy will usually reduce the raised intraocular pressure.

Hyphaema

Postoperative hyphaema (haemorrhage into the anterior chamber producing a fluid level) (*Fig. 17.4*), or vitreous haemorrhage may occur. In the case of vitreous haemorrhage, the retina must be inspected to eliminate retinal breaks or detachment.

Ⓡ Ⓢ *Management:* The haemorrhage usually clears without additional treatment.

Corneal oedema

This is known as striate keratitis when it follows surgery and affects the upper half of the cornea. It is due to prolonged operative manipulation.

Management: The oedema usually clears up. Where it Ⓢ Ⓡ persists, the medical therapy of corneal oedema will be beneficial in the first instance.

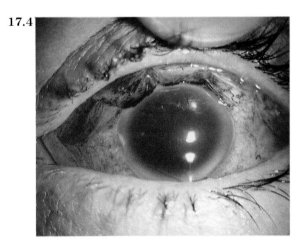

17.4

Fig. 17.4 Hyphaema following a cataract extraction

Retained crystalline lens material

Sometimes the lens cortex is retained following extra-capsular cataract extraction, which may induce post-operative inflammation in the anterior uvea (uveitis) (*Fig. 17.5*).

(R)(S) *Management:*

- The uveitis is treated with topical corticosteroid
- If it persists, residual lens matter may need to be removed

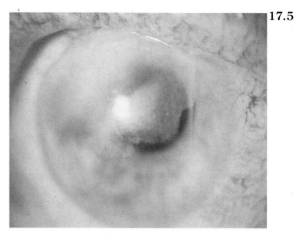

Fig. 17.5 Retained lens material following a cataract extraction

Late postoperative complications

Retinal complications

Three complications involving the retina occur:

- Retinal breaks – the incidence is increased where vitreous humour has been lost during surgery

- Retinal detachment – the symptoms and signs have been described (pp. 157–60)

- Cystoid macular oedema – more commonly seen after intracapsular cataract removal, but also seen following loss of vitreous.

Symptoms: Failure to achieve full visual potential at first eye test for spectacles, subsequent loss of vision

Signs: The cysts are radial with a petaloid distribution. The macular disease is difficult to visualise with the direct or indirect ophthalmoscope. It is best seen with a +90 D lens, Goldmann three-mirror contact lens, or by means of fluorescein angiography.

Dislocation or subluxation of an intraocular implant

Intraocular lenses are introduced into the anterior or posterior chamber, the latter being the safer.
  Dislocation of the posterior chamber lens is uncommon.

Symptoms: Sudden change in the visual acuity, or monocular diplopia.

Signs: The margin of the lens implant may pass across the pupillary region, visible against the red reflex.

Management: The lens must be recentred and may (S)(require a suture.

Opacification of the posterior lens capsule

A common complication which causes slow visual deterioration following the surgery (*Fig. 17.6*).

Management: A small opening is made using a YAG (S) laser (*Fig. 17.7*).

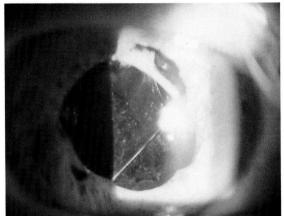

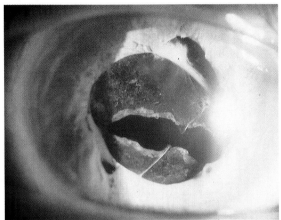

Fig. 17.6 Thickened posterior capsule following a cataract extraction

Fig. 17.7 Opening in the posterior capsule has been made using a laser

Corneal oedema

Corneal oedema, or bullous keratopathy, occurring after cataract extraction with or without an implant, is a serious complication. The following factors contribute to its occurrence (*Fig. 17.8*):

- Undue operative manipulation
- Pre-existing endothelial disease, worsened by surgery
- Injury to the endothelium by contact with the implant during or following surgery
- Excessive postoperative inflammation

Symptoms:

- Gradual reduction of vision
- Severe pain when bullae rupture

Signs:

- Corneal thickening and loss of transparency due to stromal oedema
- Formation of epithelial bullae
- Rupture of bullae, visible by staining with fluorescein or rose bengal

Management:

- Hyperosmotic agents such as saline drops (5–10%) q.i.d.
- Monitoring for bacterial flora, and antibiotic therapy when necessary
- Permanent-wear, bandage contact lens for pain when bullae rupture
- Penetrating keratoplasty to restore vision

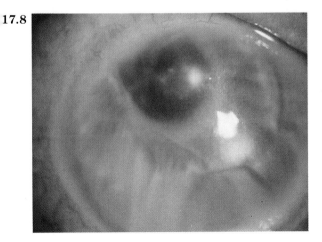

Fig. 17.8 Corneal oedema following an intraocular lens implant

Glaucoma

The types of glaucoma have been described (see pp. 119–26). The postoperative complications are described as early or late.

Acute glaucoma

Operative treatment is by peripheral iridectomy, either as a surgical procedure, or by YAG laser.

Early complications

• Elevation of the intraocular pressure due to persistence of peripheral adhesions of the iris to the cornea occluding the trabecular meshwork (peripheral anterior synechiae), or by failure to perform the iridectomy completely.

Ⓡ Ⓢ *Management:*

a. Identification of cause
b. Medical control with topical drops, such as timolol malleate 0.25 or 0.5% b.d., or pilocarpine 2–4% q.i.d.

c. Further surgery where the peripheral iridectomy is incomplete.

• Wound leakage and shallow anterior chamber

Management: Resuture of wound   Ⓢ

• Hyphaema

Management: Observation; spontaneous resolution Ⓢ occurs

Late complications

Cataract is occasionally seen. This is removed using standard methods.

Chronic simple glaucoma

Early complications after trabeculectomy

• Excessive reduction of intraocular pressure

• Flat anterior chamber and choroidal effusion, easily seen with the direct ophthalmoscope

Ⓡ Ⓢ *Management:* There is little that can be done in the emergency situation, but patients with these complications require admission. Patching and mydriatic therapy can help.

• Hyphaema

• Endophthalmitis

Ⓡ Ⓢ *Management:* According to principles outlined for cataract extraction

Late complications after trabeculectomy

• Cataract

Management: Eventual extraction is necessary   Ⓢ

• Late endophthalmitis: this is a special problem owing to the relatively easy access of bacteria into the anterior chamber through the filtration bleb and the scleral opening. The bleb (*Fig. 17.9*) must be examined for clinical signs of infection, shown by purulent reaction around and within it.

Management:

a. Admission for investigation by superficial and intra- Ⓢ ocular culture by aqueous tap.
b. Antibiotic treatment will be as outlined for endophthalmitis (see pp. 117–118).

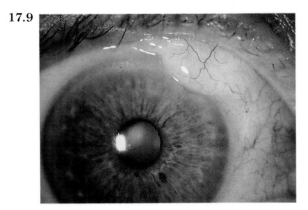

Fig. 17.9 Filtration bleb

Corneal transplantation

Corneal transplants are performed for irreversible corneal opacities which reduce vision to unacceptable levels. They may be full thickness (penetrating) (*Fig. 17.10*) or partial thickness (lamellar).

Early postoperative complications

• Wound leak: the main effect of wound leakage is a shallow or flat anterior chamber and is identified using the Seidel test. It is usually found at the interface between donor and recipient. It may be due to erosion of the suture through inflamed corneal tissue (*Fig. 17.11*).

Management:

a. Where the anterior chamber is normal or slightly shallow, no action is needed except the application of a patch dressing.
b. Where the anterior chamber is flat, the above treatment can be followed for 24 hours, but if unsuccessful, the wound must be sutured with additional interrupted sutures.

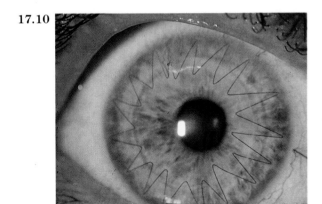

Fig. 17.10 Successful corneal graft in a patient with keratoconus

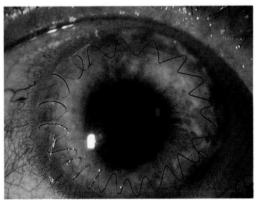

Fig. 17.11 Eroding sutures following a penetrating keratoplasty

• Anterior synechiae to the interface between donor tissue and recipient: these are usually applied to the graft interface. They may cause glaucoma by occluding the angle of the anterior chamber, or may provoke rejection of the allograft. They result from:

a. Incarceration during surgery,
b. Wound leak and inflammation during the postoperative period

®Ⓢ *Management:* Surgical separation of the synechiae will be required.

• Primary graft failure: there is persistent corneal oedema within the immediate postoperative period. It is due to damage to the endothelium during the surgery or poor quality donor tissue.

®Ⓢ *Management:* Topical corticosteroid, glaucoma medication and hypertonic saline. If the oedema persists for 7–10 days, the donor tissue must be replaced.

• Elevated intraocular pressure

• Hyphaema

• Infection

• Glaucoma

Management: It is important that it is recognised and Ⓢ treated along the usual lines. Chronic pressure elevation is the cause of visual failure in a significant number of patients.

• Corneal ulceration and endophthalmitis: produce Ⓢ clinical signs similar to those found in endophthalmitis following cataract or filtration surgery.

Management: Similar principles apply in treatment (see pp. 117–18).

Late complications

Occasionally, the original corneal disease recurs in the donor tissue (*Fig. 17.12*). Graft rejection can cause failure of the transplant with loss of sight. Early diagnosis and treatment is essential to preserve sight (*Fig. 17.13(a)–(c)*).

• Epithelial rejection with a linear defect which progresses across the graft over 3–6 days

• Stromal rejection occurs as punctate opacities or a peripheral arc of haze which progresses centrally (*Fig. 17.14*)

• Endothelial rejection presents as a thin line of keratic precipitates, originating at a zone of vascular ingrowth. The endothelium is destroyed in the wake of the precipitate which is composed of cytotoxic lymphocytes (*Fig. 17.15(a) & (b)*).

®Ⓢ *Management:*

a. Prevention: the patient must be warned about symptoms suggestive of an allograft reaction (photophobia, redness and visual blurring) and must seek immediate advice if they occur.
b. Rejection can be reversed with topical corticosteroid, best given under supervision as an inpatient.

17.12

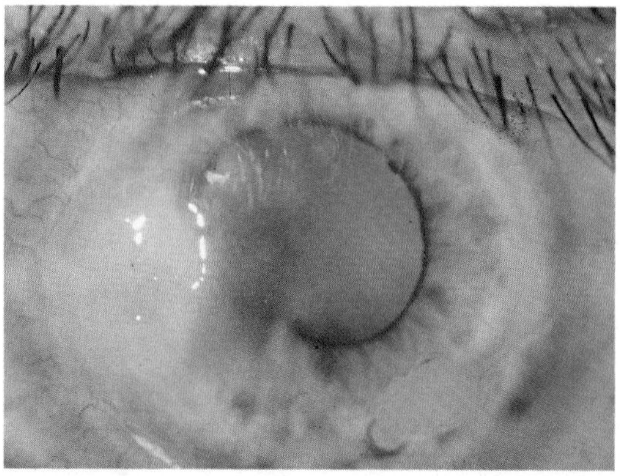

Fig. 17.12 Recurrence of herpes simplex keratitis following a corneal graft

17.13(a)–(c)

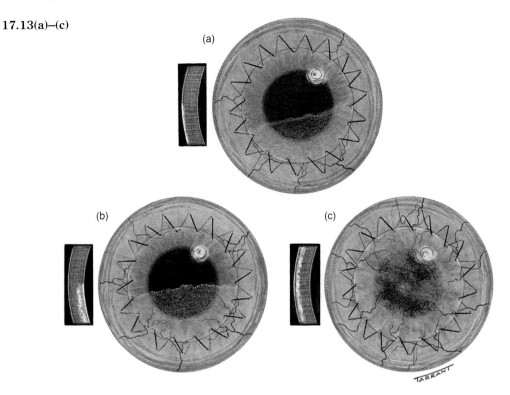

Fig. 17.13(a)–(c) An artist's impression of the three types of corneal graft rejection: **(a)** epithelial, **(b)** endothelial, **(c)** stromal

17.14

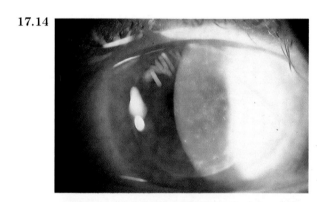

Fig. 17.14 Stromal rejection following a keratoplasty

17.15(a)

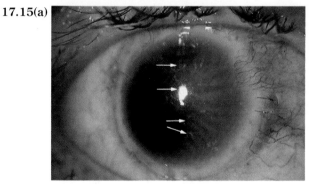

Fig. 17.15(a) Stromal oedema (arrows) due to endothelial rejection

17.15(b)

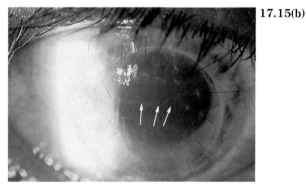

Fig. 17.15(b) Endothelial rejection (arrows)

Retinal and vitreous surgery

Retinal and vitreous surgery are intimately related and involve a large number of complex techniques.

Retinal surgery

The most important complications in retinal detachment surgery are:
- Failure of the retina to reattach
- Decrease in visual acuity in spite of a technically successful procedure
- Alterations in muscle balance
- Altered cosmetic appearance

Early complications

- Shallowing of the anterior chamber

- Choroidal detachment: shallowing of the anterior chamber is often associated with choroidal effusion and forward movement of the ciliary body. Rarely, the intraocular pressure becomes elevated and treatment will be required. More often the pressure is low.

 Management: Normalisation of the anatomy occurs over a period of 10–20 days. Where the effusion is marked and persists for longer, steps may be taken to drain the suprachoroidal fluid.

- Persisting sub-retinal fluid

- Anterior segment ischaemia: rare, most commonly seen in patients with haemoglobin SC. It is seen with circumferential cryotherapy and deep buckling, extending to the ora serrata. It is recognised by lid swelling, corneal oedema, semidilated, non-reactive pupil and progressive lens opacification.

(R)(S) *Management:* Topical and systemic steroid and loosening of the encircling buckle.

Late complications

- Macular pucker
- Cystoid macular oedema
- Change in refraction
- Muscle imbalance
- Cosmetic abnormalities
- Pain

- Infection and/or extrusion of implant (*Fig. 17.16*): implanted silicone material may become contaminated and most cases present some months after surgery.

Symptoms and Signs: The eye is red, painful and tender with chronic discharge and purulent discharge from the implanted area beneath the bulbar conjunctiva.

Management: Antibiotics are usually ineffective and (S)(R) removal of the implant is often necessary.

17.16

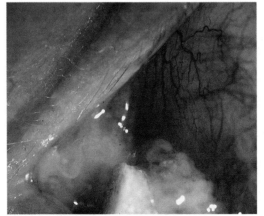

Fig. 17.16 Extruding plomb after retinal detachment surgery

Vitreous surgery

Patients who have undergone vitreous surgery are inevitably under the care of highly specialised departments. However, they may attend as emergencies because of progressive visual loss, discomfort or cosmetic reasons.

Early complications

- Corneal oedema
- Corneal epithelial deficits
- Vitreous haemorrhage
- Additional retinal tears
- Cataract

• Persistent corneal epithelial deficits: these may follow vitreous surgery in the immediate postoperative period, particularly in diabetics.

Management: Pressure dressings should be applied Ⓢ Ⓡ and topical therapy avoided until the epithelium has healed.

Late complications

• Rubeosis iridis (growth of neovascular tissue in the iris)

• Corneal oedema due to endothelial damage: may occur as a result of prolonged irrigation, the use of non-physiological solutions, direct trauma with instruments, topical epinephrine in the presence of an epithelial defect and mechanical damage from intraocular gas or silicone oil.

Ⓢ *Management:* Similar to that outlined for Fuchs' endothelial dystrophy (see p. 102).

• Phthisis bulbi (collapse and shrinkage of the globe)

• Vitreous haemorrhage: occurs as an early or late complication, particularly following procedures for retinal neovascularisation in diabetics.

Management: Patients with this complication must be Ⓢ Ⓡ admitted for bed rest in preparation for possible photocoagulation of residual areas of retinal neovascularisation.

Lacrimal duct obstruction

Obstruction at the level of the lacrimal sac or nasolacrimal duct causes chronic watering of the eye and requires dacryocystorhinostomy, the anastomosis of the mucous membrane of the lacrimal sac, to the mucosa of the nasal cavity. Secondary nasal haemorrhage is sometimes encountered and requires immediate referral for inpatient management. Sometimes, tubes are inserted to keep the passages open (*Fig. 17.17*). Occasionally, a loop protrudes from the puncta in which case they need to be restored to their original position.

17.17

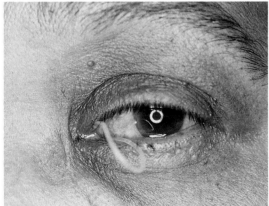

Fig. 17.17 Protruding tubes after lacrimal drainage surgery

Photocoagulation

Photocoagulation has revolutionised treatment and helped to reduce the incidence of blindness from many retinal conditions. However, occasional symptoms occur related to the treatment itself, or to complications therefrom.

Photocoagulation is used in the following ways:

- Panretinal ablation for proliferative retinopathy such as in diabetes.

- Focal treatment to seal retinal vascular and choroidal vascular leakage, as demonstrated with fluorescein angiography, such as in involutional macular degeneration.

- Focal treatment to destroy choroidal neovascularisation such as in involutional macular degeneration.

- Formation of chorioretinal adhesions around flat retinal breaks as prophylaxis against retinal detachment

- Destroy selected intraocular tumours

Complications include:

- Loss of peripheral field after panretinal photocoagulation

- Transient reduction of visual acuity

- Pain

- Exudative retinal detachment

- Choroidal detachment

- Secondary glaucoma

- Breaks in Bruch's membrane can produce choroidal or vitreous haemorrhage.

- Accidental treatment of the fovea has been recorded.

18 Contact lenses

Contact lenses may induce complications that demand immediate care, the initial management of which may concern general practitioners or casualty officers.

Contact lenses are of three types:

• **Hard** – which are now rarely used, but are indicated for high astigmatism and corneal ectasia such as keratoconus. They are generally microlenses, their edge lying well within the limbus (*Fig. 18.1*).

• **Soft hydrophilic** – composed of hydroxymethyl methacrylate, which retain 25–85% hydration. They are usually large in diameter and overlap the limbus (*Fig. 18.2*).

• **Gas permeable** – with a low water content, and high oxygen permeability.

Generally contact lenses are removed at the end of each day, but on occasions are worn for up to seven days (intermediate wear) or for periods of up to three months in (permanent wear).

The indications for contact lens wear are:
• optical
• therapeutic

18.1

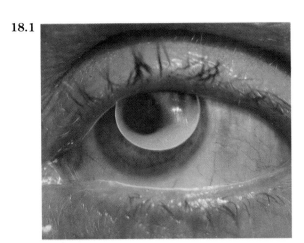

Fig. 18.1 Hard microlens – fluorescein should not be used with soft lenses

18.2

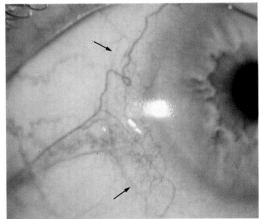

Fig. 18.2 Soft hydrophilic lens extending on to the conjunctiva. The edge of the lens can just be seen (arrows)

Complications of contact lens wear

Patients must be examined with a slit lamp, and must be referred to the care of the eye unit. The cornea, and bulbar and tarsal conjunctiva must be examined, following examination of the lens itself for damage or contamination. Patients must be asked to remove the lenses where any complication is seen, and referred to an ophthalmologist or contact lens practitioner.

Corneal complications

Vascularisation of the cornea

This occurs particularly in intermittent wear, or permanent wear. It is generally seen as superficial vessels at the upper limbus, and indicates that the patient needs to have the lens changed and refitted.

Punctate epithelial staining

This occurs in varying distributions and generally indicates that further advice is necessary. It may occur in several situations:

- Linear staining in the lower part of the cornea, induced by trauma associated with insertion or removal.

- Central corneal staining occurs in flat, fitted lenses.

- Punctate erosions in the lower part of the cornea may result from inadequate blinking.

- Peripheral arcuate staining occurs at the rim of a lens with a thickened edge, as in the case of a high minus lens.

- Hypoxia occurs in a tightly fitted lens and gives rise to diffuse or focal staining.

Small, sterile, corneal ulcers

These can occur, but generally resolve. They must, of course, be investigated in the usual way in the hospital clinic.

Bacterial infection

This results from introduction of organisms from infected lenses or lens solutions, contaminated fingers, or inadequate disinfection techniques. The patient will need admission and immediate investigation, as early treatment is essential to preserve useful vision (see p. 90) (*Fig. 18.3*).

Acanthamoeba infection

This is a rare condition occuring in contact lens wearers. It induces chronic ulcerative keratitis, which presents at the early stages with an epithelial deficit and stromal haze. It may mimic herpes simplex keratitis (*Fig. 18.4*).

18.3

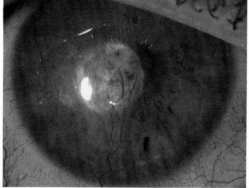

Fig. 18.3 Central scar resulting from infection following hard contact lens wear (Courtesy of Mr. R. Warr)

18.4

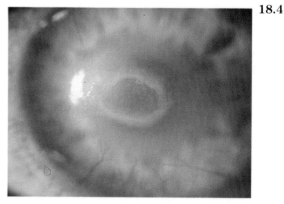

Fig. 18.4 Acanthomoeba infection of a lens leading to keratitis (Courtesy of Mr. R. Warr)

Conjunctival complications

Contact lenses induce allergic, chemical and infective conjunctivitis, and superior limbic keratoconjunctivitis.

Allergic conjunctivitis

This is occasionally seen with papillae on the upper tarsal plate. The patient has intolerance to the contact lens.

Symptoms:

- mucous discharge.
- itching and discomfort during lens wear.
- visual blurring when wearing the lens.

Signs:

- Papillae on the upper and lower tarsal plates. They are often small and have a white surface. They are always equal to each other in size.
- The tarsal plates are hyperaemic and infiltrated with inflammatory cells.
- Mucous discharge.

Management:

- Cessation of contact lens wear for a period.
- Review lens care solutions, and clean existing lenses.
- Consider changing lenses to a new type.
- Try sodium cromoglycate drops (Opticrom) 2% q.i.d.
- Where control is obtained, it may be possible to restart contact lens wear, with a gradual build-up of wearing time.

Chemical conjunctivitis

This is thought to be caused by substances carried by the contact lens such as the preservative, benzalkonium chloride.

Infective conjunctivitis

This induces typical symptoms and signs and requires immediate treatment. The patient should be advised not to wear the lenses.

Superior limbic keratoconjunctivitis

This is a persistent problem which is the result of toxicity or hypersensitivity to thiomersal, a preservative that is sometimes used in contact lens care solutions (*Fig. 18.5*).

Symptoms:

- redness
- watering and photophobia
- persistent soreness
- intolerance to contact lens wear

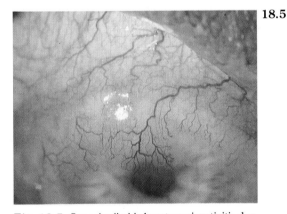

18.5

Fig. 18.5 Superior limbic keratoconjunctivitis due to thiomersal toxicity (Courtesy of Mr. R. Warr)

Signs:

- conjunctival hyperaemia and chemosis around the upper limbus

- punctate staining of the limbal conjunctiva and the upper part of the cornea with fluorescein or rose bengal

- vascularisation of the upper limbus, with dilated vessels

- opacification of the upper corneal epithelium, presenting a greyish appearance

The symptoms and signs may persist for some months and often show a poor response to treatment.

Management:

- Cessation of contact lens wear.
- Avoidance of solutions, including therapeutic eye drops, which contain thiomersal as a preservative.
- Topical corticosteroid drops may be necessary in persistent cases.
- Contact lens wear can be resumed once the condition has completely cleared.

Contact lens complications

- The lens may become damaged with splits or breakages and the help of a contact lens practitioner will be required to replace it.

- Surface film or deposits occur which should be removed with a surfactant solution (*Fig. 18.6(a) & (b)*).

- The lens may be fitted too tightly or loosely, producing immobility or excessive movement respectively. Epithelial oedema can occur in the former.

18.6(a)

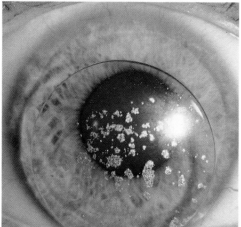

Fig. 18.6(a) Deposits on a hard contact lens (Courtesy of Mr. R. Warr)

18.6(b)

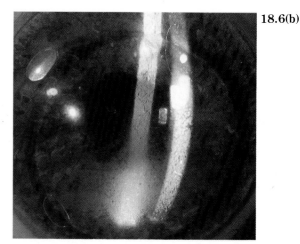

Fig. 18.6(b) Fine deposits on the surface of a soft contact lens (Courtesy of Mr. R. Warr)

19 Corneal donation

Corneal grafts are performed using tissue donated after death. As general physicians or casualty officers will sometimes be requested to remove tissue, a brief description of the technique of eye removal is presented to help the inexperienced. However, it is essential that the method has been fully demonstrated by an eye surgeon or trained eye bank technician before going ahead.

Tissue can be removed up to 12 hours after death. Eyes may be donated prior to death as a bequest, hence the involvement of the general physician. Advice about procedure should be obtained from the local eye department. Instrumentation should be available from many departments.

Although there are a number of contra-indications to donation, tissue in general must be removed when it has been donated. It is essential that donors are screened for hepatitis antigen and HIV whatever their age. Information about the previous medical history and cause of death must be supplied to the eye bank.

Absolute contra-indications to the use of donated tissue include:

- donor disease of obscure or unknown aetiology

- Jakob–Creutzfeld disease

- Alzheimer's disease

- rabies

- congenital rubella

- subacute sclerosing panencephalitis

- progressive multifocal leukoencephalopathy

- subacute encephalitis from cytomegalovirus

- septicaemia

- 'blast' forms of leukaemia

- intrinsic eye disease, including retinoblastoma, malignant tumours of the anterior segment and conjunctivitis

- Hodgkin's disease

Method for enucleation

See Fig. 19.1(a)–(f).

- The consent of the relatives must be sought, and the procedure must not be carried until this is obtained.

- A set of sterile instruments is required, together with a receptacle containing a gauze strip impregnated with saline. The procedure must be carried out under sterile conditions.

- The periorbital skin is prepared using soap solution followed by iodine solution.

- The conjunctival sacs should be irrigated with saline solution.

- A drape is placed across the eye which is to be removed. If the drape is plastic and disposable, a horizontal incision is made parallel with the palpebral fissure.

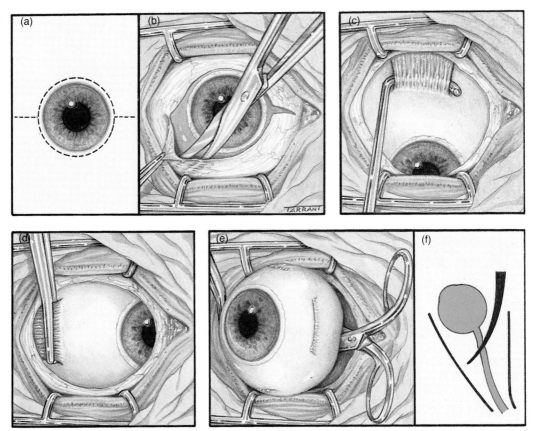

Fig. 19.1(a)–(e) Diagrammatic representation of sequence of steps required in enucleation for cornea graft donation **(a)** Conjunctival incision **(b)** Dissection of conjunctiva off globe **(c)** Each ocular muscle is isolated **(d)** Ocular muscle clamped and cut **(e)** Scissors inserted to section optic nerve

- The lids are fixed with a speculum or sutures.

- A limbal incision (peritomy) is performed and blunt dissection is used to identify the four recti muscles (*Fig. 19.1(a) & (b)*).

- A squint hook is used to identify the insertions of the four recti, which are then incised at their insertions (*Fig. 19.1(c) & (d)*).

- The oblique muscles are identified with the squint hook and transected.

- Large, curved scissors are used to transect the optic nerve (*Fig. 19.1(e) & (f)*).

- The eye is removed from the socket, transferred to a sterile container and delivered to the eye bank.

Procedure within the eye bank

The cornea and 2–3 mm of sclera are removed from the anterior segment and placed in media for storage or for transport to other centres.

The following are the methods for corneal storage:

- Moist chamber – the whole eye is retained in the sterile container and used within 48 hours of removal.

- McCarey-Kaufman (MK) medium, in which the corneo-scleral disc is stored at 4°C for short periods of up to three days prior to use.

- K sol, in which the cornea-scleral disc can be stored for about 10 days prior to use.

- Storage in medium for up to 30 days at 34°C. This allows surgery to be scheduled and avoids the need to operate as an emergency.

In the United Kingdom, information about donor eye retrieval can be obtained from the United Kingdom Transplant Service, Bristol (0272 507777), where there is a duty officer available 24 hours a day. In the USA, information is available from the local eye bank.

Further Reading

J.R.O. Collin, *A Manual of Systematic Eye Lid Surgery*, 2nd edn., Edinburgh, Churchill Livingstone, 1989

T.D. Duane (ed.), *Clinical Ophthalmology*, 5 vols, Philadelphia, Harper and Row, 1987

E.M. Eagling and M.J. Roper-Hall, *Eye Injuries: an illustrated guide*, London, Butterworths, 1986

D.L. Easty, *Current Ophthalmic Surgery*, London, Ballière Tyndall, 1990

A.R. Elkington and H.J. Frank, *Clinical Optics*, Oxford, Blackwell Scientific, 1984

A. Garner, *Pathobiology of Ocular Disease: a dynamic approach*, eds. A. Garner and G. Klintworth, 2 vols., New York, Dekker, 1982

J.S. Glaser, *Neuro-ophthalmology*, Haggerstown/London, Harper and Row, 1978

J. Kanski, *Clinical Ophthalmology*, 2nd edn., London, Butterworths, 1989

D.R. Lucas (ed.), *Greer's Ocular Pathology*, 4th edn., Oxford, Blackwell Scientific, 1989

J. Mein and B. Harcourt, *Diagnosis and Management of Ocular Motility Disorders*, Oxford, Blackwell Scientific, 1986

S.J. Miller, *Clinical Ophthalmology*, Bristol, Wright, 1987

D. Pavan-Langston, *Manual of Ocular Diagnosis and Therapy*, 2nd edn., Boston (Mass), Little, Brown; Beckenham, Distributed by Quest Publishing, 1985

M.J. Roper-Hall, *Stallard's Eye Surgery*, 7th edn., London, Wright, 1989

D.J. Spalton, R.A. Hitchings and P.A. Hunter, eds. *Atlas of Clinical Ophthalmology*, Edinburgh, Churchill Livingstone, London, Gower, 1989

M. Yanoff and B.S. Fine, *Ocular Pathology: a text and atlas*, 2nd edn., Philadelphia/London, Harper and Row, 1982

Index

All references are to page numbers.